A Physician's Handbook on Orthomolecular Medicine

Keats Publishing Titles of Relevant Interest

The Complete Vitamin E Book — Wilfrid E. Shute, M.D.

Diet and Disease — E. Cheraskin, M.D., D.M.D., W.M. Ringsdorf, Jr., D.M.D., and J.W. Clark, D.D.S.

Diverticular Disease of the Colon — Neil S. Painter, M.D.

The Heart and Vitamin E — Evan V. Shute, M.D.

Mental and Elemental Nutrients — Carl C. Pfeiffer, M.D., Ph.D.

Orthomolecular Nutrition — Abram Hoffer, M.D., Ph.D., and Morton Walker

The Poisons Around Us — Henry A. Schroeder, M.D.

Predictive Medicine — E. Cheraskin, M.D., D.M.D., and W.M. Ringsdorf, Jr., D.M.D.

The Saccharine Disease — T.L. Cleave, M.D.

Zinc and Other Micro-Nutrients — Carl C. Pfeiffer, M.D., Ph.D.

A Physician's Handbook on Orthomolecular Medicine

Edited by Roger J. Williams
and Dwight K. Kalita
with an introduction by Abram Hoffer, M.D.

Keats Publishing, Inc. New Canaan, Connecticut

A Physician's Handbook on Orthomolecular Medicine

Copyright © 1977 by Roger J. Williams and Dwight K. Kalita

Health Science edition published 1979 by arrangement with Pergamon Press

All Rights Reserved

No part of this book may be copied or reproduced in any form whatsoever without the written permission of the publishers

ISBN: 0-87983-199-5
Library of Congress Catalog Card Number: 79-65494

Printed in the United States of America

Health Science editions are published by
Keats Publishing, Inc., 36 Grove Street
New Canaan, Connecticut 06840

This book is dedicated to the physicians of the future who will be led at least to consider seriously the potentialities of orthomolecular medicine.

Roger J. Williams

It is also dedicated to my mother, Alice, Ohio Director of the Huxley Institute for Biosocial Research, and my father, Arthur, without whose love and guidance this book would not have been possible.

Dwight K. Kalita

Contents

Preface

That Orthomolecular Medicine is here to stay is the firm conviction of the Editors, and we are proud to present this collection of revealing and suggestive contributions.

This conviction is based upon a tremendous volume of cumulative evidence which reaches into the deeper recesses of the gross and microscopic anatomy, physiology, biochemistry, pharmacology, endocrinology, neurology and psychology of real people. While this evidence is diffuse and difficult to categorize and adjudicate on a statistical basis, it is nevertheless legitimate and in our opinion inescapable.

Orthomolecular Medicine is essentially the treatment and prevention of disease by the expert adjustment of the natural chemical constituents of our bodies. It places its reliance on these agents in preference to chemicals and drugs which are foreign to healthy metabolism.

Nutrition, a thoroughgoing study of which has been ostracized by traditional medicine, plays a dominant role in Orthomolecular Medicine. The development of this branch of medicine will, we believe, bring to fruition a peaceful revolution in medical thinking which has been brewing for some time. This revolution was foreshadowed by the pronouncement of Frank G. Boudreau, M.D., of the Milbank Fund of New York in 1959. "If all we know about nutrition," he said, "were applied to modern society, the result would be an enormous improvement in public health, at least equal to that which resulted when the germ theory of infectious disease was made the basis of public health and medical work.

Orthomolecular Medicine is in its infancy. Fortunately, there is no established orthodoxy to stifle creativity. The editors and individual authors cannot give unqualified endorsement to each article and each opinion expressed. We can, however, call attention to the publications as worthy of consideration and further research.

Roger J. Williams, Ph.D.
Dwight K. Kalita, Ph.D.

Contributors

DONNA BACCHI, M.S., Recently graduated from Cornell University with a major in Nutritional Science, and from the University of Cincinnati, she is a member of Omicron Nu (Home Economics Honor Society). She has done research work for Dr. Carl C. Pfeiffer and has been an administrative and teaching assistant. Her professional interest is in the application of nutritional science to the investigation, treatment and prevention of physical and mental disease.

JOHN BARON, D.O., Orthomolecular Psychiatrist, specializes in nutrition, preventive medicine and Orthomolecular Psychiatry. Dr. Baron has been practicing nutritionally oriented medicine since 1939. He is certified by the American College of Applied Nutrition and the American College of Bariatric Physicians. He is a member of the Cleveland Academy of Osteopathic Medicine and the American College of Neuropsychiatry. He has treated over 1000 hypoglycemic patients at the Baron Clinic in Cleveland, Ohio.

CHARLES BODE, Research Assistant (1973-74) Clayton Foundation Biochemical Institute, University of Texas. Pharmacist (1974): Gibson Pharmacy. He has co-authored several publications with Dr. Roger J. Williams, and his main interest is in biochemical individuality and its application to nutritional science.

EMANUEL CHERASKIN, M.D., Graduated from the University of Cincinnati College of Medicine, 1943. Has published over ten different books and over 300 scientific papers in professional journals. Presently: Professor and Chairman of the Department of Oral Medicine at the University of Alabama School of Dentistry. Listed in American Men and Women of Science and Who's Who in American Dentistry. Fellow: the American College of Pharmacology and Chemotherapy, the American Public Health Association, the American College of Dentists, the International Academy of Preventive Medicine, the American Geriatrics Society and an Honorary Member, International Academy of Metabology. Listed in Who's Who in America, 1971, 1973 and 1974. Has memberships in over 9 professional organizations including the American Medical Association and the American Academy of Oral Medicine and the American Dental Association.

ALLAN COTT, M.D., Psychiatrist, began work with Orthomolecular treatment of children with learning disabilities in 1967. He is a life Fellow of the American Psychiatric Association, a member of the Board of Trustees of the Huxley Institute for Biosocial Research, Secretary of the Academy of Orthomolecular Psychiatry, Founding Fellow of the Academy of Orthomolecular Psychiatry, Scientific Advisor to the Metropolitan Chapter of National Society for Autistic Children, Consultant to the New York Institute for Child Development, and Medical Director of the Churchill School for children with learning disabilities. He has written numerous published articles and co-authored chapters for books related to Orthomolecular therapy.

WILLIAM D. CURRIER, M.D., Graduated from the University of Nebraska College of Medicine. Taught at Harvard Medical School and at U.S.C. Medical School for over 25 years. Emeritus status at present. Founder of the International Academy Metabology, Inc., and is a member of city, county, state and national medical associations. Member of the International College of Applied Nutrition for 30 years and Medical Director of the Lancaster Foundation for Medical Research for 20 years. Has authored many scientific papers, was the physician for the research work of the Lancaster Foundation which culminated in the book: *Nutrition and Your Mind, The Psychochemical Response*, by George Watson, Ph.D. He specializes in nutritional, endocrine and metabolic diseases.

JOHN M. ELLIS, M.D., author, physician, has been associated with Titus County Memorial Hospital in Mt. Pleasant, Texas since 1956. He is Chief of Medical Staff at Titus. Dr. Ellis' clinical research with Vitamin B_6 began in 1961, and since then his work done on the subject has received international attention. He is the author of *The Doctor Who Looked at Hands*, and *Vitamin B_6: The Doctor's Report*. He has also published numerous articles in professional journals.

MRS. KAY HALL, M.A., Scheduled to receive her Ph.D. in May, 1977. Specializing in the effects of diet and general nutritional status on psychological behavior and brain physiology. Was the Texas nominee for the Outstanding Young Women of America Award in 1969. She has several scientific publications including her most recent: "Allergy of the Nervous System: A Review," *Annals of Allergy*, February, 1976. She has traveled extensively around the world, and has done psychological testing programs in such places as Saigon, Vietnam and Bangkok, Thailand. She is currently teaching human development courses to undergraduates at the University of Texas, Dallas, Texas, and to inmates in a federal prison. She has also participated in programs which use nutritional skills in the treatment of children with learning disabilities and behavioral disorders.

JAMES D. HEFFLEY, Ph.D., Research Associate, Clayton Foundation Biochemical Institute, University of Texas. Nutrition Consultant: Texas School for the blind. Self-employed as a Nutrition Consultant. He is a member of the Academy of Orthomolecular Psychiatry, and has several scientific publications in the areas of nutritional science. His research interests include the assessment of nutrient requirements for individuals and the uses of nutrients in preventive and therapeutic medicine.

ABRAM HOFFER, M.D., Ph.D., educator, chemist, psychiatrist. Received Ph.D. in Agricultural Biochemistry. M.D.: University of Toronto and specialization in psychiatry (1954). In 1955 taught at the University of Saskatchewan. In 1967 went into private practice as an Orthomolecular Psychiatrist. Developed the first biochemical hypothesis of schizophrenia and initiated megavitamin therapy. Has published over 200 scientific papers to date and is Co-Editor of *Orthomolecular Psychiatry*. Fellow of the International College of Applied Nutrition.

DWIGHT K. KALITA, Ph.D., Graduated from Bowling Green State University, 1972 with a degree in English. Interdisciplinary study of English, Theology, and Psychology. A.B. Degree from Defiance College: Major — Psychology and Philosophy. Public relations and medical speech writer (ghost writer) 1973 to present. Vocational Counselor at Bowling Green State University, 1972-73. President: Kalita Enterprises, Inc. (brokerage firm) 1974 to present. Formerly an Assistant Professor in the English Department at B.G.S.U. Has published numerous literary and scientific papers in professional journals, and is a member of several organizations including the Huxley Institute for Biosocial Research and the International Academy of Metabology. He is on the Executive Committee of the Huxley Institute for Biosocial Research of Ohio, Inc. Researcher in Orthomolecular Medicine and Human Ecology.

FREDERICK R. KLENNER, M.D., graduated from Duke University School of Medicine, 1936. Although specializing in diseases of the chest, Dr. Klenner is engaged in a limited general practice which has enabled him to make observations on the use of massive doses of ascorbic acid (Vitamin C) in virus disease as well as on other pathological syndromes. He is a Fellow of the American Association for Advancement of Science, a Fellow and Diplomate of the International College of Applied Nutrition, a Fellow of the Royal Society of Health, an Honorary Fellow of the International Academy

of Preventive Medicine. He has published 28 scientific papers and is a member of many medical and scientific organizations.

MARSHALL MANDELL, M.D., Assistant Professor, Allergy Section, Department of Pediatrics, New York Medical College, Medical Director of the New England Foundation for Allergic and Environmental Diseases. Fellow of the American College of Allergists, the International Academy of Preventive Medicine, the American Academy of Orthomolecular Psychiatry, and the Founding Fellow of the Society for Clinical Ecology. He has published many scientific papers and has given numerous public lectures. He is currently conducting clinical research in physical and mental disorders due to ecologic and addictive factors. He is a consultant to the Huxley Institute for Biosocial Research, to the Gesell Institute of Child Development, and in Allergy and Clinical Ecology for the Fuller Memorial Sanitarium, South Attleboro, Mass. He is a member of city, county, state and national medical associations.

H.L. NEWBOLD, M.D. Graduated from Duke University School of Medicine (1945). Three-year residency in psychiatry, University of Illinois. Private practice of psychiatry in Chicago and instructor in neurology and psychiatry, Northwestern University School of Medicine. At present, he is in the private practice of nutrition and psychiatry in New York. Author of numerous scientific articles in medical journals, has had eight novels published under a pen name, and has published one existential novel under his own name. A popular book on nutrition: *Meganutrients for Your Nerves* was recently published.

JOHN OTT, Sc.D., Hon., Chairman and Executive Director of the Environmental Health and Light Research Institute. In 1975 he received the Progress Medal, the highest award of the Photographic Society of America. His primary concern is with scientific research relating to the effects of light, particularly the full spectrum of sunlight on plant, animal and human life including growth, reproduction, health and disease. He has published two books: *My Ivory Cellar*: a book on time-lapse photography which includes rare pictures of plants' activities that he achieved for Walt Disney (and) *Health & Light*: a book which explores the new scientific evidence relating to full spectrum light and its effects on plant and animal health. Dr. Ott has received two additional medals for his "Exploring the Spectrum," a 16 mm film based on *Health & Light*. He has numerous scientific papers published.

LINUS C. PAULING, Ph.D., educator, Nobel prize in Chemistry (1954) and Nobel Peace prize (1962), International Lenin Peace prize (1972). Director: Institute of Orthomolecular Medicine. Professor of Chemistry at Stanford (1969-present). Honorary degrees received from over 20 different universities and colleges. Published countless numbers of articles and many books, of which *Vitamin C and the Common Cold* is most popular. First to define "Orthomolecular" medicine as the treatment of degenerative disease by "varying the concentration of substances normally occurring in the human body."

CARL C. PFEIFFER, M.D., Ph.D., Director of the Brain Bio Center, Princeton, New Jersey. Author of over 240 papers in physiology and pharmacology. President of the American Society for Pharmacology & Experimental Therapeutics, President of the Medical & Dental Staff, New Jersey Neuropsychiatric Institute. He has been a professor in the Department of Pharmacology at the University of Chicago, Wayne University College of Medicine, University of Illinois, and Emory University School of Medicine. He was the Chief Pharmacologist at Parke Davis & Company (1941-43). He has memberships in ten scientific societies and is Co-Editor of *The International Review of Neurobiology* and on the editorial board of *Clinical Pharmacology & Therapeutics*, and *Biological Psychiatry*. His present field of interest is the etiology and biochemistry of schizophrenia.

WILLIAM H. PHILPOTT, M.D., Psychiatrist, Assistant Medical Director and psychiatrist at the Fuller Memorial Hospital, South Attleboro, Mass., 1969-74. Instructor in Behaviorism: Taunton State Hospital 1972-74. Private Practice: South Laguna, California 1975. Recipient of the John Tintera Award and holds memberships in the American Medical Association, Massachusetts Medical Society, American Psychiatric Association and the Bristol County Massachusetts Medical Society. He is on the Editorial Board of the *Journal of Orthomolecular Psychiatry*, is the Second Vice President of the International Academy of Metabology, and is Editor of the *Journal of International Academy of Metabology*. He has numerous scientific publications.

THERON G. RANDOLPH, M.D. Graduated from the University of Michigan Medical School, 1933. Instructor at the University of Michigan Medical School 1935-1937. Research Fellow: Massachusetts General Hospital and Harvard Medical School 1937-39. Private Practice in Wisconsin 1939-42. Instructor in Internal Medicine and Chief of the Allergy Clinic, University of Michigan Medical School 1942-44. Private practice: Chicago 1944-present. Instructor in Internal Medicine, Northwestern University Medical School 1944-50. He is the author of over 200 scientific articles. His best known work is *Human Ecology and Susceptibility to the Chemical Environment*.

MILES H. ROBINSON, M.D. General practice: Washington State 1941. Instructor in Physiology at Vanderbilt Medical School: 1942-45. Instructor in Pharmacology at the University of Pennsylvania Medical School 1945-46. Practice of Internal Medicine, Washington State 1948-53, Baltimore 1953-58, Washington 1958 to present. Medical Advisor on the staff of U.S. Senator Paul H. Douglas of Illinois investigating the FDA from 1962-1966. Medical Advisor on staff of U.S. Senator Edward V. Long of Missouri 1966-68. He is a graduate of the University of Pennsylvania Medical School in 1938, has numerous scientific publications and is affiliated with the American Medical Association, the Montgomery County Society, and the Medical and Chirurgical Faculty of Maryland.

HENRY A. SCHROEDER, M.D. Professor of Physiology Emeritus at Dartmouth Medical School, and Director of Research at Brattleboro Memorial Hospital. He is the author of seven books, including *A Matter of Choice*, and *Pollution Profits, and Progress*, and has published hundreds of scientific papers and abstracts. One of his major contributions was the development of a low-sodium diet so widely used today for heart conditions. He also investigated the causes of hypertension from 1937 to 1956. In 1960 he was vice-chairman of the first World Health Organization symposium held in Prague, Czechoslovakia. Dr. Schroeder is well known for establishing the metal-free, environmentally controlled Trace Element Laboratory in 1960 on a remote hill in Vermont. In one of his best known books: *The Trace Elements and Man*, he maintains that life originated in the sea, and when animals — including man — became terrestrial, they brought with them a necessity for those trace elements which occur naturally in sea water. Failing to provide these trace elements in our diet can lead to serious biochemical problems.

WILFRID E. SHUTE, M.D. One of the very first medical doctors to use megavitamin treatment (1933). He is a noted heart specialist and holds that the lack of Vitamin E is directly responsible for America's number one killer: heart disease. In addition to many papers published in medical journals since 1946, this author has described the methods and results of Vitamin E treatment in a book: *Vitamin E for Ailing and Healthy Hearts*. Dr. Shute states that in the 22 years before 1969, he had treated over 30,000 cardiovascular patients. His treatment with this vitamin also includes coronary and ischemic heart disease and the accompanying angina, rheumatic fever, acute and chronic rheumatic heart disease, peripheral vascular disease, varicose veins, thrombophlebitis, arterial thrombi, indolent ulcer, diabetes, kidney disease and burns.

ROGER J. WILLIAMS, Ph.D., D.Sc., educator, chemist, discoverer of pantothenic acid. Author of the following books: *The Biochemistry of B Vitamins*, (1950), *Nutrition and Alcoholism*, (1951), *Free and Unequal*, (1953), *Biochemical Individuality*, (1956), *Alcoholism: The Nutritional Approach*, (1959), *Nutrition in a Nutshell*, (1962), *You are Extraordinary*, (1967), *Nutrition Against Disease*, (1971), *Physician's Handbook of Nutritional Science*, (1975). Professor of Chemistry (1934-71) at the University of Texas, Austin, Texas. Member of President's Panel on Heart Disease (1972). Member of American Chemistry Society (President: 1957), American Association of Cancer Research, Society of Experimental Biology and Medicine, National Academy of Sciences, New York Academy of Science, Phi Beta Kappa.

MAN-LI YEW, Ph.D. Postdoctoral Fellow (1967-69), and Research Associate (1969-present) at the Clayton Foundation Biochemical Institute, University of Texas. He has numerous scientific publications and his main research interest is in various areas of nutritional science. More specifically, he has written on Vitamin C and various dietary intake levels of Calcium.

Introduction to the Third Edition

Orthomolecular medicine and orthomolecular psychiatry have developed so quickly it is difficult even for orthomolecular physicians to keep up with newer findings. For a physician approaching it for the first time it is even more difficult. The field itself is quite complex but more important is the fact that the basic research reports are scattered throughout the medical literature, often in journals not readily available in medical libraries. For this reason this volume will be especially valuable for physicians, orthomolecular and those who would be, in bringing together some of the basic papers upon which this newer branch of medicine is based.

Orthomolecular psychiatry began when Dr. Humphry Osmond and I completed the first double blind experiment in psychiatry in 1952. We compared the effect of 3 grams per day of nicotinic acid, nicotinamide and placebo in a series of 30 acute schizophrenic patients. They were also given the standard treatment of that era, psychotherapy and electroconvulsive therapy. One year after the last patient had been treated a follow up study showed that 35 percent of the placebo group were well (natural remission rate), while 70 percent of the other two groups were well. After three more double blind controlled experiments and clinical studies on large numbers of patients we were convinced that adding this vitamin to the treatment of schizophrenia improved the number of recoveries.

By this time a small number of psychiatrists including Allan Cott, Jack Ward and David Hawkins began to confirm our conclusions. Working together we quickly expanded the use of vitamins to include pyridoxine (A. Cott), ascorbic acid and, to a lesser degree, pangamic acid. At the same time we realized that vitamin supplements without good nutrition did not work as well. Roger Williams' extraordinary work became very relevant and was incorporated into our treatment program.

Linus Pauling's classical paper in *Science* (1968) "ORTHOMOLECULAR PSYCHIATRY," provided a scientific explanation, and his term "orthomolecular" a word around which a large number of physicians could cluster. Casimir Funk's word "vitamine" marked the creation of the field of vitaminology. He coined it because he realized we humans require these key words. Linus Pauling's word has done the same.

The two final developments which round out our new medical field developed simultaneously. Carl Pfeiffer's work on minerals, especially on zinc and copper and its relation to pyrolluria made us aware that every nutritional supplement must be taken into account. W.H. Philpott working with Marshall Mandell brought into our field the basic work of Theron Randolph and other pioneers in ecology. It is now clear that cerebral allergies are a very important element in causing mental disease; if not taken into account many patients, depressions, schizophrenics, children with learning and behavioral disorders and many criminals and addicts will be denied a chance for recovery.

This volume provides for the first time a comprehensive reprinting of papers published in medical journals. Its precursor, the hardcover edition, had phenomenal success. It was a bestseller among scientific books, and deservedly so.

Every new branch of medicine must have its literature to which physicians can turn. Fortunately a large number of books are available and more are coming along. For anyone approaching orthomolecular medicine this is one of the most valuable books with which to start.

Abram Hoffer, M.D., Ph.D.
Victoria, British Columbia
June, 1979

1
Orthomolecular Medicine *
"We Command Nature Only By Obeying Her"
(Bacon)

DWIGHT K. KALITA

America the beautiful doesn't have a very beautiful health record in the year 1975. In fact, when you look at the incidence of degenerative disease in our nation, it is enough to make you sick. Ninety-three million of 213 million people in the United States (almost one-half the population) are suffering from some form of degenerative disease. Over fifty percent of those degenerative diseases are heart related. Fifteen million are arthritis victims. Approximately 347,000 die from cancer. The U.S. Department of Health and Welfare reports that 16 percent of the entire population is affected by allergies. According to hypoglycemia specialists, low blood sugar abnormalities are at epidemic stages in America. Our mental hospitals are now overcrowded, and the number of children being classified as hyperactive, retarded and schizophrenic are steadily increasing. Three hundred million man hours are lost yearly as a result of these diseases. Seventy-five billion dollars are spent yearly on the curing process, and the medical field is the 5th largest industry in the United States. A few years ago when the population was 200 million, we Americans consumed 37,273,000 pounds of aspirin in one year. We also swallowed 1,542,000 pounds of tranquilizers, 836,000 pounds of barbiturates, and 4,037,000 pounds of penicillins that year. In 1974, the retail sales for a single tranquilizer called Valium were an astounding 550 million dollars. Nearly three billion tablets were swooped up last year by what the mass media has alluded to as the "suburban junkies." Are you now convinced that our nation's health as a whole is in danger? The editors of this book are, and the following group of articles is directed at doing something constructive about it.

In his book, *University at the Crossroads*, the medical profession's eminent historian, H.E. Sigerist comments, "The ideal of medicine is the prevention of disease, and the necessity for curative treatment is a tacit admission of its failure." [1] What Sigerist, as well as other medical doctors, Nobel prize winners, Ph.D. nutritionists, and psychiatrists are saying is that a good part of America's health problems can be solved, but we can do so only by cultivating an entirely new attitude in ourselves. In the past and in the present, many physicians have been more interested in symptomatic treatment and relief rather than in curing and preventing the causes of disease. "The trouble," writes E.J. Steiglitz, M.D., "is that doctors think entirely in terms of disease, and are ignoring their opportunities for making people

healthier." [2] As a result of this attitude, the most fundamental weapons in the fight against disease are those most ignored by modern medicine. I have in mind the forty some nutrients (i.e., amino acids, minerals, trace elements, vitamins, etc.) that the cells of our bodies need to sustain and propagate themselves. Dr. Roger Williams' thesis that "the nutritional micro-environment of our body cells is crucially important to our health and that deficiencies in this environment constitute a major cause of disease," [3] has I believe, been grossly ignored by too many people. Part of the reason for this neglect is the popular emphasis on vitamin deficiency diseases. A person who has little or no vitamin C in his diet becomes sick with scurvy. A lack of B_1 causes beriberi. But these catastrophic effects of a deficiency in vitamin intake have been overemphasized; consequently, the study of the possibility of significant improvement in health of persons by going from a barely adequate intake to a vitamin intake that provides the best of health and the greatest protection against disease has been ignored. And this is where our problem begins. "Clinical nutrition is not even taught in most medical schools," writes N.S. Scrimshaw, M.D., "and not really adequately done in any of them" [4] It is only to be expected, therefore, that this "woefully weak clinical nutrition education," [5] (W.H. Sebrell, M.D., Columbia) should produce as Frederick Stare, M.D. of Harvard states, "physicians who are not well trained to identify malnutrition except for gross under- and over-weight, and this anyone can do." [6]

After glancing over the previously mentioned statistics, one can easily see why there is a growing number of physicians who are alarmed at our nation's extremely high drug consumption rate. Dr. Williams asks, "Do you really believe that you have arthritis as a result of your system's lack of aspirin?" [7] This question points to a disturbing problem. Like the ecology of our natural environment, man's inner physiological ecology can be easily upset by "alien chemical" (i.e., drugs) interference of natural processes. We have had to learn a painful lesson about introducing, for example, DDT and other contaminating chemicals into our natural environment. Similarly, there is concern among "medical ecologists" that alien chemicals (that is, chemicals not normally occurring in the human body) introduced into man's biochemical-physiological environment can also contaminate and do damage to important processes within the

*Reprinted with permission: *Journal of the International Academy Metabology*, Volume 5, #1, pp. 54-57.

body. "The basic fault of these weapons (drugs)," writes Dr. Williams, "is that they have no known connection with the disease process itself. . . . These drugs are wholly unlike nature's weapons. . . . They tend to mask the difficulty, not eliminate it. They contaminate the internal environment, create dependence on the part of the patient, and often complicate the physician's job by erasing valuable clues as to the real source of the trouble." [8] In other words, drugs are "nonbiological weapons" used in the battle against disease. Barbiturates, tranquilizers, antihistamines, anticoagulants, laxatives, pep pills, reducing pills, pain killers, anticonvulsants, etc. etc. etc., are modern medicine's arsenal of weapons. And yet, the records indicate that as many as 5 percent of all hospital admissions now are the result of adverse reactions to legally acquired prescription drugs. [9] This means that over one-and-a-half-million people are sent to the hospital each year as a result of drug therapy. And, after a patient is admitted to the hospital, his chances of falling victim of drug-induced sickness more than doubles. Drug sickness in hospitals causes suffering to well over three-and-a-half-million patients each year. [10] But the problem in today's hospitals is not only drug related. Dr. Charles E. Butterworth, Jr., M.D., Professor of Medicine and Pediatrics, University of Alabama, and Chairman of the Council on Foods and Nutrition of the American Medical Association, is alarmed by the frequency with which patients in our hospitals are being malnourished and even starved. "It seems strange that so little attention," he writes, "has been paid to the essential role of good nutrition in the maintenance of health, and particularly in recovery from acute illness or injury. Stranger still, however, is how frequently one sees the hospital stay prolonged and the patients' suffering made worse by what we are now recognizing as frank mismanagement, if not downright neglect, of the patients' nutritional health in our hospitals. I am convinced that iatrogenic malnutrition (physician-induced) has become a significant factor in determining the outcome of illness for many patients. . . . I suspect, as a matter of fact, that one of the largest pockets of unrecognized malnutrition in America, and Canada, too, exists, not in rural slums or urban ghettos, but in the private rooms and wards of big hospitals." [11] Certainly, this terrible "skeleton in the hospital closet" should be the first evidence of neglect that we must all seek to remove!

In the light of these disturbing facts, we must now turn our attention to the etiology (root causes) of degenerative disease. It is the opinion of some physicians that cellular malnutrition, biological nutrient deficiencies, and an inferior diet are the major causes of degenerative disease in America today. They insist that the top priority in the battle against disease should always begin with weapons which are most similar to nature's own biological weapons, and that we should be very cautious about introducing "alien chemicals" into any human body. The term "Orthomolecular Medicine" was first coined by Dr. Linus Pauling in 1968. Very simply stated, the term means "right molecule." The implication is that treatment of disease is a matter of "varying the concentration of substances (right molecules) normally present in the human body." [12] Instead of being concerned about the minimum daily requirement of nutrients, Orthomolecular physicians center their attention on the *optimum* molecular environment that each cell in our body needs for optimum health and resistance to disease. "If our body cells are ailing," writes Dr. Williams, "as they must be in disease, then chances are excellent that it is because they are being inadequately provisioned. The list

of the things that these cells may need includes not only all amino acids and all the minerals, plus trace elements, but about fifteen vitamins and probably many other coenzymes, nutrilites, and metabolites." [13] And as we shall see, the nutritional quality of the food we consume determines to a great extent the adequacy or inadequacy of the internal cellular environment of our bodies. And, of course, this internal environment is crucial to human health and vitality. Witness to the fact that when we become ill in some way or another, our internal cellular environment becomes deranged. This derangement at the microscopic level is no small matter. Each cell — and there are trillions of cells in each of us — is, as Dr. Williams has said, like a factory complex:

> Every cell has its own power plant from which it derives its energy. The burning process from which energy is derived is a highly ordered, many-step process in which many different catalysts are involved. Each catalyst (enzyme) is protein in nature and is made up of hundreds of amino acids (and often vitamins) put together in exactly the right way. The power plant makes it possible for every cell to be highly dynamic. Something is happening every microsecond. Complex chemical transformations — filtering, ultrafiltering, emulsifying, dispersion, aggregating, absorption — are continually in progress. Tearing down, building up, and repairing are constantly going on.
>
> Cells have their own ways of designing and making blueprints; "printing" and duplicating are very much in evidence. Cells also have their own versions of assembly lines. They have transportation systems; sorting, pumping, and streaming; and molecules riding piggy-back on others are common processes. Intricate mechanisms, including feedbacks, are used by cells to regulate their numerous activities.
>
> Cells have communication systems — messages and messengers. They have the equivalent of both an intercom system and devices for sending and receiving messages to and from the outside. Electrical activities are continually manifest. Cells are equipped with sewage and disposal systems. They even have in effect pollution-control mechanisms whereby toxic molecules are converted into others which are relatively harmless. [14]

Obviously, every single cell is a miraculous creation unto itself. However, because it is complex, each part of the mechanism is subject to disorder. Indeed, should the cell become deranged, its entire function may be seriously impaired. And if you multiply one deranged cell times a couple hundred million cells, you experience what modern medicine calls degenerative disease. To understand the root causes of disease, we as scientists must recognize that all sorts of cellular derangements are possible. We must also see that there is little hope of control unless the fundamental mechanisms of cellular activity are thoroughly understood. Orthomolecular medicine seeks such an understanding by postulating that if the biochemical individual integrity of each cell is nourished with the optimum nutrients necessary for its proper functioning, then our internal environment can be brought into line with individual human needs, and all forms of disease will eventually be controlled. To be sure, the list of necessary nutrients may be the same for every human being, but the relative amounts needed may be distinctively different for each person. And this is where Orthomolecular physicians come to the front lines in the battle against disease. Many medical men, including psychiatrists, are beginning to clinically observe positive results when patients are treated at the cellular level with "biological weapons" (nutrients) that nature has provided in her own structure of defense for millions of years.

It is important to realize that the greatest enemy of any science is a closed mind. We must always ask impertinent questions so as to shake our complacency and thus challenge our minds to look deeper into the farthest reaches of that great mystery called the human body. The contributors in this book have all accepted this challenge. Indeed, some have spent an entire lifetime researching one particular nutrient and its bio-chemical reactions in the body. It should be kept in mind, however, that no one nutrient or vitamin by itself cures or prevents any disease. Like your friendly "doctor of motors" (automobile mechanic) knows, you do not necessarily fix your car's breakdown by exchanging one spark plug. You must look at all the parts as they relate to each other, and you must also examine the fuel supply to see if your car has enough octane to run efficiently. So it is with your Orthomolecular physician. He looks at all the nutrients of the body and gives an in-depth examination of your fuel supply (diet). Your biochemistry may be "knocking" because the octane level of your diet is too low. But be assured, an Orthomolecular physician will never say, "put two aspirins in your tank, and call me in the morning." What he will say is that like your automobile's preventive maintenance program, your body also needs a preventive health program (i.e., supplying each cell of the body all the optimum nutrients which that cell needs for optimum health) that must begin in the mother's womb and continue all the days of your life. For a preventive nutrition-health program is the one safe weapon that can be used in the battle against your body's breakdown into degenerative disease.

Finally, I would like to emphasize that since teamwork among nutrients is essential, so is teamwork among researchers necessary. This book's editorial team wishes to thank all the writers for the contributions of their thoughtful and critical research papers. In fact, the future of Orthomolecular Medicine depends upon all of our critical opinions being pooled into a unity of honest dialogue, open-minded research and clinical implementation of discovered truths. But we must begin now — in our medical schools and throughout all our medical clinics — to cease dabbling in nutritional areas of science and to implement programs of intensive research. If we do, it will be an unparalleled accomplishment for all mankind.

REFERENCES

1. Sigerist, H.E. *The University at the Crossroads.* New York: Shuman, 1946, p. 114.
2. Steiglitz, E.J. *Time,* July 23, 1956.
3. Williams, R.J. *Nutrition Against Disease.* New York: Pitman, 1971, p. 4.
4. Scrimshaw, N.S. *Hunger U.S.A.* Washington, D.C.: The New Community Press, 1968, p. 40.
5. Sebrell, W.H. "Changing Concepts of Nutrition." *Am. J. Clin. Nutr.,* 15:111, 1964.
6. Stare, F.J. *Hunger U.S.A.* p. 40.
7. Williams, R.J. *Nutrition Against Disease.* p. 11.
8. Williams, R.J. *Nutrition Against Disease.* p. 11.
9. "Important Prescribing Information from FDA Commissioner Charles C. Edwards, M.D.," U.S. Department of Health, Education and Welfare, 1971.
10. Gross, M. *The Doctors.* New York: Random House, 1966.
11. Butterworth, C.E. "The Skeleton in the Hospital Closet." *Nutrition Today,* April, 1974.
12. Pauling, Linus. "Orthomolecular Psychiatry." *Science,* 160, 265, 1968.
13. Williams, R.J. *Nutrition Against Disease.* pp. 13-14.
14. Williams, R.J. "Medical Research Leading to the Acceptance of the Orthomolecular Approach." *Journal of Orthomolecular Psychiatry,* Vol. 4, No. 2, p. 99.

2

A Renaissance of Nutritional Science is Imminent*

ROGER J. WILLIAMS, JAMES D. HEFFLEY,
MAN-LI YEW AND CHARLES W. BODE

INTRODUCTION

There is a wide spectrum of uninformed inexpert opinion regarding the practical importance of quality nutrition in our daily lives. At one extreme are the food enthusiasts, including faddists; at the other is the majority of practicing physicians who through the fault of their medical school training tend to ignore all but the most elementary aspects of nutrition, and to avoid becoming involved in a field so characterized by intricacies, uncertainties, and ignorance.

Those who have medical training are in a unique position; they alone have the background necessary to grasp fully the deep-seated significance of nutrition in relation to health and disease. Unfortunately, however, medical science has not developed and nurtured nutritional science [1], and the public has all too often discovered that those who should know the most about nutrition know very little.

There have been, of course, far-sighted physicians who have been interested in nutrition and have contributed a substantial part of what is presently known. They have often chided their colleagues — generally, but not always, with soft voices — largely to no avail. These physicians who are really interested in nutrition often lack prestige and tend to operate outside the mainstream of medicine. In addition, an increasing number of those who are medically trained carry out investigations which impinge strangely on nutrition, yet because of their training they are not nutritionally oriented.

As a result of decades of neglect of nutritional science by medical science, what we would regard as sophisticated well-rounded nutritional science does not exist. Senator Schweiker, a layman, has recognized this severe deficiency and has introduced a bill authorizing the appropriation of $5 million annually to provide nutritional education in medical schools.

Expert sophisticated nutritional science necessarily involves a basic understanding of biochemistry, physiology, and pathology and an ability to deal in depth with the functioning and inter-relationships of all the nutrients — minerals, trace minerals, amino acids, vitamins, etc. Not only this, but it must also encompass the biological nature of the human beings who are to be nourished, including the inheritance factors which affect their nutrition. As

*Reprinted with permission: *Perspectives in Biology and Medicine*, Vol. 17, No. 1. Autumn 1973.

with other branches of science, its development must depend on interdisciplinary interest and intercommunicating specialized experts. Many tools, including those of mathematics, are now available with which to study human beings and their biological uniqueness. What is needed is the incentive, interest, and support of such investigations.

Sophisticated nutritional science, when developed, will recognize four basic facts which have not entered the mainstream of medical thinking. These four facts will be presented briefly, not with the claim that they are completely new or previously unheard of, but rather that they are crucial to the development of nutritional science and are commonly neglected.

I. Food is a Part of our Environment

Once stated, the above proposition becomes so obvious as not to require defense. We get oxygen from the air we breathe, water from the fluid we drink, and an assortment of about 40 or more essential nutrients from the food we consume. These all become a part of our internal environment, the *milieu interieur* that Claude Bernard talked about in the last century.

The mere recognition of this fact raises serious questions. What happens to cells and tissues if this nutritional environment is not well adjusted? May not the quality of the nutritional environment have a profound effect on health [2]? Can we afford to monitor carefully and scientifically other aspects of our environment like air and water, at the same time giving inexpert stepmotherly attention to the most complex part? From a practical standpoint, in what ways is this complex nutritional environment most subject to damaging deterioration?

II. Suboptimal Nutrition Prevails in Nature

Because nutritional science has been neglected, another crucial consideration has not been grasped. It is the fact that it is very common indeed for organisms in nature to live continuously under suboptimal nutritional conditions. This may happen during embryonic stages of development, but is most certainly the rule during postembryonic stages of life.

Among higher organisms, those receiving the best nutrition

are the very young, the sprout nurtured by the seed, the embryos of mammals and fowls, and the suckling young. Nature has ordained it so that good nutrition is often furnished; otherwise the young would not survive. When, however, organisms pass from these early stages to become corn growing in a field, partially grown fowls or mammals, children of school age or younger, there is no automatic way in which they get what they need, and suboptimal nutrition prevails.

That suboptimal nutrition is common throughout the biological kingdom can be made clear by a few examples. A half-ounce cake of compressed yeast, if given good nutrition continuously, will yield in 1 week over a billion tons of yeast. This kind of nutrition is not supplied to yeast cells in nature. Corn growing in a field may produce all the way from less than 1 bushel up to 150 or more bushels per acre, depending on the quality of the environment furnished. Practically speaking, this environment is always suboptimal. Young weanling rats fed grain diets which were thought "normal" 50 years ago develop slowly, gaining weight at the rate of 1-2 grams per day. Now, when we know more about rat nutrition, they may be expected to develop rapidly and gain, if well fed, 5-7 grams per day. Some organisms commonly get in nature better nutrition than others, but in general adult organisms do not get nutrition of such high quality that it could not be improved.

No doubt the same principles apply to human beings. Large segments of the world population subsist on nutrition which is very far from optimal. The cells and tissues of our bodies (like those of other species, including all plants and animals) commonly compete for food essentials, and it certainly cannot be assumed that even in more advanced countries these cells and tissues automatically get precisely the right assortment of individual nutrients. This is a particularly dangerous assumption when applied to a highly industrialized culture in which processed and preserved foods are consumed and scientific nutrition is neglected.

We often get passable nutrition for the cells and tissues of our bodies because we are surrounded by plants and animals which furnish us food. These plants and animals have in their metabolic machinery the very same building blocks — minerals, amino acids, and vitamins — that we have in our cellular machinery. The removal of some of these building blocks during processing and preservation can only cause damage, and this damage cannot be repaired by partial replacement.

The acceptance of the idea that suboptimal nutrition is universal is enough by itself to change one's entire outlook. Nutrition now becomes something that is always subject to improvement. "Normal nutrition" becomes a relatively meaningless expression; if it means anything, it is some level of suboptimal nutrition. If nutrition were optimal, it certainly would not be "normal."

III. Individuality is a Crucial Factor in Nutrition

A third vital consideration neglected by a backward nutritional science, in spite of its tremendous practical importance, is individuality in nutrition. Lucretius wrote about 2,000 years ago: "What is one man's meat is another's poison," but medical science in its general neglect of realistic nutrition has not sought to explore the roots and determine the full significance of this ancient saying.

The bearing of individuality on the practical application of nutrition can be indicated by this illustration. The following five statements are probably true. (1) The majority of adults require 750 mg or less of calcium per day. (2) The majority of adults require 10 mg or less of iron per day. (3) The majority of adults require 800 mg or less of lysine per day. (4) The majority of adults require 1 mg or less of thiamine per day. (5) The majority of adults require 1.5 mg or less of riboflavin per day.

If we attempt to collect and tabulate these five bits of information, we may arrive at the following table. This, however, is completely spurious.

Daily Needs of the "Majority of Adults" (Spurious)

Calcium	750 mg or less
Iron	10 mg or less
Lysine	800 mg or less
Thiamine	1 mg or less
Riboflavin	1.5 mg or less

To explain how this collective tabulation is invalid and that the collective data do not necessarily apply to not more than about 3 percent of the supposed population, we may start with an imagined population of 1,000 adults. If the first statement regarding calcium needs is strictly and literally true, 499 out of the 1,000 adults may have calcium needs higher than 750 mg and, hence, strictly speaking must be excluded from the tabulation. If the second statement is likewise strictly true, 250 more may have iron needs above 10 mg and, hence, cannot with strictness be included. If the third, fourth, and fifth statements are likewise true, 125, 62, and 31 additional individuals may be successively eliminated from the collective estimates, leaving a residue of only 33 out of 1,000 to whom all five estimates must apply.

If our illustration had included a large number of nutrient items, the percentage for whom the collective estimates certainly apply would decrease to the vanishing point, regardless of the exact method of calculation. If 30 nutrients were involved, for example, calculating on the same basis as above shows that all but about five members of the entire estimated world population would be excluded from the collective estimates. If the five original estimates were correct for "80 percent of adults" instead of the "majority of adults," the collected estimates would apply not to "80 percent of adults" but to about 33 percent. If in this case there were 30 nutrient items involved, the collected estimates would apply to only one adult in 806 instead of "80 percent of adults."

Those who neglect this principle may concern themselves unwittingly with the nutrition of a minuscule part of the whole population — those whose needs are about average in each of dozens of respects.

This discussion would be merely academic if individual needs were clustered around narrow limits, but this is very far from the case. When the Food and Nutrition Board considered several years ago the desirability of publishing the ranges of human needs, they were confronted by the fact that these ranges were not known. The studies essential to such determinations had not, in many cases, been made.

The situation is about the same at the present time. We have found definitive, though not necessarily ample, evidence with respect to range of needs of 10 nutritional items as presented in Table 1.

Table 1.   Ranges of Daily Human Needs for Certain Nutrients

Nutrient	Range	No. Subjects	Reference
Tryptophan	82-250 mg (3-fold)	50	3, 4
Valine	375-800 mg (2.1-fold)	48	3, 5
Phenylalanine	420-1,100 mg (2.6-fold)	38	3, 6
Leucine	170-1,100 mg (6.4-fold)	31	3, 7
Lysine	400-2,800 mg (7-fold)	55	3, 8, 9
Isoleucine	250-700 mg (2.8-fold)	24	3, 10
Methionine	800-3,000 mg (3.7-fold)	29	3, 9
Threonine	103-500 mg (4.8-fold)	50	3, 11
Calcium	222-1,018 mg (4.6-fold)	19	12
Thiamine	0.4-1.59 mg (3.9-fold)	15	13

For 10 other items — magnesium, iron, copper, iodide, vitamin A, vitamin D, vitamin E, ascorbic acid, pyridoxine, cobalamine — there is some indirect evidence about differences in requirements but little about ranges. In the cases of vitamin A [14, pp. 143-146; 15; 16], vitamin D [17, 18, 19], ascorbic acid [20, 21, 22], and pyridoxine [23, 24, 25], the evidence is that the ranges are probably very wide if the entire population is included. For 16 other nutrients, about which there can be no serious question, we find no information whatever regarding ranges of human needs. The presumption, on the basis of the definitive information available, is that the needs for all nutrients vary on the average over a fourfold range.

These data cannot be neglected in any intelligent realistic approach to human nutrition. To do so can result only from living in a dream world where the "hypothetical average man" is of most vital concern and real individuals are banished.

An inspired writer in the *Heinz Handbook of Nutrition* wrote 13 years ago as follows:

> Individual organisms differ in their genetic makeup and differ also in morphologic and physiologic aspects, including their endocrine activity, metabolic efficiency, and nutritional requirements. . . . It is often taken for granted that the human population is made up of individuals who exhibit average physiologic requirements and that a minor proportion of this population is composed of those whose requirements may be considered to deviate excessively. Actually there is little justification in nutritional thinking for the concept that a representative prototype of *Homo sapiens* is one who has average requirements with respect to all essential nutrients and thus exhibits no unusually high or low needs. In the light of contemporary genetic and physiologic knowledge and the statistical interpretations thereof, the typical individual is more likely to be one who has average needs with respect to many essential nutrients *but who also exhibits some nutritional requirements for a few essential nutrients which are far from average.* [26] [Italics supplied]

This statement, however, has barely rippled the waters of the dyed-in-the-wool nutritionists. The time has come, we believe, when far more serious attempts will be made not only to know more about the ranges of human needs, but also to determine for individuals what needs they may have which are "far from average." In the case of some nutrients, this can be done now, but to make substantial progress in this area will require a major effort. Medical science must come to the rescue, applying to the job a substantial proportion of the resources it has been furnished. Automated equipment and computerized techniques will be widely used in this effort.

Acceptance of the facts of individuality greatly magnifies the possibilities of improving the suboptimal nutrition which is so widespread. People who are regarded as in relative good health may be living with suboptimal nutrition in a generalized sense; more pointedly, however, they are very likely to be functioning at a low level of efficiency because their nutrition is suboptimal in specific ways which can be not only determined but also corrected.

These considerations lay the groundwork for a grand eye-opening with respect to the importance of expertly monitored nutrition for people in general as well as the tremendous role it can play in medical practice. Instead of assuming, as physicians are prone to do, that patients automatically are well nourished, it will become accepted as common knowledge that generally speaking they are not, even if they do escape beriberi, pellagra, scurvy, and kwashiorkor. It will be realized that with human beings as with experimental animals [27], there is an enormous variability on the part of individuals to subsist on diets of mediocre or poor quality.

The genetotrophic concept, now 23 years old, is of vital concern in this discussion [28]. The basic idea may be simply expressed as follows: Diseases which have hereditary roots (this may be a widely inclusive category) may exist because the individuals concerned have unusual nutritional needs that are not easily met. If this is so, then meeting these needs should abolish the diseases in question.

It is well recognized in biological science that specific organisms require suitable environments if they are to thrive. The genetotrophic concept is an application of this principle. Certain individuals, it proposes, must have special nutritional environments if they are to thrive.

In spite of the fact that genetotrophic diseases may well include most noninfectious diseases, the validity or nonvalidity of this postulate has received practically no attention. The word genetotrophic is in medical dictionaries, but that is about as far as the matter has progressed. This could not possibly have happened if medical science were alert to the principles of nutrition. The soundness of the genetotrophic idea has never been questioned; it simply has not been tested for its applicability to any common disease.

It has been found inadvertently to be valid in some cases. In phenylketonuria, for example, fully adequate diets low in phenylalanine are not found naturally, but when these are compounded and furnished children suffering from phenylketonuria, the difficulty is controlled.

Certain rats with a hereditary need for high levels of manganese develop on ordinary diets severe inner ear difficulties. When these animals are artificially furnished high manganese diets, the inner ear difficulties do not appear [29-31]. There are probably a number of other isolated examples that could be cited, but what medical science needs to ascertain, by using expertise that is not generally cultivated, is whether individuals who are peculiarly susceptible to heart disease, obesity, arthritis, dental disease, mental disease, alcoholism, muscular dystrophy, multiple sclerosis, and even cancer, can be benefited by nutritional adjustments. How can we possibly know if medical science, taking the vital facts of individuality into account, does not try seriously to find the answer?

IV. In Nutrition, Teamwork is Essential

The fourth basic fact in nutrition which has been sadly neglected by medical science is that of the essential "teamwork" among nutrients. Because this principle has been neglected, a wholly unscientific concept has been widely accepted with respect to what a nutrient may be expected to do.

The basic error, tacitly accepted, may be expressed as follows. Nutrients – amino acids, minerals, and particularly vitamins – are potential "medicines," and should be tested accordingly, using statistical methods and suitable placebo controls to determine their efficacy in combating diseases. If they prove to be "specifics" for particular diseases, well and good; if not, they must be regarded as medically worthless. In defense of this way of thinking is the historical fact that individual nutrients have in some cases acted like medicines – thiamine for beriberi, ascorbic acid for scurvy, niacinamide for pellagra. However, the parallel between these vitamins and "medicines" is more apparent than real, as careful consideration will show.

Following this erroneous reasoning, it is concluded that since specific individual nutrients are ineffective when tested in this way against specific common ailments, these nutrients are worthless for combating disease. It is easy to conclude also that there should be no substantial concern regarding the intake of these nutrients on the part of patients.

The joker in the argument is that while no nutrient by itself is an effective remedy for any common disease, the nutrients acting as a team are probably effective in the prevention of a host of diseases. Against infective diseases, the teamwork may serve to increase resistance. The reasonableness of this broad claim becomes apparent if we accept the postulate that when the environment of our body cells and tissues is adequate and perfectly adjusted, the cells and tissues will perform all their functions well, and a disease-free condition will be promoted.

It must be emphasized that adequate nutrition must involve the complete chain of nutrients. If a diet is missing one link in the nutritional chain, it may be as worthless for supporting life as if it were missing 10 links. One nutrient – mineral, amino acid, or vitamin – added as a supplement to a food can bring no favorable effect unless the food contains some of all the other nutrients or unless they are available from the reserves of the person being nourished.

It is now well recognized, for example, that while thiamine does act as a remedy for beriberi, it does so because in the diet of polished rice the weakest link in the chain is its thiamine content; thiamine alone will do no good if the other members of the nutrition chain are absent. It is a well-authenticated fact that to bring back health to a victim of beriberi, pellagra, or scury, complete nutrition – the complete chain or team – is essential. Manifestly, the nutritional chain is as strong as its weakest link. Every nutrient in the list acts like a gear in a complicated machine. There are no nutrients (or gears) which are dispensable.

To seek to educate the public as the Wheat Flour Institute has done [32, p. 14] by teaching that vitamin A, thiamine, niacin, riboflavin, vitamin C, vitamin D, protein, calcium, and iron are the "key nutrients" is to miseducate. Is there any evidence to suggest that phosphate, magnesium, zinc, vitamin B_6, vitamin B_{12}, and pantothenic acid are not key nutrients? Actually, the list of key nutrients is a long one. Every essential nutrient is a separate key which operates only when the other keys are also available.

The development of nutritional science will reveal, we believe, a clear-cut distinction between medicines and nutrients. The physiological effects of medicines can be ascribed to their ability to enter into metabolic machinery and interfere with enzyme systems. This can happen to the detriment of parasites, and presumably in a beneficial way when the host tissues are concerned. Nutrients, on the other hand, act constructively as building blocks for enzyme systems. If a medicine were to act constructively, it would cease to be medicine. It would be a nutrient.

Those who would lightly dismiss the teamwork principle as exemplifying the "shotgun approach" fail to appreciate that biologically every kind of organism in existence derives from its environment all of its nutritional essentials as a team. An organism typically derives whatever nutrients it needs simultaneously, not *ad seriatim*. If the teamwork principle exemplifies the "shotgun approach," it can hardly be condemned on this basis. This approach has a very long and honorable history. It has been used consistently and universally ever since life on earth began.

It is no coincidence that those nutrients so often stressed in elementary "nutritional education" of the past include conspicuously those which have historically acted like "medicines." These are undeniably important, but to think of them as *the* key nutrients" is to deny the teamwork principle.

Nutrients as physiological agents must be judged on the basis of how they participate in teamwork. A substance suspected of being an indispensable nutrient cannot be excluded on the basis of its ineffectiveness when tested as a "medicine." Nutrients can be extremely valuable, particularly in preventive medicine, but not unless they are used with intelligent appreciation of how they work as members of a team.

Those who recognize fully the validity of the teamwork principle cannot be complacent about the possible existence of nutritional "unknowns." If there are still unrecognized cogs, they must be identified before the operation of the whole machinery can be adequately controlled and studied. Unless there are important alternative ways in which organisms bring about metabolism, the furnishing of each of the nutrients we know about depends upon all the other nutrients being available. Laboratories that are pharmaceutically oriented tend to be interested in any new "medicine," but the search for unknowns in human nutrition is relatively quiescent. That these may exist is suggested by our inability to grow cells at will in chemically defined media in tissue culture. If medical science were fully alert, it would be very much concerned with the problem.

A reflection of the lack of appreciation of the teamwork principle is the reliance placed upon food composition tables. These tables as ordinarily presented in government publications and elsewhere give no hint of the existence of a large indispensable team of coordinated nutrients. They give only fragmentary information which is easily misleading. Judgments as to the nutritional value of a food based on such tables are subject to serious error, especially when processed foods are involved and when nutrient items listed include prominently those which have commonly been added as fortification — thiamin, riboflavin, niacin, and iron.

"Nutrition surveys" [33] reflect the same neglect of the teamwork principle. The nutritional adequacy of the food consumed in different localities cannot be judged adequately on the basis of its content of thiamin, riboflavin, niacin, and iron, particularly when these are the nutritional elements used to "enrich" bread and cereals.

In our laboratories we have recently studied an alternative criterion for judging food values [34]. This is by measuring what we call the "trophic" or beyond-calorie value. Experimentally we ascertain how much new tissue the food in question can produce, beyond that produced in control animals where carbohydrate is supplied in place of the tested food. This method, which inevitably involves biological testing, measures the effective presence of the entire team necessary for tissue building and repair, including the unknowns if they exist.

BROAD SIGNIFICANCE OF THESE FOUR CRUCIAL FACTS

The four facts we have outlined — food is a part of our environment; suboptimal nutrition is ubiquitous; individuality is crucial in nutrition; and teamwork is essential in nutrition — cannot be seriously disputed, and they are far from trivial. When they are accepted, as they must be, there will be a revolution not only in nutritional science, but also in all of medicine, particularly when it is concerned with prevention.

When these four facts are duly considered and nutritional science developed, many currently accepted ideas will be weighed in the balance and found wanting, as either meaningless or misleading and essentially false. Such statements as the following are often made or tacitly accepted. "People in America get good nutrition." "Food contains an abundance of all the minerals, vitamins, etc. that are needed." "Food composition tables adequately reveal food values." "Nutrition surveys will tell us wherever there is malnutrition." "The recommended daily allowances of the Food and Nutrition Board are a safe guide to all nutrient needs." "If you want nutritional advice, ask your physician."

In the light of the four facts we have emphasized, these statements are puerile and are accepted only in ignorance. The fact, which must be faced, is that nutrition is an involved and intricate matter, and at present no one knows just what optimal nutrition is or how precisely to find out. Abundant incentives exist for attempting to reach this goal [35]. Such an objective must await the further development of nutritional science.

The general acceptance of the four facts we have outlined will result in far more intelligent regulations on the part of the Food and Drug Administration. This body is naturally influenced greatly by current medical opinion, and it will change its attitudes as medical thinking changes. At present the Food and Drug Administration credits physicians with an expertise they should possess but do not. Their regulations too often reflect the backwardness of nutritional science.

The four facts we have discussed are simple ones. They can be and need to be understood even by adolescents. The menace of faddism and charlatanism can only be overcome by education,

but it has to be education at a much higher level than has been customary. When the public is reasonably well informed, and medical science has adopted nutritional science as its own, faddism will tend to disappear, and people can get dependable nutritional advice from their physicians.

The prevention of disease, an objective which is inherent in better nutrition and the development of nutritional science, is as old as Hippocrates, who advocated nutrition first, then drugs, then surgery.

Prevention of disease — by every means at our disposal — is the wave of the future in medicine. The expertness medical science has developed in preventing infectious disease will spread to the prevention of non-infective disease. The economics resulting from prevention in terms of health and wealth will be enormous [36]. Prevention of a disease in an individual, when the means are known, may cost only a few cents or a few dollars, while if the disease is allowed to strike, the cost in money alone may easily run into the thousands of dollars. A gram of prevention is worth a kilogram of cure. The development of nutritional science is the principal highway that will lead to the prevention of noninfective disease.

Scientifically, nutritional science is a mere shadow of what it will be when medical science throws its weight behind its development by promoting a health-oriented instead of a disease-oriented discipline.

One relatively open area for scientific investigation is that of intercellular symbiosis [37]. There are probably many substances, of which glutamine, other "nonessential" amino acids, inositol, lipoic acid, and coenzyme Q are examples, which are considered nonessential for the "normal human being" who produces them endogenously. In the light of our discussion of individuality and the genetotrophic concept, however, these nutrients may be crucially needed by certain individuals whose endogenous processes may be somewhat impaired. It appears, for example, that victims of heart disease often are unable to produce enough coenzyme Q to keep their heart muscle unimpaired [38].

All the nutrients we have mentioned above, as well as others, are potential additions to the armamentarium of future physicians who wish to prevent and treat disease by sophisticated nutritional means.

A well-developed nutritional science which recognizes the hard facts of individuality will also delve into many other problems such as the matter of imbalances, the role of intestinal microorganisms in the nutrition of individuals, the question of the incidence and importance of defective enzymatic systems in the digestive tract [2, pp. 189-190], the large problem of malabsorption as it relates to the nutrition of individuals, and the broad question of the overall effects of slow or rapid development during youth on future health and well-being during adulthood.

Another area of great concern to those who would embrace sophisticated nutritional science is that of the basic functioning of some of the well-established nutrients like vitamin A, vitamin A acid, vitamin E, and vitamin C. Because enzymology is a relatively active field, the functioning of many of the B vitamins is relatively well understood, but the physiological function of the vitamins which were originally designated by the first, third, and fifth letters of the alphabet, still presents serious enigmas.

Another area of great scientific interest is the relationship of nutrition to hormone production. It is well known, for example, that thyroid hormone production may be limited by the availability of dietary iodine. Is insulin production, for example, ever limited by dietary lack of sulfur-containing amino acids, or are there other hormones the building of which may be impaired because of nutritional lacks? Development of sophisticated nutritional science will inevitably help solve the major problem of the biochemical functioning of hormones and the general problems of endocrinology.

Of great practical interest is the question of how expert nutritional adjustments can come into play in protecting against pollution. The well-recognized fact that ascorbic acid protects animals against lead poisoning and the recent finding that vitamin E protects animals against atmospheric pollutants [39, 40] call attention to this important potentiality. The broad problem of pollution includes iatrogenic pollution of the internal micro-environments and that produced by self-medication and self-indulgence in tobacco, marijuana, caffeine, and alcohol. All of the foreign elements which enter into the *milieu interieur* are capable of affecting the nutritional status of the individual concerned.

Still another area of great practical interest and one that cannot be explored without regard for the facts of individuality and the other facts we have discussed is that of the self-selection of food.

Some nutritionists have stated dogmatically that there is no instinct which guides one in his choice of food. This extreme position in our opinion is just as untenable as the opposite one, namely, "instinct always guides us to select the right food." Somewhere between these two extremes lies the truth, and it needs to be ascertained. It is known that in healthy animals total food consumption (also water consumption) is often well controlled by internal forces. It is also known that impairment of the adrenals greatly affects salt consumption and the ability to taste salt [41, 42]. Some recent studies show that rats have a mechanism in which the brain is involved for selecting essential amino acids [43, 44]. Their food consumption is also affected by the amino acid levels in the blood [45]. It is known that in humans excessive sugar or fat or salt consumption may lead to nausea and rejection.

Experiments have shown that healthy young children given a wide selection of wholesome foods will provide themselves with reasonably good nutrition. Such experiments beg the question of how well the selection will work if some of the foods are not so wholesome! It is a common observation that if children are given a choice of beverage — milk, sweetened chocolate milk, or a cola drink — a large percentage will choose most unwisely. It seems probable this unwise selection is based, in part at least, upon previous poor nutrition of that portion of the brain which plays a role in food selection. Body wisdom is probably not fostered by the consumption of deficient foods. The whole problem of whether and to what extent human beings have internal mechanisms which help them select food wisely needs exploration, along with the question of whether nutritional adjustments can improve faulty choice mechanisms.

The problem of prenatal nutrition requires, in our opinion, special attention, taking into account all of the four facts we have stressed. Nutrition during the reproductive period is more exacting than at other times. It has been found consistently that diets which will successfully maintain adult animals may not be adequate for reproduction. This has been demonstrated in rats, mice, dogs, cats, foxes, monkeys, chickens, turkeys, and fish. For this reason one might suspect that in a world where suboptimal nutrition generally prevails, pregnant women are often inadequately nourished. Nature tries to provide growing fetuses with good environments, but it is powerless to do so if the necessary raw materials are absent from the food consumed. Prenatal nutrition merits extensive and careful study because for reasons we cannot detail here it is probable that infertility, miscarriages, "spontaneous" abortions, premature births, birth deformations, minor birth defects, and mental retardation often have their roots in the suboptimal environment pregnant women furnish the embryos when they eat carelessly or follow inexpert advice [2, chap. 4]. Even if the hereditary cards are stacked somewhat against one, this does not mean in the light of the genetotrophic concept that expert nutritional help could not obviate the potential difficulty.

SUMMARY AND PROSPECTS

Up until recent years interest in nutrition had been waning, but there is now evidence of resurgent interest. In 1967, for example, there was a projected national nutrition survey which resulted finally in a 10-state survey (1968-1970). This indicated a substantial interest on the part of what we may call "the establishment."

There is also a rapidly growing grass roots interest in better nutrition on the part of millions of people as is evidenced by the multiplication of health food stores, the sale of food supplements, and the publication of numerous books and magazine articles dealing with health and nutrition. Misinformation is common, of course, but how could it be otherwise when the majority of physicians are themselves so untutored. Faddism has its roots in interest, accompanied by inadequate basic knowledge. It cannot be corrected by lack of interest accompanied by inadequate knowledge. It will be corrected when more physicians are both interested and reasonably competent in the area of nutrition.

Thousands of physicians and medical students are becoming interested in nutrition and in the possibilities which have been missed up to the present. This groping on the part of physicians and medical students, of course, leads to error, but in the end the groping will pay off. Four new medical societies have been formed in the past year or two, all of them leaning strongly toward nutrition and its use in the prevention and treatment of noninfective disease. They are the International Academy of Preventive Medicine, the Academy of Orthomolecular Psychiatry, the Society of Biologic Psychiatry, and the International Academy of Metabology.

Many encouraging signs indicate that at long last a renaissance of nutritional science is imminent.

REFERENCES

1. Williams, R.J., *Persp. Biol. Med.,* 14:608, 1971.
2. Williams, R.J., *Nutrition against disease.* New York: Pitman, 1971.
3. Rose, W.C., *Nutr. Abstr. Rev.,* 27:631. 1957.
4. Leverton, R.M., Johnson, N., Pazur, J., and Ellison, J. *J. Nutri.,* 58:219, 1956.
5. Leverton, R.M., Gram, M.R., Brodovsky, E., Chaloupka, M., Mitchell, M., and Johnson, N. *J. Nutr,* 58:83.1956.

6. Leverton, R.M., Johnson, N., Ellison, J., Geschwender, D., and Schmidt, F., *J. Nutr.*, 58:341, 1956.

7. Leverton, R.M., Ellison, J., Johnson, N., Pazur, J., Schmidt, F., and Geschwender, D. *J. Nutr.*, 58:355, 1956.

8. Jones, E.M., Baumann, C.A., and Reynolds, M.S., *J. Nutr.*, 60:549, 1956.

9. Tuttle, S.G., Bassett, S.H., Griffith, W.H., Mulcare, D.B., and Swendseid, M.E., *Amer. J. Clin. Nutr.*, 16:229, 1965.

10. Swendseid, M.E., Williams, I., and Dunn, M.S., *J. Nutr.*, 58:495, 1956.

11. Leverton, R.M., Gram, M.R., Chaloupka, M., Brodovsky, E., and Mitchell, A., *J. Nutr.*, 58:59, 1956.

12. Steggerda, F.R., and Mitchell, H.M., *J. Nutr.*, 31:407, 1946.

13. Pett, L.B., *J. Public Health*, 36:69, 1945.

14. Williams, R.J., *Biochemical individuality*. New York: Wiley, 1956.

15. Williams, R.J., and Pelton, R.B., *Proc. Nat. Acad. Sci.*, 55:125, 1966.

16. Rodriguez, M.Z., and Irwin, M.I., *J. Nutr.*, 102:909, 1972.

17. Spies, T.D., and Butt, H.R., *In:* G.D. Garfield (ed.). *Diseases of metabolism*, p. 473, Philadelphia: Saunders, 1953.

18. Albright, F., et al. *Amer. J. Dis. Child.*, 54:529, 1937.

19. Reed, C.I., et al. *Vitamin D.* Chicago: Univ. Chicago Press, 1939.

20. Kline, A.B., *J. Nutr.*, 28:413, 1944.

21. Williams, R.J., and Deason, G. *Proc Nat. Acad. Sci.*, 57:1638, 1967.

22. Yew, Man-Li, *Proc. Nat. Acad. Sci.*, 70:969, 1973.

23. Malory, C.J., and Parmelle, A.H., *J. Amer. Med. Assn.*, 154:405, 1954.

24. Hunt, A.D., et al. *Pediatrics*, 13:140, 1969.

25. Rosenberg, L.E., *New Eng. J. Med.*, 281:145, 1969.

26. Burton, B.T., (ed.) *The Heinz handbook of nutrition.* New York: McGraw-Hill, 1959.

27. Williams, R.J., and Pelton, R.B., *Proc. Nat. Acad. Sci.*, 55:126, 1966.

28. Williams, R.J., Beerstecher, E., Jr., and Berry, L.J., *Lancet*, 1:287, 1950.

29. Hill, R.M., et al *J. Nutr.*, 41:359, 1950.

30. Asling, C.W., et al. *Anat. Rec.*, 136:157, 1960.

31. Hurley, L.S., and Everson, G.J., *Proc. Soc. Exp. Biol. Med.*, 102:360, 1959.

32. *Eat to live.* Chicago: Wheat Flour Institute, 1970.

33. Interdepartmental Committee on Nutrition for National Defense. *Manual for nutritional surveys.* 2d ed. Bethesda, Md.: Nat. Inst. Health, 1963.

34. Williams, R.J., Heffley, J.D., Yew, M.-L., and Bode, C.W., *Proc. Nat. Acad. Sci.*, 70:710, 1973.

35. Williams, R.J., Paper presented to Nat. Acad. Sci., October 1971.

36. Weir, C.E. An evaluation of research in the United States on human nutrition. Benefits from nutrition research. Washington, D.C.: U.S. Dept. Agr., 1971.

37. Williams, R.J., Tex Rep. *Biol. Med.*, 19:245, 1961.

38. Folkers, K., et al. *Inter. J. Vitamin Res.*, 40:380, 1970.

39. Goldstein, B.D., Buckley, R.D., Cardenas, R., and Balchum, O.J., *Science*, 169:605, 1970.

40. Roehm, J.N., Hadley, J.G., and Menzel, D.B., *Arch. Intern. Med.*, 128:88, 1971.

41. Richter, C.P., *Amer. J. Psychiat.*, 97:878, 1941.

42. Supplee, G.C., Bender, R.C., and Kahlenberg, O.J., *Endocrinology*, 30:355, 1942.

43. Rogers, Q.R., and Harper, A.F., *J. Comp. Physiol. Psychol.*, 72:66, 1970.

44. Leung, P.M.B., and Rogers, Q.R., *Life Sci.*, 8:1, 1969.

45. Peng, Y., and Harper, A.F., *J. Nutr.*, 100:429, 1970.

3

"Supernutrition" as a Strategy for the Control of Disease*

ROGER J. WILLIAMS

INTRODUCTION

Aside from the frank starvation there are three levels of nutrition that human beings have experienced: poor, fair and good. "Supernutrition" (total nutrition in the most sophisticated sense) is above and beyond all these. It is concerned with the quality of nutrition, and is antithetical to calorie overnutrition.

Poor nutrition brings about in human populations severe underdevelopment of the young as well as deficiency diseases: beriberi, scurvy, pellagra, rickets, kwashiorkor and all the ill-defined combinations and variations of these afflictions.

Fair nutrition is good enough to prevent the well-recognized deficiency diseases but is not good enough to promote positive good health and excellent development. Certainly our present nutrition is not above suspicion when an official government report indicates "one of every two selective service registrants called for preinduction examination is now found unqualified," (One-Third of a Nation [1]). Mediocre nutrition is unfortunately the kind which medical practitioners have generally been taught to regard as satisfactory. Many nutritionists have tended to accept the same doctrine, namely, if everyone gets the minimum daily requirements of certain specified nutrients ("recognized by the U.S. government!") and are free from overt deficiency diseases, the major aims of nutrition have been achieved.

Good nutrition is best exemplified by what we often give our cats and dogs, as well as chickens and pigs being raised for the market. Such nutrition provides the animals not only with energy but with an abundance of protein of high quality, as well as a good assortment of minerals and vitamins far above the danger line. In accordance with extensive evidence presented in a current book (Williams [2]), good nutrition is probably experienced by no more than a minority of the population such as ours in the United States; for many are satisfied if their nutrition is fair and the physicians, who are typically ill-trained in this area (Williams [3]), often concur.

SUPERNUTRITION

Supernutrition exists at present only as an idea — a potential strategy for promoting health and preventing disease. It is a valid

*Reprinted with permission: *Orthomolecular Psychiatry*, Volume 1, # 2.

concept because there are many loopholes even in good nutrition. If all individuals had perfect digestive systems and about average needs in every respect, then the loopholes would be minimal; but such individuals are probably so rare that they need not be considered, Burton [4]. If medical education had not been remiss in its attention to nutrition during the past six or eight decades, supernutrition would not by now be a strange idea, nor would seeking to attain it be an unusual goal.

The idea of supernutrition is based on two biological observations which can hardly be challenged: First, living cells, in our bodies and everywhere, practically never encounter perfect optimal environmental conditions; second, living cells when furnished with wholly satisfactory environments, including the absence of pathogenic organisms, will respond with health and vigor.

An ideal optimal environment for the cells in our bodies would include not only water and oxygen and a suitable ambient temperature but also an impressive team of about 40 nutrients all blended in about the right proportions and working together. It is no wonder that cells usually have to put up with environments which fall short of ideal.

OPTIMAL ENVIRONMENTS

If living cells commonly lived under optimal conditions, with no room for substantial improvement, then there would be no room for supernutrition. As it is, there is vast room for a serious attempt (which has never been made) to provide the cells and tissues comprising our bodies with highly favorable environmental conditions.

One of the crucial factors involved in any attempt to give our cells and tissues something like optimal environments is the teamwork which has so often been neglected, Williams [2]. If any link in the environmental chain is weak or missing, then the cells cannot remain healthy. The weak link may be something well-recognized like oxygen, tryptophan, thiamin or iron or it may be something more obscure like molybdenum, folic acid or selenium. The result is the same: an impoverished environment which leads to functional impairment.

At one time nutritionists used to speak of major and minor nutrients and of the major and "lesser" vitamins. It is true that some nutrients and some vitamins were discovered before others but once a nutrient is found to be indispensable, it can no longer be regarded as minor or "lesser." Any nutrient which is absolutely indispensable is a link in a chain and is a major nutrient regardless of quantitative relationships.

Another factor which may be crucial in attempting to give every cell and tissue what it needs is the existence of many barriers within our bodies. It cannot safely be assumed that the mere presence of a nutrient in our food insures its delivery to the cells and tissues that need it.

Digestion, absorption and transportation are not automatic processes that always take place with perfection. Even if certain nutrients get into the blood, this does not mean that all cells and tissues automatically receive an adequate supply. As Pauling [5] has pointed out, the "blood-brain barrier," for example, not only may protect the brain cells against unwanted metabolites, but it may also act imperfectly in the direction of excluding needed nutrients. For all we know, there may be in our bodies other barriers comparable to the "blood-brain barrier."

A complicating factor, which makes it not a simple matter to provide human tissues with optimal environmental conditions, is the consistent presence of microorganisms in intestinal tracts which may help (or hinder) the attainment of the goal.

BIOCHEMICAL INDIVIDUALITY

Another complication is the high probability that human needs are distinctive and appreciably different from those of other animals. The detailed needs of different species are not well-enough known to yield a definitive and adequate answer to this question.

Still another complication is the undeniable fact that each individual human being has nutritional needs which, from the quantitative standpoint, are distinctive, Williams [6]. The facts of biochemical individuality point to the possibility that computerized techniques will have to be employed before refined supernutrition can be applied to individual human beings, Williams and Siegel [7].

It becomes obvious in the light of these observations that scientific expertise has not arrived at the point where we know definitely how to provide any human being (or animal) with supernutrition. This is clearly no playground for amateurs. If supernutrition is to be used to combat disease, experts must be engaged in the undertaking.

RAISE THE QUALITY OF NUTRITION

Despite the inherent difficulties which make attainment of the goal difficult or impossible, there are many measures which can be taken to help raise the quality of nutrition up toward the "super" level. First, we can be as sure as possible that every recognized essential nutrient is supplied in something like suitable amounts. This can be accomplished with a measure of success by consuming milk, eggs and the cells and tissues of other organisms. The same building blocks — the amino acids, minerals (including trace minerals), and many of the vitamins — are universal and present in the metabolic machinery of living cells regardless of their origin. The energy storehouses (e.g., degerminated grains,

fats, oils, sugar) of plants and animals are different; they do not contain all the nutritional essentials, and if we depend largely upon them for nutrition, the result will be an impoverishment of the environment of our cells and tissues.

We cannot safely assume that furnishing high-quality nutrition to an individual will inevitably provide adequate amounts of all the essential amino acids. There are numerous enzymes in our digestive juices, and strong evidence indicates that the patterns possessed by different individuals are distinctive, Williams [2]. Feeding amino acids as such would be a reasonable move in specific cases to help insure the adequacy of the amino acid environment of the cells and tissues.

Providing suitable minerals is difficult, partly because, as was shown in the investigations of Shideler [8], mineral balances are highly distinctive for different healthy young men. As shown by the research of Schroeder and others (Schroeder [9], Schroeder et al. [19]), the trace elements situation is complicated in that the amounts needed are imperfectly known and the supplies are uncertain.

CONSIDER ALL KNOWN VITAMINS

One relatively easy step which may be taken to move in the direction of supernutrition is to provide generous amounts of all the vitamins, especially those which have been demonstrated to be harmless at higher than usual levels. This is relatively safe because in general vitamins which are provided in moderate excess are physiologically inactive. This is less true in the case of amino acids and minerals. Trace minerals in general cannot be tolerated at high levels. Supernutrition assuredly involves not only supplying enough of every nutrient but also avoiding excesses and imbalance, Williams [2].

Several years ago in a different context we carried out an experiment (Pelton and Williams [11]) related to "supernutrition." A group of mice already receiving a commercial stock diet (supposedly well-supplied with all nutrients, including pantothenic acid) were given an extra supply of calcium pantothenate in their drinking water. The result was an increased longevity of about 19 percent. If this result is achieved by strengthening only one link in the chain, one can legitimately expect the result to be even more striking if one attempted to strengthen all the links.

EVERY LINK IN ENVIRONMENT ESSENTIAL

Secondly, in addition to furnishing all the known nutrients, we must have concern for those nutrients which are presently unknown. That such exist is evidenced by the hard fact that cells in tissue culture cannot in general be cultivated in "synthetic" media. The presence of significant unknown nutrients in uncooked food has long been suspected, and Schneider [12] has partially isolated an unusual unknown nutrient for mice.

An attempt to supply supernutrition would involve a deep concern for all unknowns. Scientists whose work impinges on medicine need to identify these unknowns because they may constitute indispensable links in the nutritional chain. If so, their inclusion in attempts to supply supernutrition will spell the difference between success and failure. *Every link in the environment is essential.*

A third step in the direction of supernutrition is to supply nutrients which ordinarily are of endogenous origin but which, under some circumstances, are produced endogenously in suboptimal amounts. The list of such substances may be long. Certainly to be considered are inositol, glutamine, lecithin, lipoic acid and coenzyme Q.

What can we hope to accomplish by attempting to supply supernutrition? The results will obviously depend on how successful we are in reaching for the goal. It is equally obvious, if we assume that healthy cells and tissues spell healthy bodies, that the potentialities are vast.

GENETIC FACTORS

Critics may immediately point out that there are genetic as well as environmental (including nutritional) factors to be thought of. This limitation becomes less severe when we realize, for example, that PKU babies have a genetic defect which, however, can be corrected at least to a considerable degree by special nutritional measures. Rats may have a genetic defect (it causes severe inner ear difficulties) which involves defective manganese utilization. The symptoms can be duplicated in other rats by depriving them of manganese, and can be eliminated from the afflicted rats if the animals having the genetic defect are given an abundant supply of this element, Daniels and Everson [13], Hurley and Everson [14], Hurley [15]. These observations exemplify the genetotrophic concept which was set forth in 1950 (Williams et al. [16]) and in more detail in 1956, Williams [17]. The possibility that genetic defects may be involved does not cancel out the potentialities of supernutrition.

It seems unthinkable that medical science will be inclined to reject, without trial, the hypothesis that promoting the health of all body cells and tissues will result in general health and that the total environment of these cells and tissues is of far-reaching significance in connection with maintaining their health. There may be cells and tissues that are so defective genetically that they cannot be reached by environmental (nutritional) means but this should not be assumed to be true until serious attempts have been made to reach them by this means.

A PREVENTATIVE APPROACH

I have presented elsewhere evidence, hitherto unassembled, which supports the conclusion that supernutrition, or something approaching it, has the capability, if expertly applied, of preventing, (Williams [2]):

1. The birth of defective, deformed and mentally retarded babies.
2. The development of cardiovascular disease and premature aging.
3. The high incidence of dental disease.
4. Metabolic disorders, obesity, arthritis, etc.
5. Mental disease with all its accompanying ramifications.

A CHALLENGE TO MEDICAL SCIENCE

All of the stresses to which we as human beings are subject can be withstood with far greater ease if all our cells and tissues,

including those in the brain, are provided with excellent environments. This is a hypothesis eminently worth extensive trials.

It seems probable that even "incurable" diseases such as muscular dystrophy and multiple sclerosis can be prevented by expert application of supernutrition, especially if it could be started with vulnerable individuals at an early age.

AN UNPARALLELED OPPORTUNITY

This evidence offers an unparalleled opportunity to the medical profession. To the comment "it is all untried," my retort is a legitimate one: "Why hasn't it been tried?" I believe it will be and that the result will be even more impressive than that suggested by the physician, Frank G. Boudreau [18], who said in 1959, "If all we know about nutrition were applied to modern society, the result would be an enormous improvement in public health, at least equal to that which resulted when the germ theory of infectious disease was made the basis of public health and medical work."

It is my considered belief that medical science has taken an extremely important and unfortunate wrong turn in its neglect of nutrition and that this wrong turn is evident in connection with the thinking about all diseases, including cancer.

Cancer is very much in the public mind these days and in the area of medical science treatments and cures are of the utmost concern. Prevention draws little attention and is thought of in a very restricted way.

Here again supernutrition merits serious consideration. There is certainly room for the hypothesis that cells will not go wild (become cancerous) if they are continuously supported by strong environmental conditions. Several studies have shown that cancer incidence in animals is decreased when their nutrition is improved in specific ways, Engel et al. [19]; Antopol and Unna [20]; Sugiura [21]; Kensler et al. [22] No one has taken the trouble to see whether attempts to strengthen every link in the nutritional chain will result in the decreased incidence or disappearance of cancer. This seems a lot to hope for, but available evidence points to the conclusion that if supernutrition can be successfully furnished, cancer initiation may be stopped. Friction, light, carcinogens and viruses are all environmental agents which cause cells to become cancerous. There is an excellent possibility that cells which are provided excellent environments will increase their resistance to all these outside influences, Williams [2].

If we spend money on cancer research wisely, we will certainly not forget about the ounce of prevention.

CONCLUSION

I most respectfully urge that every section of the National Research Council which has to do with human health join with the leaders and investigators in the National Institute of Health and the National Cancer Institute in giving more than cursory study to "supernutrition" and its possibilities. The biological principles on which it is based are, I submit, irrefutable.

REFERENCES

1. One-Third of a Nation: A Report on Young Men Found Unqualified for Military Service. Compiled by the President's Task Force on Manpower Conservation, Jan. 1, 1964.

2. Williams, Roger J. *Nutrition Against Disease: Environmental Prevention.* New York (and London), Pitman Publishing, 1971.

3. Williams, Roger J. How can the climate in medical education be changed? Perspectives in Biology and Medicine, 14:608, 1971.

4. Burton, B.T., Executive Editor. *The Heinz Handbook of Nutrition.* New York, McGraw-Hill, pp. 137, 1959.

5. Pauling, Linus. Orthomolecular psychiatry. *Science,* 160:265, 1968.

6. Williams, Roger J. *Biochemical Individuality.* New York, John Wiley & Sons, (Science Editions), 1963. Austin, Tex., Univ. of Texas Press, current paperback edition.

7. Williams, Roger J. and Siegel, Frank L. "Propetology," a new branch of medical science? *Am. J. Med.* 31:325, 1961.

8. Shideler, Robert W. Individual Differences in Mineral Metabolism. Doctorial Dissertation. Austin, Tex., Univ. of Texas, 1956.

9. Schroeder, H.A. Losses of vitamins and trace minerals resulting from processing and preservation of foods. *Am. J. Clin. Nutr.* 1971.

10. Schroeder, H.A., Balassa, J.J. and Topton, I.H. Essential trace metals in man: Manganese: A study in homeostasis. *J. Chronic Dis.* 19-545, 1966.

11. Pelton, R.B. and Williams, R.J.: Effect of pantothenic acid on longevity of mice. *Soc. Exp. Biol. Med.* 99:632, 1958.

12. Schneider, H.A. Ecological ectocrines in experimental epidemiology. *Science,* 158:597, 1967.

13. Daniels, A.L. and Everson, G.P. The relation of manganese to congenital debility. *J. Nutr.* 9:191, 1935

14. Hurley, L.S. and Everson, G.J.: Influence of timing of short-term supplementation during gestation on congenital abnormalities of manganese-deficient rats. *J. Nutr.* 79:23, 1963.

15. Hurley, L.S. Studies on nutritional factors in mammalian development. *J. Nutr. Sup. 1,* 91:27, 1967.

16. Williams, Roger J., et al. The concept of genetotrophic disease. *Lancet,* 1:287, 1950.

17. Williams, Roger J. Biochemical Individuality. (also see ref. 7).

18. Boudreau, Frank G. Food, Yearbook of Agriculture, 1959. Washington, D.C., U.S. Dept. of Agri. Publ.

19. Engel, R.W., et. al. Carcinogenic effects associated with diets deficient in choline and related nutrients. Ann. N.Y. *Acad. Sci.* 49:49, 1947.

20. Antopol, W. and Unna, K. The effect of riboflavin on the liver changes produced in rats by p-Dimethylamino-azobenzene. *Cancer Res.* 2:694, 1942.

21. Sugiura, K. On the relation of diets to the development, prevention and treatment of cancer, with special reference to cancer of the stomach and liver. *J. Nutr.* 44:345, 1951.

22. Kensler, C.J., et. al. Partial protection of rats by riboflavin with casein against liver cancer caused by p-Dimethylamino-azobenzene. *Science,* 93:308, 1941.

4

Supernutrition*

A. HOFFER

INTRODUCTION

Life consists of the interaction between cells and the environment, each having modified the other. It is impossible to consider either the cell or its environment in isolation unless one is content with the artifacts produced by death. As higher, more complex forms of life evolved the relationship naturally became more complex, and eventually the environment consisted of two main types, (a) the chemical environment which includes the interaction between cells and every chemical in the environment whether airborne, contact, or ingested, and the physical interaction with light, radiation, pressure, temperature, humidity, and so on, and (b) the psychosocial environment. There is a continual interaction between the organism and the chemical and psychosocial environments. This is so complex and its recognition so recent that it is virtually impossible at this time to analyze the entire situation. To do so one would have to integrate all the information we have, imperfect and incomplete as it is, in chemistry, physics, biology, psychology, sociology, and so on, obviously an impossible task.

In this discussion of supernutrition I will therefore ignore the psychosocial environment and consider only the interaction of the organism to a major aspect of the chemical environment, its food supply. I will ignore the role of all airborne chemicals and of all physical variables already listed. Nutrition is the science which deals with the interaction between an organism and its nutrient environment.

Supernutrition is a term used by nutritionists who recognize that each organism has unique requirements. Roger Williams has clearly established the individuality of man. This should not be surprising since it has been recognized for a long time that we are psychologically unique, we seldom look alike, our fingerprints are different, and our blood types are not alike. It would be surprising indeed if our biochemical systems which produced these well-known individual differences were not equally unique. It then follows that the concept of minimal, average, and optimal requirements for people has limited usefulness only. If for every nutrient there is a normal range of variation of need (the usual bell-shaped frequency distribution curve), there would still be left

five to 10 percent of that population which would require much more or much less than the calculated average. This would apply equally to minimum, average, and optimum requirements. There is thus a basic contradiction between a consideration of means and a consideration for the unique individual. Supernutrition is nutrition for the unique individual. This means that nutritional rules can be used only as very rough guides. Following that, only individual studies by the person and, if necessary, with the help of his physician or any other nutritionally sophisticated person can lead to a nutritional program labelled supernutrition.

Those who are unaware of supernutrition are apt to fall into two main types of error, (a) the error of the means and (b) the error of the extremes. Both are equally misleading and dangerous. The errors of the first sort are perpetuated chiefly by physicians and nutritionists. They adhere firmly to mean requirements, lay down general food rules, and advise everyone to adhere to them. They adopt a statistical point of view in which all human uniqueness vanishes. Perhaps it is this view which has turned physicians away from nutrition, because the physician is confronted with a unique individual who is ill, who has already shown by his illness that general rules of health have been of little value.

The second type of error is made by people who have discovered that a certain type of diet is best for them and immediately conclude that this must then be the best type of diet for everyone. Thus a person discovers that he feels much better if he avoids red meats, or dairy products, or certain fats, and promptly develops an insight that this is the ideal diet for everyone. It is comical how perpetuators of both errors attack each other so vigorously when both are wrong because they have ignored the uniqueness of the individual. Recently I was engaged in a brief letter-writing debate with a Minister of Health, meaning with his nutrition department. He wrote that the biggest food fraud was the position put forth by organic food faddists. I had to disagree with him vehemently, claiming instead that much more fraudulent were the claims of many of the food-processing industries. The food industries were dealing with averages considering everyone had identical needs (usually for their product), while the organic food faddists were convinced everyone required only organic foods. I consider the errors of both sorts equally pernicious, but I am much more critical of nutritionists because as trained individuals they should know better. In the long run

---

the food faddists (and I do not consider faddist a derogatory term) will have done more for the health of people than our nutritionists who perpetuate errors of the first sort, for they have helped establish the wide range of needs for nutrition.

Supernutrition tries to avoid both errors. It is optimum nutrition for the individual.

WHY SUPERNUTRITION IS REQUIRED

Man has never been free of his need for food. Throughout the ages there have been major fluctuations both in the quantity and quality of food ranging from severe famine which is still present and growing in many parts of our globe to super-abundance, especially of calories. The term malnutrition is applied to any individual suffering from any inadequate provision of nutrients. When there is a shortage of food in general resulting in too few calories, this is described as starvation. I will use the term malnutrition for the situation where the total intake of calories is adequate but when there is a serious deficiency of one or more essential food nutrients.

Starvation is due to an inadequate intake of calories and leads to weight loss and eventually death. The more serious the lack of food the more quickly will the individual die. Patients are seriously, even critically, ill if they lose more than one-third of their body weight, assuming they were not too fat to begin with.

Malnutrition is produced when there is an excess or deficiency of any nutrient. It is therefore possible to have the following situations:

(a) Starvation alone. There is an inadequate amount of food, but what food is available is of a good quality. There is no imbalance between nutrients. Before food processing became highly developed this was a common problem for every part of the world, but it is rare in highly industrialized nations which have adequate distribution facilities. The word starvation is more apt to strike terror into people and nations, because its aftermath is dramatic and frightening. Governments are much more worried about starvation than they are about other forms of malnutrition.

(b) Starvation and malnutrition. This is more likely to be the case, since under starvation conditions the variety of foods is sharply restricted, leading both to starvation and usually severe malnutrition.

(c) Malnutrition alone. This is much more prevalent today than ever before, particularly in highly industrialized nations. There is an adequate quantity of food, more than enough calories are available, but the food is of such a poor quality that a variety of diseases of malnutrition develop.

Malnutrition alone became more prevalent after the development of cereal crops which provide an abundance of carbohydrate-rich foods, but it began to flourish only in the past century. With the introduction of modern food technology not only did we develop rapid transportation of food, refrigeration, sanitation which are essentially good, but we also developed highly processed food-like materials which do not provide calories, protein, fat, carbohydrate, minerals, or vitamins. It is possible to eat attractively packaged food-like substances which look good, taste good, but which contain no nourishment of any sort and provide us with chemicals foreign to the body, are difficult to deal with, and perhaps are responsible for some of the current plague of degenerative diseases.

It is this synthetic addition of palatability to food-like materials which has created a major problem for modern nations. When unprocessed foods only were available, the high-protein foods were generally more palatable and, where there was a free choice, were selected. Sweetness was relatively rare, being confined to honey and a few fruits. Refined sugar was not available, but it became increasingly available over the past 300 years and now has reached an average consumption of about 120 pounds per person per year in the Western nations. Today it is difficult to purchase prepared foods which are free of sugar. Our mass palate has been so conditioned to sweetness that, to many, unprocessed foods taste flat. Many children no longer look upon water as a thirst-quenching liquid and prefer sucrose-enriched beverages whenever they are given a free choice, and too often demand their sucrose solutions and obtain them from parents who are too weak to resist or too ignorant to know how dangerous these habits are.

About 40 years ago the variety of foods was limited mainly to unprocessed foods. A random selection of food from such a store of that era was less apt to provide an unbalanced diet than a random selection of foods from a supermarket today. At one time our palate alone was a pretty good guide for nutrition, but today, with the ubiquitous use of sugar, salt, and a variety of additives, our palate has become as unreliable as flying a modern jet by the seat of one's pants. This is why we must develop the science and art of supernutrition for we must replace the use of our palate by the use of our intelligence. The answer to the rapidly growing processing industry is supernutrition. When a substantial number of our population practise supernutrition, our food industries will rush in their direction and provide the foods demanded. Until then it may be necessary once more to prepare our own foods. The art of supernutrition cooking must be revived. For only when supernutrition overcomes the malnutrition produced by food processing will there be a halt in the increasing incidence of the diseases of malnutrition and hopefully a reduction.

ELEMENTS OF SUPERNUTRITION

Since supernutrition is based upon the uniqueness of man, there will be no discussion of minimal or optimal standards. For the individual these are meaningless standards. However, the practitioner of supernutrition must be aware of the major components of food and how they are related to each other.

It has been helpful in studying the chemistry of foods to isolate the various components such as proteins, fats, carbohydrates, and so on. This is a valuable way of determining the relationship of foodstuff to our needs and does no harm as long as we remember that these are chemical artifacts. In nature none of these constituents exist alone and in pure form. There is always a complex mixture of all the food constituents. From a knowledge of the properties of these food constituents we infer that in the natural state they have the same properties. This is probably only partially true.

Protein

Proteins are nitrogen-containing foodstuffs. They are made up of smaller molecules or units called amino acid. Of the two dozen or so amino acids, eight are considered to be essential since they cannot be made in the body. The others can be synthesized from other substances. However, a deficiency of any amino acid, either because there is too little in the food or because too little can be made in the body, will produce some interference in metabolism.

The quality of a protein is determined by the quantity of the essential amino acids. A high-quality protein therefore has more of these amino acids than a low-quality protein. Two low-quality proteins may be consumed together to provide a high-quality meal if the deficiency in essential amino acids in one is made up by an adequate quantity in the other.

The quality of a protein may then be inferred from an amino acid analysis of the protein. However, the quality of foods rich in protein cannot so readily be determined, and one must resort to feeding tests. The best assay of a food's ability to support life is its ability to grow young and growing animals at their natural growth rate.

The quality of a protein can be lowered by excessive heat treatment which changes the chemical nature. The protein is said to be denatured, and its biological quality is decreased. Of course heating meat makes it safer and for many people more palatable, but there is an accompanying loss of quality. Proteins provide the amino acids which are used by the body to synthesize tissue, enzymes, and so on. They are not primarily calorie sources. Each gram provides four calories (120 calories per ounce of pure protein). However, protein can be the only caloric source. It is impossible to obtain protein only as very few foods consist of protein only, but it is possible to live on a combination of protein and fats. This was the staple diet of Eskimos, for example, until they came into contact with and adopted the more typical North American diet. Excessive consumption of pure protein could be undesirable. Recently, for example, it has been reported that on high-protein intake there is an increased loss of calcium. Generally, the problem of too much protein rarely exists.

Too little protein is much more common as a cause of malnutrition, and as the world's population continues to outstrip protein production, this will become even more a serious problem. If the pregnant mother consumes too little protein not only is she more apt to develop diseases such as eclampsia, but her child may be formed underdeveloped and stunted both physically and mentally. An infant raised on too low protein intake may also be retarded. Once the brain has been fully developed, protein deficiency is much less dangerous to the brain. But protein deficiency may prevent full development of the physical body, leading to a stunting of the body. Protein deficiency in an adult will, of course, cause muscle wasting which must have a steady supply of amino acids.

Protein requirements vary with state of health, with physical activity, and so on. The optimum quantity of protein will provide the essential amino acids to provide for growth and repair. Too little is dangerous. Too much is wasteful. Each subject should determine from his own sense of well-being what is the optimum requirement for him.

Fats (also known as lipids)

The fatty portion of foods is free of nitrogen but contains carbon and hydrogen. They range from short chain fatty acids to long chain acids and are combined with other constituents. Fats are not soluble in water. They have three main functions: (1) to provide supportive structures, (2) to participate in chemical reactions in the body, and (3) to store extra calories. Each gram provides nine calories. If the same quantity of energy were stored as protein or carbohydrate, twice as much volume would be required. Extra sugar is converted into fat and stored in the fat depots of the body. When required, the fats are released and metabolized. Fats are therefore the reserve depots in the body and buffer the body against variations in food intake.

Quality of fats is judged by the degree of unsaturation. A saturated fat has no double bonds. An unsaturated fat does contain double bonds. Unsaturated fats are liquid at room temperature. The liquidity of the fat therefore is a measure of the degree of unsaturation. Beef and lamb fats are more saturated than chicken or pork fats. If hydrogen is added to unsaturated fats, it becomes less unsaturated (more saturated) and less liquid. Vegetable fats (oils) are converted into solid fats at room temperature by the hydrogenation of some of the double bonds, thus making margarine, etc.

Quality is also determined by the length of the chain. Essential fatty acids are long chain molecules containing 18, 20, and 22 carbon atoms per molecule (arachidonic acid, for example). They are related to the prostaglandins. Quality of the foods containing fats is, therefore, determined by the proportion of all the fats which are unsaturated and by the essential fatty acid content. There are other fats, such as lecithin, which play an important role as well.

The relation between fats in the diet and cardiovascular disease has been examined seriously for the past 20 years. Generally individuals who have too much fat in their blood (cholesterol and triglycerides) are more prone to develop arteriosclerosis. It is not clear whether these elevated fat levels arise from the fats in our diet as many physicians believe, or whether they arise from excessive intake of sucrose and other carbohydrate foods. Probably both factors are operative. This would be expected. What is not clear is what portion of the responsibility should be allocated to each factor.

As a result of the interest in fats, the relationship between unsaturated and saturated fats has been implicated. There is some clinical evidence that saturated fats are more apt to be a factor than the unsaturated fats, and strenuous efforts have been made to increase the amount of unsaturated fats in our diet. This, it was hypothesized, would half and perhaps decrease the prevalence of cardiovascular disease. However, there is a danger that too much unsaturated fat will increase the formation of free radicals, oxidize very reactive fragments of molecules, which are very toxic. Substances such as vitamin E destroy there free radicals and prevent their build up in the body. As a result there is a marked depletion of vitamin E in the body, and this may lead to changes such as accelerated aging. There is probably an optimum ratio of unsaturated to saturated fats for each individual, but there is no way this can be determined by chemical tests. As a rough guide it has been recommended that about 20 percent of the total fat intake should be unsaturated.

Too much fat in the diet will lead to obesity and perhaps to elevated fat levels in the blood. But this seems to be infrequent, perhaps because it is more difficult to overconsume fat compared to sugar. When too much fat is present in the diet, one quickly becomes satiated. Furthermore fat tends to decrease the emptying time of the stomach and gives one a sense of fullness which lasts for many hours. This effectively deters the subject from continuing to overconsume fats. This is the basis of the popular Atkins diet, which for a portion of the program emphasizes high-protein and -fat foods. Later carbohydrate is added to the dietary program.

Too little fat in the diet is also very rare and makes the diet very unpalatable for most people. The stomach empties quickly, and the person suffers from excessive hunger. This is one of the unpleasant complications of the low-fat diet used to treat heart disease. Excessive hunger increases the intake of carbohydrate, which may counteract the fat-lowering effect desired by the prescriber of the low-fat diet. It may also increase the amount of hunger for sugars and make increasingly difficult the weight-reduction program.

Another problem with too little fat in the diet is that fat-soluble vitamins such as vitamin D_3 are also either in short supply or not readily absorbed. Generally excessive quantities of pure fats such as butter, margarine, and oils should be avoided, but there should be no avoidance of high-fat foods such as eggs or milk provided they are consumed in moderation.

Carbohydrates

Carbohydrates are short and long chain molecules much richer in oxygen than are proteins and fats. The long chain fibrous polymers make up cellulose, pectins, and, in animals, glycogen. The basic units are simpler sugars which may have from two to six carbon chains. Glucose, fructose, and galactose are simple six carbon sugars or hexoses. Two hexoses combined form disaccharides such as lactose and sucrose. Long chains make up the complicated carbohydrates such as starch and glycogen.

All carbohydrates must be broken down in the digestive tract into the simple sugars which are then absorbed into the blood. In some people the enzymes which split the disaccharides, such as galactose and sucrose, are lacking, and these sugars are not absorbed. Remaining in the intestines, they tend to retain water there and provide a medium for bacteria, with generally undesirable effects. It is for this reason that some people cannot digest milk. They lack the enzyme which digests lactose (milk sugar).

The carbohydrates have a minor structural role in animals in contrast to plants where cellulose is one of the major structural components. Their main role is to provide calories. Each gram provides four calories.

Pure carbohydrates, especially sugars, are not found free in nature. When plants lay down starch in the wheat kernel, it is associated with smaller quantities of protein and fat but also with minerals and vitamins. The enzymes required to convert the sugars into starch are not removed when the process is completed. Germination reverses the chemical reaction and converts starch into the simple sugars, using the same enzymes which were used to synthesize the starch. When this starch in its original form is consumed, the same vitamins and minerals are available to be used by the body.

When man refines the carbohydrates and sugars, he produces chemical artifacts, i.e., carbohydrates (starches and sugars) free of the other nutrients with which they are normally associated. This is one of the reasons why excessive consumption of sugar generally depletes the body's stores of vitamins.

The result of too much carbohydrate depends upon the type of carbohydrate being overconsumed. The greatest danger arises from overconsumption of the refined sugars; of these the chief villain is sucrose, followed by alcohol.

There is increasing evidence that excessive consumption of sugar is responsible for a condition termed the saccharine disease. The consumption of sugar has increased over the past 300 years from under five pounds per year to well over 100 pounds per year. This is an average figure and includes infants and people who wisely eat very little sugar. This means that a large number of people eat over 200 and even 300 pounds of sugar per year. A person who eats half a pound of sugar per day is consuming 900 calories of sugar, or around 40 percent of his total caloric intake.

The availability of sugar in pure form and its general use as an additive to many foods is usually accompanied by a decreased intake of fiber, a decreased intake of protein, and of course a substantial decrease in minerals and vitamins. The symptoms of the saccharine disease include obesity, diabetes, and diseases of the mouth such as caries and paradontal disease due to a simple overconsumption of sugar. An apple contains about the equivalent of one teaspoon of sugar. Because of the bulk of apple it is rather difficult to consume six apples in two or three minutes. Yet it is a simple matter to dissolve six teaspoons of sugar to consume them in a couple of minutes. Sugars are so dilute in natural sources, even in the natural sugar cane, that it becomes difficult to eat enough of this raw material and to overconsume the sugar portion of it.

A second set of symptoms include peptic ulcer and dyspepsia due to the release of gastric juice when there is too little protein in the stomach. A drink of a sugared beverage increases secretion of gastric juice, and, lacking protein, there is little in the stomach to bind the acid which is then free to act as a stomach irritant. A third set of symptoms is believed due to a decrease in fiber intake. This results in sluggish passage of food through the intestines and constipation. Chronic constipation leads to hemorrhoids, varicose veins, diverticulitis, and perhaps to cancer of the colon. At least populations who consume a lot of fiber are spared these conditions.

Excessive intake of refined sugars also leads to disturbances of carbohydrate metabolism which may express themselves in a variety of carbohydrate irregularities. When the ingestion of a challenge dose of glucose decreases blood sugar more than 20 mg over the next five hours relative hypoglycemia is said to be present. This must be distinguished from absolute hypoglycemia which may arise from pancreatic tumors. Relative hypoglycemia has been considered a disease, but I believe it is more appropriate to consider it an abnormal laboratory test indicative of a disturbance of carbohydrate metabolism. I consider it a symptom of the saccharine disease. In the same way I do not consider hypercholesterolemia a disease. It, too, indicates a disturbance in fat metabolism. Therefore one does not treat the abnormality but the more basic cause. In the same way one does not treat the high blood sugar of the diabetic, but one does treat the body so as to remove the factors leading to elevated glucose levels in the blood.

In my opinion the treatment of the saccharine disease is to markedly lower the intake of refined sugars. The total elimination of sucrose and a moderate reduction in other refined carbohydrates will provide the corrective measures for restoring the carbohydrate metabolism to normal, and this should reverse or prevent the saccharine disease. An absolute elimination of sucrose is obviously impossible, but one should strive for a reduction to under 40 pounds per person per adult per year (about 1½ ounces per day or 160 calories).

Too little carbohydrate is seldom a major problem and, for the majority of people, a rare luxury. However, such a diet throws an increased burden upon protein and fats to provide the calories and tends to be too low in fiber or bulk. A moderate consumption of unprocessed starchy foods can do no harm and does have the virtue of making the diet more palatable and attractive. The proportion of carbohydrate in the diet can easily be determined by the degree of over or underweight. The overweight individual should reduce his carbohydrate intake, while the underweight individual may need to increase it. Most of the effective and safe reducing diets recommend a major decrease in the sugars and a moderate decrease in the starchy foods.

Vitamins

Vitamins are defined as essential substances which cannot be made in the body. However, a couple of vitamins by this definition would be excluded. Thus vitamin D_3 is made in the body and should be classed as a steroid hormone, and nicotinic acid made in the body from the amino acid tryptophane should be classed as an amino acid. However, long usage determines that they will continue to be looked upon as vitamins.

Vitamins are not used as sources of energy but are used to form enzymes which catalyze reactions in the body. When they are not present in sufficient quantity, metabolism ceases or is deranged.

There is an enormous range in vitamin requirements. About 1 mcg. of Vitamin B_{12} is required by most people each day, but there are a few who require 1,000 times as much, i.e., 1 mg per day. When a person with an average range of requirement consumes a diet which does not supply this amount, he will develop a vitamin-deficiency disease. A few classical conditions are scurvy due to a deficiency of ascorbic acid (vitamin C), pellagra due to a deficiency of vitamin B_3, and beriberi due to a deficiency of vitamin B_1. If, however, that person has a much greater need for any vitamin, even a good diet cannot provide this amount. The same deficiency condition may develop. The patient is said to be vitamin dependent. There is no sharp demarcation. When sensitive tests are developed, I suspect that there will be a substantial number who fall in between these two groups. About 20 vitamin-dependent conditions have been described.

Not every vitamin deficiency causes a definite deficiency disease. For this reason it is much more difficult to establish a clear-cut relationship. Conversely, vitamins have beneficial properties which are totally unexpected. Thus nicotinic acid is a broad-spectrum hypolipidemic agent when 3 - 6 grams per day are used. Before my colleagues and I established this finding in 1955, no one could have predicted from any of the known properties of this vitamin that it would have this fat-lowering property. Similarly no one could have predicted before it was first used that megadoses of ascorbic acid would have anti-cold properties. Because of the long-accepted vitamin-deficiency theory, many physicians automatically rejected the early findings that vitamins in larger doses would have these unexpected properties.

When we first published our data showing that nicotinic acid lowered cholesterol levels in the blood, *Nutrition Reviews* carried an abstract written by a physician who was so incredulous of our

work that he misread our table of data and, using our data, proved that nicotinic acid could not lower cholesterol levels. A corrective letter I wrote many months later was published in the same journal.

Most will recall the massive emotional assault on Dr. Linus Pauling's suggestion that vitamin C had anti-cold properties. Since then controlled studies have provided additional support for his conclusions. I have yet to see an apology or retraction from any of his vociferous critics.

Vitamin E is under similar attack even though there are a large number of good clinically controlled studies which establish its beneficial cardiovascular effects. Vitamin B_3 has a unique role in the treatment of schizophrenia and allied conditions, but, as with the other vitamins, these claims are incredulous to those who have not used it as described in the medical literature. However, there is an increasing awareness of the importance of these vitamins in the prevention and treatment of conditions usually not accepted as vitamin deficiencies. The narrow definitions of vitamins and their role in health and disease is slowly widening.

I do not consider that the minimum or optimum recommended daily doses have any serious meaning for the individual. The uniqueness of each person determines his optimum requirement. These standards are crude guesses, are subject to change at the whim of a few people, and even change when one crosses the border into a different country.

The question arises whether every person should supplement his diet with vitamins. In my opinion when a person has the degree of optimum health with which he is content, he need not modify his diet nor be concerned about vitamin or mineral supplementation. Good health I define as a condition in which a person is free from physical and mental symptoms and signs, is able to enjoy his life most of the time, and has adequate reserves of energy to cope with the stresses which we all must unavoidably face now and then. This fortunate individual does not require vitamins or minerals as supplementation in the same way that he does not require penicillin, insulin, antidepressants, or tranquilizers. It is obvious his dietary pattern is good and this contains adequate vitamins and minerals for him or her.

Other individuals not so fortunate probably will require dietary modification and may require nutrient supplementation.

If a patient consults me about the question of supplementation, I first advise that the diet be examined and, if it does not conform to the principles described here, should be modified. If after a reasonable period of time, say three to six months, there is no improvement or too slight an improvement, then I advise a consideration of vitamin supplementation. If this becomes necessary, then it is economical to start with a few basic ones, such as ascorbic acid, vitamin B_3, pyridoxine, and vitamin E, and try to work out the minimal quantity which will produce the optimum feeling of well being.

Several years may be required to work out one's optimal vitamin supplementation. This can be substantially shortened if it is done under the care of a nutritionally oriented physician, nutritionist, or any other person sophisticated in nutrition.

As this review is not meant to be a primer on megavitamin therapy, I will list some of the vitamins which have been proposed by physicians, some of the indications which have been proposed by physicians, and some of the side effects which may occur in some of the people who take these vitamins. It would

Table 1. Megadoses of vitamins which have been recommended by physicians who have worked with these vitamins for many years. For supplementation for people who are not made well by good nutrition only.

Vitamin [2]	Indication [2]	Dose [3]	Side Effects [4]
Thiamine (B_1)	depression Korsakoff-Wernicke Syndrome polyneuritis multiple sclerosis	100 mg to 3000 mg	nausea

Nicotinic Acid	high blood fats
	coronary disease
	schizophrenia
	learning and behavioral
	  disorders
	anti-allergy
	senility
	arthritis
		usually 2 to 6 grams per day.
		Sometimes much more is
		  required
			nausea
			transient flush,
			occasional brown pigmentation of skin

Nicotinamide	as above but does not
	  have any fat lowering action
		same	as above,
			  no flush is produced

Ascorbic Acid	Anti-allergy anti-stress anti-cold constipation anti-infection	over 2 grams per day	diarrhea and gas if dose is too high
Pyridoxine	premenstrual tensions malvaria schizophrenia learning and behavioral disorders	250 mg to 3000 mg per day	nausea

Vitamin E	antisenility
	to promote healing of ulcers
	  and burns for cardiovascular
	  conditions
		400 to 3000 mg (I.U.)	?

Combination of Vitamins A and D_3			
Calcium Pantothenate	to prolong life anti-allergy	250 to 1000 mg	none

Notes:
[1]   See suggested reading list.
[2]   One indication may apply to several vitamins.
[3]   The dose must always be optimum for the individual.
[4]   The vitamins are relatively nontoxic so there is very little literature on toxicology.

only be fair to state that there is a good deal of controversy about these recommendations which will in time be resolved.

The vitamins are generally recognized as relatively safe or nontoxic. However, such a statement has little meaning for the average person. To make such a statement have some meaning, it is important to compare the relative danger of vitamins against the relative danger of other common substances, such as salt, sugar, and aspirin. No chemical, including water, is entirely and wholly safe when taken in huge quantities. This is a self-evident conclusion. But is the substance safe when used within the recommended dose range? With these considerations I have concluded that the vitamins are as safe as sugar and salt, much safer than aspirin, and infinitely safer than tranquilizers, anti-depressants, insulin, antibiotics, and a whole range of synthetic drugs used in medicine. The reason is fairly simple. The toxicity of a drug depends upon the body's familiarity with it. If it is a strange chemical, there are no enzymes for dealing with it; it may build up in the body and thus cause grave harm. But vitamins, being nutrients, are not foreign to the body. They are rapidly metabolized, extra quantities are rapidly excreted, and dangerous levels cannot build up. In addition, the B vitamins, when taken in excess, cause nausea and eventually vomiting. This effectively deters continual abuse. Living organisms have been in contact with vitamin molecules since before life began. There is evidence that the primeval soup (from which life is believed to have sprung) contained nicotinic acid molecules with the other amino acids. The cells of the body react to vitamin molecules as old friends. At times they may be crowded, but excess numbers are quickly carried away and do not harm the cells.

There is a highly emotional attempt to frighten people away from vitamins by pointing to actual and potential hazards. When vitamin supplements, if needed, are used as recommended with skill and caution, they are nontoxic.

It is a truism that not every side effect after ingesting a vitamin tablet is a side effect of the vitamin, for these tablets contain additives, excipients, fillers, and so on to which an individual may be allergic. The best vitamin preparations are free of starch and sugar. This decreases the incidence of side effects.

The question also has been raised whether vitamin supplementation should be taken by normal individuals in order to prevent disease later in life. This question cannot be answered as there is little research designed to test this idea. I see no reason why individuals should not conduct such research on themselves. But I would expect that it would be better to increase the amount of all the vitamins perhaps to 10 times the minimally recommended doses, with special emphasis on vitamin C and vitamin E. It is better to provide a wide spectrum of vitamins rather than just one or two. Perhaps one day Departments of Nutrition will conduct these important experiments.

Mineral Metabolism

If life originated in the sea, it is not surprising we have in our cells the same minerals which are in the sea, having washed in from the land. Every chemist knows how difficult it is to prepare a solution which is free of mineral contamination. It requires an extraordinary amount of work to achieve less than total purity. Life was faced with similar problems. It would make good evolutionary sense to incorporate these minerals into the cell and to make use of them in the construction and function of the cell. In fact, that is what life has done.

The elements which are present and required are called trace elements. There are substances such as iron, magnesium, zinc, copper, manganese, and so on.

In contrast to the vitamins, the range of need of the minerals is not as wide as it is for the vitamins. As with the vitamins, the optimal needs will vary from person to person and must be individually determined.

I will not list and describe the minerals and their function in the body. This information is available in the list of recommended reading.

As with the vitamins, it is preferable to obtain our minerals from our food and only if there are special needs to look to mineral supplements. This can be achieved in most cases by eating whole grain cereals and by avoiding water which is too rich in minerals like copper and lead. Minerals are not evenly distributed throughout cereal grains. In the wheat kernel the lowest concentration of minerals is lowest in the middle, in the endosperm. This is the starchiest portion of the grain and is used for making white flour. The richest source of mineral is near the outer coating of the kernel in the bran and wheat germ portion. If one eats whole grain cereals or enriches the diet by the addition of bran then it is much more likely that minerals will be supplied in adequate quantities.

An advantage only now becoming apparent is that minerals available in foodstuff are bound as organic compounds from which they are released slowly in the body. This is preferable to the pure salts which then have to be bound in the body. For example, it has been found that pure iron salts, when ingested, may increase susceptibility to infection, since this form of iron is available to bacteria to meet their own requirements. Iron already bound to protein cannot be used by bacteria, which will then be less apt to grow.

TRANSLATING PROTEIN, FAT, CARBOHYDRATES, VITAMINS, AND MINERALS INTO FOOD WHICH WE EAT

We don't buy protein, fat, carbohydrates, vitamins, and minerals, we buy food. If we had to translate our needs of the various nutrients into food, it would require a computer for each one of us. Fortunately nature has already turned our needs to a variety of foods available to us. We do not need to worry about these nutrients provided we consume foods which contain the correct quantities of the nutrients. We should improve upon nature and not go backward by destroying the nutritive quality of our foods.

A few simple rules will provide a good diet for most of us. These are:

(1) Eliminate or markedly reduce the consumption of individual food components. These include sugars, especially sucrose, salt, and other pure chemicals.

(2) Reduce the consumption of refined foods such as white flour or polished rice.

(3) Markedly reduce the consumption of processed foods which are rich in additives (colors, preservatives, flavors, and so on).

(4) Increase the intake of roughage, foods which provide bulk in the diet.

(5) Diversify one's food intake. This will decrease the possibility of developing various food allergies.

These rules may be simplified even further into one rule — the no-junk rule. Junk is defined as any food which contains added sugar, refined flour, polished rice, and alcohol. This simple rule will eliminate most processed foods such as prepared cold cereals, pastry, candy, chocolate, white bread, ice cream, soft drinks, and so on. It is the diet which is recommended for the saccharine disease, and for the correction of that form of carbohydrate pathology measured by the five-hour glucose-tolerance curve and called relative hypoglycemia.

Any person who approximates the no-junk rule will be well on the way toward supernutrition.

DAILY PATTERN OF SUPERNUTRITION

The only real objective of eating is to provide the cells of our bodies with all the nutrients they require. The nutrients must be delivered to the fluid surrounding each cell, the extracellular environment. Ideally all the nutrients should be present at about the same time. The cells can then absorb what they need, reject the rest, and excrete into the fluid what they do not require. The ideal situation is seldom met. There is usually a wide variation in the amount of nutrients in the extracellular fluid, but we should at least strive toward the ideal. The most practical method is to eat three well-balanced meals per day with a few small snacks in between. This will allow the body to deliver the nutrients to the cells without too much variation in the concentration of the nutrients.

The term balance should apply to the entire food pattern. There should be a balance over the whole day. All the essential nutrients in optimum amounts should be provided over a 24-hour period. Daily needs will of course vary, depending upon the level of stress, upon the presence of disease, and so on. Generally, stress increases the need for certain nutrients, if not for them all. Certainly there is an increased need for vitamins and for some of the minerals.

There should also be a balance over a meal. It is inappropriate, as an extreme example, to eat all the protein for breakfast, all the fat for lunch, and all the carbohydrates for supper. Each meal should contain a proper combination of the essential foodstuff described.

Finally each food should be as balanced in itself as possible, i.e., one should use the whole kernel rather than only its inner endosperm (whole wheat flour rather than white flour). It is being argued that it is perfectly permissible to eat a totally unbalanced food if during the same meal a balanced food is used. Thus cornflakes, it is said, is consumed combined with milk and therefore the nutrient value of the mixture only should be considered. Roger Williams has highlighted the fallacy of this argument by pointing out that sawdust and milk is a better food than sawdust alone. When nutritionally inadequate foods are consumed, the essential protein, vitamins, and minerals necessary to metabolize these inadequate foods must be taken from the nutritionally adequate foods. As a result there is a net reduction in total vitamin and mineral intake, since foods generally do not contain extra quantities of these essential nutrients.

Supernutrition demands whole unprocessed foods for each meal and over the entire day.

FOOD ALLERGIES OR FOOD INTOLERANCE

Supernutrition takes into account not only the beneficial aspects of food but also the food intolerances or food allergies. It is possible to become allergic to any food, but usually allergies develop to foods consumed frequently and in large quantities. Thus in children milk allergies are common, in adults less frequently.

Food allergies can produce any form of neurosis, psychosis, or behavioral disorder. Often these are the patients who do not respond to megavitamin or tranquilizer therapy. Over the past year there has been a marked increase in interest in food allergies as a factor in psychiatric illness.

There are several ways of determining food allergies, and there will be undoubtedly more. The methods under investigation include, (a) skin testing, the most accurate are intracutaneous tests; (b) provocative oral tests, using food or extracts of foods following a four-day fast or a period of abstinence from that food; (c) rotation food tests; (d) elimination diets. Treatment includes the food, but this may be impossible if multiple food allergies are present.

Desensitization techniques may be used specially prepared, using specific food extracts. These have to be prepared by skillfull allergists. After a course of desensitization which may last a year,

the subject will often be able to consume the food in small amounts. At least he need no longer be concerned about eating small quantities of that food.

Supernutrition will prevent or decrease allergy formation. The probability of allergy formation is greatly decreased if a large variety of foods are consumed in a randomized manner. The greater the variety of foods, the smaller will be the intake of each, and the less likelihood there is allergies will develop.

REFERENCES

Abrahamson, E.M., and Pezet, A.W. *Body Mind and Sugar*. Holt, Rinehart and Winston, New York, 1951.

Adams, R. and Murray, F. *Body, Mind and The B Vitamins*. Larchmont Books, New York, 1972.

Bailley, H. *The Vitamin Pioneers*. Rodale Books, Inc. Emmaus, Pennsylvania, 1968.

Blaine, Tom R. *Mental Health Through Nutrition*. The Citadel Press, New York, 1969.

Blaine, Tom R. *Prevent That Heart Attack*. The Citadel Press. Secaucus, New Jersey, 1972.

Cheraskin, E., and Ringsdorf, W.M. *Diet and Disease*. Rodale Books, Emmaus, Pennsylvania, 1968.

Cheraskin, E., and Ringsdorf, W.M. *New Hope for Incurable Diseases*. Exposition Press, New York, 1971.

Cheraskin, E., and Ringsdorf, W.M. *Predictive Medicine*. Pacific Press Publishing Association. Mountain View, California, 1973.

Davis, Adelle. *Let's Eat Right to Keep Fit*. Harcourt Brace Jovanovich, Inc. New York, 1954, 1970.

Davis, Adelle. *Let's Have Healthy Children*. The New American Library of Canada, Ltd. Scarborough, Ontario. 1972.

Fredericks, C. *Eating Right for You*. Grosset and Dunlap, New York, 1972.

Fredericks, C., and Bailey, H. *Food Facts and Fallacies*. The Julian Press Inc. New York, 1965.

Fredericks, C., and Goodman, H. *Low Blood Sugar and You*. Constellation International, New York, 1969.

Hawkins, D.E., and Pauling, L. *Orthomolecular Psychiatry*. W.H. Freeman and Co. San Francisco, California, 1973.

Hoffer, A., and Osmond, H. *The Hallucinogens*. Academic Press. New York, 1967.

Hoffer, A., and Osmond, H. *New Hope for Alcoholics*. University Books, New Hyde Park, New York, 1968.

Pauling, Linus. *Vitamin C and the Common Cold*. W.H. Freeman and Co. San Francisco, California, 1970.

Pfeiffer, C.C., Ward, J., El-Meligi, M., and Cott, A. *The Schizophrenias: Yours and Mine*. Pyramid Books, New York, 1970.

Pfeiffer, C.C. *Neurobiology of the Trace Metals Zinc and Copper*. International Review of Neurobiology. Academic Press, New York, 1972.

Pugh, K. *Mental Illness: Is It Necessary?* Carlton Press Inc., New York, 1968.

Roberts, Sam E. *Exhaustion: Causes and Treatment*. Rodale Books, Inc. Emmaus, Pennsylvania, 1967.

Shute, W.E., and Taub, H.J. *Vitamin E for Ailing and Healthy Hearts*. Pyramid House, New York, 1969.

Steincrohn, P.J. *Low Blood Sugar*. Henry Regnery Co., Chicago, 1972.

Stone, Irwin. *The Healing Factor. "Vitamin C" Against Disease.* Grosset and Dunlap, New York, 1972.

Szent-Gyorgyi, A. *The Living State*. Academic Press, New York, 1972.

Underwood, E.J. *Trace Elements in Human and Animal Nutrition*. Academic Press, New York, 1971.

Watson, G. *Nutrition and Your Mind*. Harper and Row, New York, 1972.

Williams, Roger J. *Biochemical Individuality*. John Wiley and Sons, New York, 1963.

Williams, Roger J. *You Are Extraordinary*. Random House, New York, 1967.

5

On Sugar and White Flour
...the dangerous twins!*

*How, with the best of intentions, we have managed
to process natural foods into appetite-tempting,
disease-breeding trouble-makers...*

MILES H. ROBINSON

Dr. Robinson, who has served as Medical Advisor on the staffs of two United States Senators during six years of their investigations of the Food and Drug Administration, here documents in fascinating detail the research that has led to realization of the damage we have done to important foods during their processing ... and what the resulting lack of their dietary fiber and excess of sugar is doing to our health. — Richard Stanton, Publisher, *Executive Health*

The importance of fiber (roughage) in the food we eat has been much in the news lately, mostly in connection with new evidence that a lack of it in the diet causes cancer of the colon. Less well known is the evidence that fiber also protects against other important diseases found principally among people who eat the Westernized diet of refined foods low in fiber.

Around 1920, when the startling epidemic of coronary heart attacks began, it soon became clear that some factor in our environment or life style had broken through our resistance to this disease. In recent years, it seemed to be an excess consumption of saturated fat and cholesterol accompanying an affluent diet of meat and dairy products, but this has turned out to be highly controversial, and at best only a partial answer.

There are now strong indications that fiber deficiency has been a major missing link in our understanding, not only of coronary thrombosis, but also of a strange collection of other diseases, ranging from hemorrhoids and varicose veins to gall-bladder disease and diabetes. And sugar, that seductive charmer, the taste of which we love so much, appears to have been an even more powerful link, which has collaborated with fiber deficiency to strike the health of modern man a punishing one-two punch.

An explanation of how these diseases, and others, could have the same basic cause was set forth in a medical article entitled "The Neglect of Natural Principles in Current Medical Practice," by Surgeon Captain Thomas L. Cleave [1], published in 1956 in the *Journal of the Royal Naval Medical Service*. He pointed out that the refining of carbohydrates inflicted concentrated products on the body which it was never designed to handle, particularly white flour and sugar, which have been stripped of the diluting roughage which naturally occurs in both grain and sugar cane or sugar beets.

Eighteen years later, in his latest book, *The Saccharine Disease* [2], Dr. Cleave now shows in detail how the removal of roughage from these foods greatly slows the passage of the bowel contents, which produces diverticular[1] disease, and is a strong factor in cancer of the colon. In addition, the relatively stagnant accumulation of feces pressing on the great pelvic veins raises the pressure in them, slows the flow of blood draining from the area of the rectum and legs, and the end results can be hemorrhoids, varicose veins, and femoral thrombosis (which Mr. Nixon had).

At the same time, the lack of bulky roughage in these concentrated foods causes the stomach to be less distended, so that the satiety mechanism is not fully utilized, and over-consumption of food occurs. Both the abnormal quantity of food and its concentrated nature then subtly disrupt the digestion, and lead to diseases of over-consumption, such as obesity, diabetes and the dreaded coronary thrombosis. Sophisticated methods of analysis are now being used to detect disturbances in body chemistry, which develop under these conditions and ultimately affect many other parts of the body.

Thus, all the diseases mentioned, and others, although appearing to be separate diseases, become only the manifestations of a single master disease, consisting of the over-consumption of refined carbohydrates, showing up in the various digestive, circulatory and other bodily systems. Dr. Cleave has named this parent condition the saccharine disease, meaning related to sugar, whether eaten as table sugar or transformed into glucose during the digestion of white flour and other refined carbohydrates.

Widespread interest in this new explanation of civilized diseases had to wait until Dr. Denis P. Burkitt, of the British government's Medical Research Council and world-renowned for his studies linking viruses to lymph gland cancer, took up the cause about three years ago. Burkitt is actively expanding Cleave's epidemiological documentation, especially regarding cancer of the colon, and he gives full credit to Cleave for his "original hypothesis" and "brilliant conception."

Before considering in more detail the various conditions which Dr. Cleave believes are merely symptoms of a master disease, we should look briefly at the history of attempts to link ill health to the refining of flour made from grains.

---

[1] An outpouching or sac protruding from the intestinal lining into the intestinal wall.

*Reprinted with permission: *Executive Health*, Volume XI, #6.

THE LONG HISTORY OF REFINED FLOUR

The refining of flour made from cereal grains, which removes the outer coats (husk) of the kernel, has been practiced since the time of the early Egyptians. The object was to obtain a white flour which, when made into bread or cake, had a more luxurious taste than that made from the coarse whole flour. The flour was filtered through a sieve of cloth, a process called bolting. The extra cost of the labor generally restricted its use to the upper classes, while the poor ate their grain unrefined. In 13th century England, bread made from the finest particles of sieved flour was called "paindemaine," from the French meaning "bread of the lordly." About 1870, the roller mill was invented, and this achieved a far more rapid, cheap and precise separation of the bran, germ, and white inner substance than ever before.

But not until 1920 was it known that most of the vitamins and minerals are carried in the outer layer of the bran and germ. Given the still used opprobrious name of "offals," these were fed mostly to animals. The full importance of the discarded fiber (roughage) is only now being investigated by modern methods, although the laxative effect of unbolted flour has been known ever since Hippocrates (460-359 B.C.)

For three hundred years, when the Roman soldier was the most physically energetic and mentally ingenious fighting man the world had ever seen, the only bread he ate was made from coarse wheat flour. Wrestlers "ate only coarse wheaten bread to preserve them in the strength of their limbs," and the Spartans were famous for it.

WHAT GRAHAM FOUND . . .

American interest in unrefined flour arose over a century ago, and was due primarily to the efforts of one man, Sylvester Graham (1794-1851), for whom graham crackers and graham flour are named. In 1837, his remarkable little book, *Treatise on Bread and Bread-Making*, was published in Boston.

Graham very concisely gave the history of bread, the virtues of not discarding any part of the grain, details on the chemistry and technique of bread-making, and vigorously attacked the use of noxious ingredients by the bakers. The facts that he assembled, the force of his logic, and the apparent success of those who followed his advice made converts on a wide scale.

Graham was a careful observer. He cited the fact that livestock could not be healthy without bulk along with grain. He stated that whole grains would relieve many cases not only of constipation, but also of diarrhea. This recognition of the dual action of whole grain anticipated by over a hundred years the clinical findings published last year by English doctors, that bran can normalize rapid as well as slow intestinal transit times. He recognized the initial irritation which may occur during the first few weeks of a return to whole grains. He emphasized that diet alone cannot counteract the ill effects of other bad habits, and urged the necessity of exercise and the avoidance of overeating.

The impact of Graham's views can best be understood from the era in which he lived. On the one hand, it was a period of exceptionally able leaders, working in a society receptive to vigorous and independent ideas such as Graham's.

On the other hand, it was also a period when the practice of medicine was in a low state. Clinical thermometers and blood pressure machines did not exist. No one knew anything about cells or bacteria. Dr. Holmes' great paper on the strange contagiousness of childbed fever was not published until six years after Graham's book. Appendicitis was treated with the deadly procedures of purging and morphine, and not until 1848 was the first appendix surgically removed by Dr. Hancock of London.

Ignorance about drugs, and their abuse, prompted Dr. Holmes' famous remark: "I firmly believe that if the whole *materia medica* as now used could be sunk to the bottom of the sea, it would be all the better for mankind — and all the worse for the fishes." Note that this comment was made in his address to the Massachusetts Medical Society in 1860, after Holmes had been professor of anatomy and physiology and later dean of Harvard Medical School!

FROM VALLEY FORGE TO WORLD WAR II . . .

Baron Steuben, the German officer who trained the American soldiers at Valley Forge and throughout the Revolutionary war, said that the peculiar healthfulness of the Prussian soldiers was due to their unbolted "ammunition bread." Another example occurred near the end of the 18th century. During the war with France eighty thousand English soldiers in Essex were fed on bread made from unbolted flour, following an act of Parliament designed to stretch the supply of grain. After a few weeks of initial dislike, the soldiers came to prefer it; and so great was the improvement in their health that whole grain bread became widely popular in England. But when the law expired and cheap refined flour came in from America, white bread gradually came back into use.

Much the same sequence occurred in England during both world wars, with the same general improvement in health. Reasons given by the government for the reversion to white flour after the wars were that it spoiled less easily, was needed by bakers to make more artful products, the bran and wheat germ were needed by farmers to nourish the livestock, and other foods would supply the nutrients lost in the refining of flour.

In Denmark, when a combination of a severe drought and the Allied blockade threatened to cause massive starvation in 1917, essentially the same experiment was repeated on a very large scale. Dr. M. Hinhede, superintendent of the State Institute for Food Research in Copenhagen ordered 80 percent of the pigs and 66 percent of the cows slaughtered. The cereals thereby saved were fed to the population in the form of whole rye bread to which was added 12-15 percent of wheat bran.

The results were striking. The mortality from all causes fell in the first rationing year by 17 percent to the lowest level ever seen in any country up to that time. When the great world-wide pandemic of influenza struck in 1918, Denmark was the only country in Europe without an increase in mortality. The Danish death rate from all causes actually decreased, while in other European countries it rose by as much as 46 percent.

Sir Arbuthnot Lane (1856-1943) was probably the most eminent advocate of whole grains down to the present time. One of the great surgeons of England, he invented the use of metallic plates fastened directly to fractured bones, and specialized in surgery on the colon. From his extensive experience with diseases of the colon, Lane appreciated the importance of whole grains, and they became a crusade of major importance to him. He founded The New Health Society to promote his views on the prevention of disease, and was editor of its journal.

In his book, *The Prevention of the Diseases Peculiar to Civilization*, Lane wrote:

> "The greatest of all physicians, Hippocrates, used to urge upon the citizens of Athens that it was essential that they should pass large bulky motions after every meal, and that to ensure this they had to eat abundantly of wholemeal bread, vegetables and fruits. . . . On this I can only comment that the modern doctor is not following the precepts and practice of his great predecessor, and that knowledge of diet has not formed an integral part of his education."

But again, the hard-earned lessons of the past were fading, and Sir Arbuthnot Lane had little support for his dietary views from orthodox medicine. He died in 1943 at the age of 87, just at the time when a great new wave of medicine swept in — the era of genuine wonder drugs: sulfa, penicillin and the other antibiotics. Ever since, we have been inclined to seek relief from our puzzling chronic diseases in pill bottles rather than in life styles. We drifted back into the luxurious assumption that it mattered very little what kind of food we ate.

THE RENAISSANCE OF NATURAL FOOD

As we have seen, intelligence and dedication have not been lacking over the last hundred and fifty years, in the attempt to settle the question of the apparent benefits of unrefined foods to the health of man — particularly whole grains with their full quota of vitamins, minerals, protein and fiber. Yet, no one had been able to get enough facts together, examine them free from the blandishments of medical innovations and special interests, and interpret them carefully enough to establish a principle which would not perish with its advocate.

That brings us back to Surgeon Captain Cleave, and his concept that our degenerative diseases are caused by concentrated foods, especially white flour and sugar, which have had the fiber refined out of them. For his 1956 article, Cleave compiled a graph showing that the per capita intake of sugar increased from about 15 pounds per year in 1815 to the present figure of about 120 pounds. This enormous increase of sugar in the diet, unknown to man through millions of years of his evolutionary development, facilitated by a breakdown of the satiety mechanism dependent on fiber, and exacerbated by an instinctive and overcultivated taste for anything sweet, may have approached a "critical mass" (to use nuclear language) around 1920, thus touching off an explosion of disturbed body chemistry and coronary heart attacks. (EDITOR'S NOTE: This occurred at the same time the automobile came into mass production and as Dr. Paul Dudley White warned: "It has taken men off their feet." So the lack of sufficient daily walking combined with the excess of sugar and the lack of sufficient fiber in our diet seem at least three of the key causes of the modern epidemic of heart disease in Western civilization.)

Dr. Cleave began his work on the problem of refined foods by combating constipation in families of navy men under his care. Since about 1931 he had been prescribing crude unprocessed wheat bran as received straight from the flour mills. Then, while Senior Medical Officer on the battleship, *King George V* during the second world war, he gave this bran to thousands of sailors aboard ship to relieve the rampant constipation caused or exacerbated by the unavoidable scarcity of fresh fruits and vegetables at sea. The dose was a tablespoon of bran per day, washed down with a glass of water.

From the success of this simple treatment, Dr. Cleave moved steadily into his present conception, correlating clinical, anatomical and epidemiological evidence, and showing how the interrelated effect of fiber deficiency and sugar excess could produce the following:

(1) OBESITY . . .

Dr. Cleave believes that salvation in over-weight lies basically in taking carbohydrate foods in their natural unconcentrated state, that is, with the original fibre still in position, and not in calculations involving calories. At first sight it seems so logical to work out things calorifically. Thus, if the 5 oz. of sugar now consumed by the average person per day in Westernized societies is contained in some 2½ lb. of sugar beet, it would appear to make no difference calorifically whether one consumes the former or the latter. But, this entirely ignores the all-important factors of appetite and satiety. It is easy enough to take down the 5 oz. of sugar in sweets, but taking it down in the form of a 2½ lb. sugar-beet, or the equivalent amount of raw fruit, such as some 20 average apples is a very different affair. And similarly with puffy white bread, as against dense wholemeal bread. No wild animal such as a rabbit in a whole field of grass, ever eats too much; it knows nothing about calories, but appetite and satiety, acting on unconcentrated carbohydrates, protect it infallibly. There are no wild fat rabbits! But due to our concentrated carbohydrates, appetite and satiety no longer protect us. No wonder the average, desk-bound executive is overweight — or just plain fat.

Please remember you should try to avoid all refined carbohydrates, since all are absorbed as mono-saccharide sugars from the intestine, en route to constituting the sugar (glucose) of the blood. It would obviously be open to serious error to forget the maltose you consume if you drink beer, since many men prefer "bitters" to sweetstuffs, yet both are equally capable of causing obesity and other diseases based on over-consumption.

(2) DISEASE OF THE VEINS . . .

It can be shown anatomically that constipation tends to overload the colon, which then presses on the great veins of the pelvis carrying blood back from veins in the rectum, leg veins and scrotum. The resultant sluggish circulation in these parts can be expected to cause hemorrhoids, varicose veins, femoral thrombosis, and varicocele (scrotal swelling). Statistics from around the world show that the incidence of these conditions is negligible in primitive tribes which are still on unrefined diets high in roughage, with rapid intestinal transit times . . . about half that of Western man.

Thrombosis (clotting) in the femoral vein can be fatal, if the clot comes loose and lodges in the heart or lungs. It is particularly dangerous after operations, and the incidence of this has quadrupled in hospitals in recent years, associated with the decline of preoperative enemas and other attention to the bowel. But clinical research is now going forward in England showing that when fiber in the form of bran is put back in the diet preoperatively, the bowel does not clog and press on the pelvic veins, and the incidence of femoral thrombosis after surgery is prevented or decreased.

(3) PEPTIC ULCER, GALLBLADDER DISEASE APPENDICITIS AND E. COLI INFECTIONS . . .

Refining removes from wheat a significant amount of protein (about 11 percent), which is also of a higher quality. Protein buffers the hydrochloric acid secreted by the stomach, and tends to protect the stomach from being ulcerated by the acid.

Regarding gallbladder disease, both animal and human experiments have shown that fiber deficiency and sugar excess impair the function of bile and cholesterol. Gallstones formed from cholesterol are common in people on refined diets, but almost unknown in primitive tribes.

As for the appendix, this is a little blind alley easily clogged and infected under stagnant conditions produced by a lack of fiber. Epidemiologically, appendicitis is almost unknown where unrefined foods are eaten.

Urinary tract infections can occur by the migration of bacteria from the intestine through the lymphatic system. This is more likely to occur if the bacteria become virulent, which tends to happen if over-fed by sugar. Again, such infections are rare in populations which do not refine their food.

Of course, mere association of two factors, such as refined food and a disease, does not prove a causal relationship. Civilization is also characterized by other things, such as stress, inadequate exercise, etc. But the incrimination of fiber deficiency and sugar excess in the diet is building up.

(4) CANCER OF THE COLON . . .

Chemicals with a potential for causing cancer are found in the intestine, either ingested in the food or formed by undesirable reactions of the intestinal bacteria. In either case, a slow transit time caused by fiber deficiency permits such chemicals to lie longer against the intestinal lining, injuring its cells and risking the development of cancer. In the United States, cancer of the colon is second only to lung cancer as a cause of death, and our commonest affliction of the colon is diverticulosis. Both of these conditions are exceedingly rare in the primitive tribes of Africa, but become common when this same racial stock eats refined foods.

(5) DIABETES . . .

According to the Cleave conception, over-eating of concentrated refined food puts an unnatural strain on the pancreatic production of insulin, although it may take as long as twenty years to culminate in diabetes. It is both the rate at which the food energy hits the pancreas, as well as the quantity, which

does the damage. While sugar does provide quick energy, which may be useful in an emergency, it is like burning gasoline in a home furnace. It will burn, but it wrecks the machinery. (The design of the body resembles not a gas but a diesel engine, which is more efficient, and gets its more powerful stroke from a slower burning of a cruder fuel.)

The decrease of diabetes during wars when sugar was scarce and foods less refined (in order to make them go farther), and the virtual absence of the disease among primitive tribes eating unrefined food, both tend to support the thesis that fiber deficiency and sugar excess are important factors, if not the main cause, in diabetes. (EDITOR'S NOTE: As you read last month in our report *"Trace Minerals, Part I . . . On Chromium Deficiency and Atherosclerosis,"* lack of this trace mineral, too, is important in fomenting diabetes and heart disease. It is startling to realize as Henry A. Schroeder, M.D., a world authority on trace minerals points out in his important new book, *"Trace Elements and Man"* [3]: "The milling of wheat into refined white flour removes 40 percent of the chromium, 86 percent of the manganese, 76 percent of the iron, 89 percent of the cobalt, 68 percent of the copper, 78 percent of the zinc and 48 percent of the molybdenum, all trace elements essential for life or health. Only iron, and that in a form poorly absorbed, is later added to flour. The residue, or millfeeds, rich in trace elements, is fed to our domestic animals. And by the same process, most of eight vitamins are removed from wheat, three are added to make the flour enriched; millfeeds are rich in vitamins. Similar depletion of vitamins and essential trace elements occurs when rice is polished and corn meal is refined. Likewise, most of the bulk elements are removed from wheat: 60 percent of the calcium, 71 percent of the phosphorus, 85 percent of the magnesium, 77 percent of the potassium, 78 percent of the sodium, which appear in the millfeeds.

"Refining of raw cane sugar into white sugar removes most (93%) of the ash, and with it go the trace elements necessary for metabolism of the sugar: 93 percent of the chromium, 89 percent of the manganese, 98 percent of the cobalt, 83 percent of the copper, 98 percent of the zinc and 98 percent of the magnesium. These essential elements are in the residue molasses, which is fed to cattle.")

(6) CORONARY HEART DISEASE . . .

This disease is only part of a more general degeneration of the arteries, called atherosclerosis, which is responsible for more death and disability than any other disease. For example, atherosclerosis produces strokes in the brain, nephritis in the kidneys, and loss of sight in the eyes. The reason arterial degeneration has such dramatic effects in the heart is simply because its main arteries are relatively few, small in diameter, and indispensable to life. The relation of diet to arterial damage has long been inescapable. At first, the main cause was thought to be an increased intake in the more affluent Western civilizations of foods high in cholesterol and saturated fat, especially dairy products and meat. This fitted the facts that the damaged arteries have abnormal deposits of cholesterol and fat, which can be produced in various animals by a high intake of these substances. Furthermore, a low intake of them in some groups of people was associated with less arterial disease. This theory, however, has become very controversial because other human studies show no such correlation.

Before we consider the new light thrown on this controversy by sugar and fiber, it helps to know something about cholesterol. Most of what we use does not come from food, but is manufactured in our liver and intestinal lining. Cholesterol is a complicated four-ring alcohol which, despite its structural complexity, our body easily makes out of simple acetic acid, the main constituent of ordinary vinegar. Although cholesterol is one of the most important constituents of cells, its function is still mysterious, being somehow involved in their structure and permeability. It is also a major ingredient of bile and of gallstones. From it are made the bile acids, the vitamin D synthesized in the skin by sunlight, and the sex and adrenal hormones.

These last include the cortisone group which strongly affect, among other things, the metabolism of proteins, fats and carbohydrates, immune and inflammatory responses, wound healing, permeability of blood vessels, and muscle integrity.

Much of the controversy about the relation of food cholesterol, blood cholesterol and associated disease may be due to emphasizing cholesterol intake, while neglecting other ways blood cholesterol can be affected. The blood level really depends on a balance between many factors, among them the different amounts of cholesterol which the body (1) ingests, (2) manufactures, (3) converts into bile acids, (4) recirculates in the blood from the bowel back to the liver, and (5) excretes in the feces. Unless the last four factors are in balance, cholesterol can pile up in the blood regardless of the amount eaten in food. Conversely, if the internal machinery of cholesterol is in good shape, the amount eaten becomes less important, and possibly of little importance. For example, the African Masai have phenomenally low blood cholesterol, remarkably healthy arteries and almost no coronary attacks, in spite of a high consumption of saturated fat and cholesterol, on their unusual diet of meat, blood and sour milk. But they get a great deal of exercise as nomadic herders, seldom eat sugar, and their machinery for balancing cholesterol metabolism is wonderfully efficient.

It has been found that adding sugar to the diet of both men and animals will raise the blood cholesterol, and adding fiber will lower it. One of the ways fiber seems to work is that substances in it such as pectin and lignin combine with bile salts (which contain the cholesterol nucleus), and thus maintain a healthy excretion in the stool of cholesterol.

THE RESULTS OF TOO MUCH SUGAR

Too much sugar in the diet has several bad effects associated with arterial damage. First, the body easily converts it into fat and raises the level of blood fats, which, along with cholesterol, are abnormally deposited in diseased arteries. Second, as mentioned, the blood cholesterol is also raised by excess dietary sugar. Third, both an excess of sugar and a lack of fiber tend to derange the normal bacterial flora of the intestine. These bacteria break apart bile salts into a variety of bile acids which are mostly recycled back to the liver. A certain amount of them are bound to bacteria and to fiber, which carry them off in the stool as a sort of overflow safety mechanism. (You may be amazed to know that one-third of the normal stool by dry weight consists of bacteria, and that the number of bacteria in a single stool is usually 1,000 times greater than the population of the world.)

In this way, the bacteria strongly influence the internal balance of cholesterol and the biliary compounds made from it. Current research is actively investigating this role of the bacteria, on the reasonable assumption that a derangement of it could be a factor in arterial damage.

WHAT GOES ON IN OUR COMPOST HEAP?

It may be a little shocking at first to think of the many bacterial inhabitants in our intestines. But this is only a good example of the remarkable cooperation between species, which is just as necessary as their competition, in the world of living things. For example, the complex chemical and bacterial activity in the intestine is surprisingly like that which takes place in a compost heap such as gardeners use. In both, fiber acts as a dispersal agent, and serves as food for the bacteria. In both, there is a variety of micro-organisms in great numbers; in garden compost, around 100 million per cubic inch. In soil, these organisms break down fiber to form acids which help make the nutrients in the earth available to plants. In the intestine, fiber and bile salts are likewise broken down into acids, presumably for useful purposes. In grass eating animals, the intestinal bacteria break down fiber in such large amounts that the resultant acids (chiefly acetic acid) becomes a major source of food energy. But in man this happens only to a small extent, perhaps just enough for the health of our bacteria and as part of the delicate balance of cholesterol which we make from acetic acid.

In addition to their function in the cholesterol-biliary system, our intestinal bacteria make significant quantities of vitamins: niacin, riboflavin, K, B_{12}, folic acid, biotin and para-aminobenzoic acid. It has been shown that antibiotics like penicillin may kill off so many of these useful bacteria that a vitamin deficiency develops and persists until the flora re-establishes itself or supplementary vitamins are given.

It is important that the intestinal bacteria be properly fed (and not overfed), because a new generation occurs about every four hours, and it is characteristic of all bacteria to develop unsuitable and even virulent strains depending on how they are fed. Both a lack of fiber and an excess of sugar appear to produce an abnormal bacteria flora, which may be a factor in the known rise of blood cholesterol on such a diet.

We should recognize that the intestine is one of our most vulnerable frontiers. It amounts to a highway through our personal city, crowded with a great many things from the outside world, pushing against the marvelous barrier of the intestinal lining, much of which has a myriad of tiny fingers projecting into the bowel. In the cells of this velvety lining, an incredible number of chemical reactions are constantly taking place, absorbing what is wanted out of the food, and manufacturing substances such as cholesterol, essential to the life of cells throughout the body.

In thinking about this frontier, it is worth remembering the ancient policy of the Romans along their frontier of the Rhine. They encouraged the settlement on their side of the river of half-wild but friendly tribes to keep the barbarians at bay. Likewise, on our intestinal frontier, we need to encourage by proper food the presence and health of our normally friendly bacteria. These deny living space to harmful varieties, which are always capable of arising in the population and dominating it.

THE SOUTH AFRICAN BABOONS

Early in 1974, a year-long experiment in South Africa showed the remarkable benefits of a natural diet free of sugar. Thirty baboons (which are very close to man physiologically) were divided into five groups: a control group; and four experimental groups, each of which was fed as its only carbohydrate either glucose, fructose, sucrose (table sugar), or starch. All the four experimental groups were also given an elaborate vitamin and mineral mixture, and fluffy cellulose as a source of fiber.[2]

The four experimental groups, each fed a different kind of refined carbohydrate, all developed varying degrees of substantial damage to their aortic arteries, together with an approximately 35 percent rise in blood cholesterol. Note that arterial damage is rare in animal primates, including baboons, although occasionally found in baboons kept in zoos.

But the group of baboons on the control diet, consisting of bread, bananas, yams, oranges and carrots, showed practically no damage to their aortas, and no average rise of blood cholesterol. The latter stayed at the original figure of 113.

From this experiment we gain the useful information that the 3 kinds of sugar or the starch diet can cause serious damage in the arteries of our close animal cousins. But if we want to have healthy arteries, we should be even more interested in a complete chemical analysis of the diet of bread, bananas, etc., eaten by the control baboons which enjoyed arterial health. Exactly what kind of bread, fiber, protein, carbohydrate, fat, minerals, vitamins, and so forth was in their diet? The report does not say!

THE RISK OF MEDICAL DOGMA

The ever present risk in medical research and practice is that we may accept as basically normal a common practice of today (for example, the eating of sugar and other refined food) and then build a massive structure on top of this premise which never gets to the bottom of the problem. In the case of the digestive diseases, this would be particularly regrettable, because they are so widespread. Figures from the National Center for Health Statistics show that these diseases account for one out of every six illnesses in the United States, affect half of all Americans, and rank third as the cause of death in the nation. But these figures do not include diseases of the arteries or diabetes which, as we have been describing, are caused, or strongly influenced, by the kind of food we send down to our digestive machinery.

ON GIVING YOURSELF ENOUGH FIBER

One way to increase the roughage in your diet is to eat more vegetables and fruits. This presents no special problems. But whole grain bread and bran are a little different, because for some people there may be a temporary unsettling effect, from the more powerful fiber in them, until the intestinal factory rearranges the bacteria, enzymes and production lines to handle more roughage. Oddly, this may occur when eating homemade, freshly baked, whole wheat bread for the first time ... or when you start

[2] Reference to fiber in this report refers to cereal fiber from wheat, rice, etc ... not to synthetic cellulose.

breakfast with hot oatmeal to which you have added a tablespoon or two of plain, unrefined, unsugared, untreated bran. There may also be a weakening of the intestinal lining due to many years of inadequate fiber, vitamins or minerals. In any event (however poor your past diet has been) the recuperative powers of your body are enormous, if it gets what it was designed for. One thing more. Remember that you need to drink more water. At least six glasses a day in addition to any other fluids. For roughage absorbs and requires more liquids.

To Sum Up:

Physicians and scientists are increasingly suspicious of the modern Western diet and have been paying particular attention to the dramatic decrease in cereal fiber and increase of sugar in the diet. Nondigestible plant fibers are being called the essential but forgotten nutrient.

Sugar and white flour can be taken easily and quickly into the body in the form of soft drinks, candy, soft white bread and pastries. These foods are easy to chew and digest, so the body secretes less saliva and gastric juice than when roughage is eaten. These secretions are needed for digestion and also to distend the stomach and give the sense of satiation. More of the highly refined foods, therefore, must be eaten before one feels full.

Fibrous foods such as wholemeal breads and cereal (such as oatmeal) on the other hand provide physiological barriers to energy intake. Undigestible plant materials take up space in the bowel and stomach. The same amount of sugar in a candy bar is found naturally in three pounds of apples, but most persons would find it impossible to eat this natural equivalent at one sitting. Fibrous foods require more chewing than refined foods, induce more saliva and gastric juice secretion, and thus give a quicker sense of satiation. Fiber also reduces the absorptive efficiency of the small intestine, making only about 92 percent of the calories available, compared to 97 percent with refined foods.

A diet high in fibers, including bran, can be used to prevent and treat diverticular diseases. One of five Western adults has this disease of the colon, due apparently to years of eating refined foods. A low fiber diet results in a small, viscous stool that requires forceful contractions and pressure to dispel. After years of this pressure, small outpockets can form in the colon wall, and these often get infected and require surgery. A bulky, fibrous diet is easier on the colon, increasing stool frequency and decreasing transit time.

The retention time may be an important factor in cancer of the colon. Some researchers think viruses may be the cause of colon cancer. Others think the carcinogen may be a by-product of the action of intestinal bacteria on food, digestive or excretory material. Still others think colon cancer may be caused by carcinogenic chemicals which contaminate foods. Regardless of the cancer-causing agent, the consensus is that the longer it takes for foods to travel through the alimentary tract, the more exposure the colon will receive to the harmful agent.

A high incidence of colon cancer usually is found in the same population groups with high incidences of obesity, diabetes, heart and certain other vascular diseases, peptic ulcer, gallbladder disease, appendicitis and e.coli infections of the urinary tract. All these separate diseases may be only the manifestations of a single master disease, since the most consistent feature of all of them is an over-consumption of concentrated carbohydrates lacking their natural quota of vitamins, minerals and fiber.

So, there is every reason for you to experience great benefit from more fiber and from a reduction or elimination of sugar in your diet. Indeed, sooner or later, it may mean the difference between a long healthy life and a lingering death brought on before your time by cancer of the colon, diabetes or a damaged heart.

And, finally, be sure to keep exercise on your team for health. The habit of a brisk hour's walk a day is the safest and best exercise. It makes the body sing with joy, when the food is right.

REFERENCES

1. Cleave, T.L., M.R.C.P. (London) Surgeon-Captain Royal Navy (Retd.). Formerly Director of Medical Research, Institute of Naval Medicine.

2. Keats Publishing, Inc., New Canaan, Conn., 06840. Two editions are in print: Hardcover ($7.95) and Paperback ($4.95). Either edition can be ordered directly from the publisher.

3. *The Trace Elements and Man: Some Positive and Negative Aspects* ($7.95), The Devin-Adair Company, Publishers, Old Greenwich, Conn., 06870. Also *The Poisons Around Us* by Henry A. Schroeder, M.D., ($4.95) published by Keats Publishing, Inc., New Canaan, Conn. 06840.

6

The Nutritional Teamwork Approach: Prevention and Regression of Cataracts in Rats*

(galactose-induced cataracts/toxicity resistance/suboptimal nutrition/nutrient testing)

JAMES D. HEFFLEY AND ROGER J. WILLIAMS

We have taken advantage of a newly assimilated principle in nutrition: no nutrient by itself should be expected to prevent or cure any disease; nutrients as such always work cooperatively in metabolism as a team.

By feeding galactose-containing diets to young rats, cataracts are regularly produced. When, however, we furnished galactose-fed animals with what may be considered a well balanced, full team of nutrients, cataract prevention was accomplished. On four galactose-containing diets supplied with a full team of nutrients, not a single cataract developed in 24 rats (48 eyes). On four diets using the same dietary galactose challenge, accompanied with inadequate nutritional teams, 47 out of 48 eyes developed cataracts. Diets of intermediate quality induced the development of intermediate numbers of cataracts. Cataracts once formed were regressed slowly and incompletely by shifting the animals to a diet similar to that which had previously been found to protect against cataract formation.

The significance of these findings for nutritional research and for attacks on the problems of human cataracts and other ailments is discussed.

The nutritional teamwork approach to the prevention or treatment of a diseased condition has been at least partially justified in earlier writings [1, 2]. Many nutritional investigations of past decades support the teamwork concept, notably the very early finding that the deficiency of one amino acid (tryptophan) alone will cause cessation of growth in young animals, and the clear-cut early demonstration that calcium, phosphate, and vitamin D are implicated together in the etiology of rickets. Despite many supporting evidences, however, the teamwork idea has not, until very recently, been clearly expressed and what is far more important, it has not been accepted and applied as a working principle. Instead, there is the widely accepted idea, certainly not openly endorsed by more sophisticated investigators, that single nutrients, especially vitamins, act like drugs or medicines, and

their effectiveness, if any, resides in their ability to prevent or cure some specific diseased condition.

While this criterion of effectiveness is satisfied in some cases, e.g., thiamin-beriberi, niacinamide-pellagra, ascorbic acid-scurvy, it is fundamentally an erroneous criterion because it overlooks a basic universal fact, namely, that unlike drugs, single nutrients always act constructively like parts of a complicated machine, and are effective as nutrients only when they participate as members of a team. This does not prevent nutrients from having drug-like actions when used in amounts higher than the physiological levels.

When particular vitamins appear to cure specific diseases, it is because they round out the team, transforming a limping incomplete team into one that is complete enough to function with some degree of physiological adequacy. In order to bring a victim of beriberi, pellagra or scurvy back to health, it is required that the victim receive continually every one of the essential nutrients. While in one sense such nutrients as thiamin, pantothenic acid, manganese, zinc, or threonine have nothing to do with rickets, a victim of rickets must have all these nutrients (and others), in addition to proper amounts of calcium, phosphate, and vitamin D, in order to be brought back to health.

Testing nutrients for their effectiveness is thus entirely different from testing drugs. Unless a nutrient is tested under conditions which allow it to participate in teamwork, the results are likely to be seriously misleading.

Galactose-induced Cataracts in Rats

Mitchell and Dodge [3] showed in 1935 that rats, receiving a very high level of lactose in the diet, developed cataracts in their eyes with considerable regularity. Subsequent experience has demonstrated that galactose is a crucial agent involved in cataract formation in rats. A considerable literature related to this phenomenon has accumulated, as evidenced by two reviews [4, 5]. In the latest review, van Heyningen concludes her discussion with the statement, "Although it is comparatively easy to find methods of causing cataracts in animals, prevention and cure of cataracts is a long term aim ... I can think of no systemic treatment that has been proved to alter the course of cataract formation without also altering the level of blood galactose."

*Reprinted with permission: Proc. Nat. Acad. Sci. USA, Vol. 71, No. 10, pp. 4164-4168, October 1974.

Table 1. Number of cataracts produced in groups of six Holtzman rats on different galactose-containing diets

| Diets (numbers are % of total calories) | Number of cataracts | | | | Weight (g) |
	3 Weeks	5 Weeks	7 Weeks	9 Weeks	9 Weeks
1. 20 Gal, 80 L.C. + V.M.	0	0	0	2	372
2. 20 Gal, 80 L.C.	0	0	0	1	379
3. 20 Gal, 40 L.C., 40 Glc	0	0	2	2	323
4. 20 Gal, 20 L.C., 60 Glc	0	6	10	11	193
5. 20 Gal, 10 L.C., 70 Glc	5	12	12	12	108
6. 20 Gal, 80 Egg + V.M.	0	0	0	0	353
7. 20 Gal, 80 Egg	0	0	0	0	356
8. 20 Gal, 40 Egg, 40 Glc	0	2	6	6	240
9. 20 Gal, 20 Egg, 60 Glc	0	10	11	12	193
10. 20 Gal, 10 Egg, 70 Glc	0	5	10	12	122
11. 20 Gal, Syn. I(+)	0	0	0	0	294
12. 20 Gal, Syn. I	0	0	0	0	296
13. 20 Gal, 80 M. Milk + V.M.	0	0	1	1	332
14. 20 Gal, 80 M. Milk	0	1	6	8	330
15. 20 Gal, 40 M. Milk, 40 Glc	0	8	12	12	286
16. 40 Gal, Syn. II(+)	0	0	5	7	281
17. 40 Gal, Syn. II	0	11	11	12	229
18. 0 Gal, 100 L.C. (Control)	0	0	0	0	379

Abbreviations: Gal = galactose; L.C. = Purine Laboratory Chow; V.M. = vitamin mixture (see Table 3); Glc = glucose; Syn. I & Syn. II = semi-synthetic diets; Syn. I (+) & Syn. II (+) = supplemented semi-synthetic diets; (see Table 2); M. Milk = mineralized milk (dry whole milk + 0.014% $FeCl_3 \cdot 3H_2O$ + 0.1% $MnCl_2 \cdot 4H_2O$ + 0.006% $Cu(C_2H_3O_2)_2 \cdot H_2O$).

With this information as a background, we confirmed in preliminary experiments that galactose-induced cataracts are easy to produce, and then set out to study their nutritional control. We accepted as a working premise that no single nutrient would be able, by itself, to prevent cataracts, but that a complete team of nutrients might be effective. Since high levels of galactose are metabolically toxic to the lenses of the eyes of rats, we sought to find out: Can high quality nutritional teamwork successfully counteract such a metabolic poison?

EXPERIMENTAL

Eighteen different diets were fed *ad libitum* respectively to 18 groups of rats; each group consisted of six matched male weanlings. The diets, except the control diet, all contained high levels of galactose which in most cases comprised 20 percent of the calories in the diet. The diets, as summarized in Table 1, were compounded so that some would furnish a relatively adequate team of nutrients; others, for comparison, often furnished the same nutrients but at inadequate levels. All rats were examined daily for cataracts during the 9 weeks of the test.

Of the 18 diets, nos. 1, 2, 6, 7, 11, and 12 were judged in advance to contain relatively well proportioned amounts of all the essential nutrients needed by rats — a complete nutritional team. In addition, there were two other diets, nos. 13 and 14, which also contained a good assortment of team members, but were not comparable to the other relatively good diets because these diets contained a high proportion of mineralized milk, an additional source of metabolic galactose. Diet nos. 1 and 2 contained 80 percent of a commercial "lab chow" and were judged to be reasonably adequate. Diets nos. 6 and 7 were regarded as probably adequate because they contained 80 percent whole egg which we have found by itself to be an unusually complete diet for rats [6]. The basic semi-synthetic diets (nos. 12 and 17) were formulated variously to be relatively complete, but were further supplemented (diets nos. 11 and 16) with the vitamin mixture to see if they could be improved. Detailed information regarding the composition of diets nos. 11, 12, 16, and 17 and the vitamin mixture is presented in Tables 2 and 3.

Table 2. Composition of semi-synthetic diets (g/kg)

	Casein	Galactose	Glucose	Triolein	Salt mix*	Vitamin mix†
Diet 11 Syn. I(+)	200	234	496	50	50	60
Diet 12 Syn. I	130	197	561	50	50	12
Diet 13 Syn. II(+)	200	437	227	50	50	60
Diet 14 Syn. II	130	427	302	50	50	12

*Salt mix: Briggs-Fox (11) + 0.01% $CoCl_2 \cdot 6H_2O$ + 0.05% NaF + 0.005% $NaMoO_4^4 \cdot 2H_2O$ + 0.002% $NaSeO_3 \cdot 3H_2O$.
†Vitamin mix: see Table 3.

Table 3. Nutrient amounts (per 100 calories) furnished by vitamin mixture in diets nos. 1, 6, 11, 13, and 16
(Nutrients furnished in diets nos. 12 and 17 at 1/5th these amounts)

Vitamin A acetate	(I.U.)	1333	Pyridoxine·HCl	(mg)	0.8
Vitamin D$_2$	(I.U.)	66.7	Cobalamine	(μg)	3.3
dl-a-tocopherol	(mg)	40	Folic acid	(mg)	3.3
Menadione sodium bisulfite	(mg)	0.13	Biotin	(μg)	70
Thiamine·HCl	(mg)	0.83	Choline	(mg)	50
Riboflavin	(mg)	1.67	Inositol	(mg)	33.3
Niacin	(mg)	10	Linoleic acid	(g)	1.3
Calcium pantothenate	(mg)	5.3	Short chain fatty acid mix*	(g)	1.3

*Short chain fatty acid mix: 30% tributyrin, 30% capric acid, 10% caproic acid, 10% tricaprylin, 20% lauric acid.

Diets nos. 3, 4, 5, 8, 9, 10, and 15 were qualitatively similar to more complete diets, but were quantitatively deficient in varying degrees, because the relatively complete food was diluted in each case with various amounts of glucose which furnishes only energy.

A second experiment involved feeding 13 male weanling rats a deficient cataract-producing diet (diets no. 4, Table 1) until at least one eye of each rat exhibited a cataract. The second day after the initial appearance of a cataract, each rat was shifted to an excellent diet for 9 weeks to see if there would be regression of the cataracts. The diet used was the same as no. 6, Table 1, except that the galactose was absent. In every animal, a second cataract developed within a week even though the diet had been changed, so that a total of 26 cataracts were under observation.

Table 4. Cataract scores of individual rats on supplemented diets after induction of cataracts by galactose feeding

Rat no.		3 Weeks Diam.	Dens.	Score	5 Weeks Diam.	Dens.	Score	10 Weeks Diam.	Dens.	Score	% Decrease in Score 3rd to 10th week
1	R	4.0	4	16.0	3.6	4	14.4	3.0	4	12.0	25
	L	3.0	4	12.0	1.2	4	4.8	1.4	4	5.6	53
2	R	3.6	4	14.4	3.6	4	14.4	1.6	4	6.4	56
	L	3.4	4	13.6	3.4	4	13.6	2.0	4	8.0	41
3	R	3.0	4	12.0	1.2	4	4.8	1.4	4	5.6	53
	L	3.4	4	13.6	1.2	4	4.8	1.8	4	7.2	47
4	R	3.6	4	14.4	3.6	4	14.4	1.4	4	5.6	61
	L	3.6	4	14.4	3.6	4	14.4	1.8	4	7.2	50
5	R	2.8	3	8.4	3.0	1	3.0	2.6	1	2.6	69
	L	2.8	4	11.2	2.8	2	5.6	2.8	2	5.6	50
6	R	2.8	3	8.4	2.2	3	6.6	2.0	4	8.0	5
	L	3.0	4	12.0	3.0	4	12.0	2.0	4	8.0	33
7	R	3.2	4	12.8	2.6	4	10.4	1.4	4	5.6	56
	L	3.2	4	12.8	3.4	4	13.6	1.4	4	5.6	56
8	R	3.6	4	14.4	3.2	4	12.8	2.2	4	8.8	39
	L	3.4	4	13.6	1.6	4	6.4	1.8	4	7.2	47
9	R	2.6	3	7.8	1.8	4	7.2	1.4	4	5.6	28
	L	2.8	4	11.2	1.2	4	4.8	2.2	4	8.8	21
10	R	2.8	4	11.2	3.0	1	3.0	1.8	1	1.8	84
	L	3.0	4	12.0	3.0	4	12.0	1.4	4	7.6	37
11	R	3.6	4	14.4	1.2	4	4.8	1.6	4	6.4	56
	L	2.8	4	11.2	1.6	4	6.4	2.0	4	8.0	29
12	R	4.0	4	16.0	3.6	4	14.4	3.6	4	14.4	10
	L	4.0	4	16.0	3.6	4	14.4	20.0	4	8.0	50
13	R	2.8	4	11.2	3.2	4	12.8	2.6	3	7.6	32
	L	2.6	4	10.4	2.6	4	10.4	2.6	1	2.6	81

R, L = right and left eyes, respectively. Diam. = estimated diameter of cataract in mm. Dens. = estimated density of cataract, with 1 = least and 4 = most dense. Score = product of Diam. and Dens.

RESULTS

The results of the preventative experiment are summarized in Table 1. They are clear-cut and require little explanation. Although the dietary galactose challenge was the same in diets nos. 1 through 12 (20 percent of the total calories), no cataracts whatever appeared in animals on four of the superior diets (nos. 6, 7, 11, and 12) and on four diets we knew to be poorer (nos. 4, 5, 9, and 10); 47 of the 48 eyes involved were cataractous. Diets of intermediate quality yielded intermediate numbers of cataracts. In one of the two diets in which the galactose level was raised to 40 percent of the total calories, the supplemented semi-synthetic diet afforded some but not complete protection. Also, the increased level of whole milk in diet no. 14 afforded some protection in spite of the increased lactose challenge. When this diet was supplemented with a vitamin mixture, diet no. 13, the protection was almost complete. Each basal diet appeared to have some distinctive properties with respect to its ability to protect against cataracts. The diluted lab chow diet, no. 5, seemed to induce cataracts the most rapidly of all; even when the lab chow was at the 80 percent level, diets nos. 1 and 2, protection from cataract formation was not complete.

The results of the second experiment, in which animals were placed on good diets after cataracts had been produced on a poor diet, designed to determine if there would be regression, were not as clear-cut as the experiment involving prevention. The results on 26 cataracts are summarized in Table 4. Of the 26 cataracts observed, 16 showed an improvement in their "scores" of from 40 to 80 percent. In general the regressions were slow and incomplete, though improvement in many cases was clearly manifest.

DISCUSSION

It is difficult to discuss our experimental study and findings adequately and in proper perspective. On the one hand our strategy, once it is described, seems so simple, if not obvious, that it appears to require little comment. On the other hand, so far as galactose-induced cataracts are concerned, it is a new, untried strategy; if it had ever been tried at any time during the past 3 or 4 decades it would have been successful. The potential value of our findings rests on the probability that this same strategy, if broadly followed, may yield highly important unforeseen benefits in the realm of medical science.

Although our success in preventing galactose-induced cataracts in rats was complete on four diets for 9 weeks, this was not an "all or none" process. Other diets protected almost completely, and some yielded only very partial protection. If the galactose challenge had been less severe, it seems probable that diets of mediocre quality would have sufficed to give protection; if the challenge had been more severe, it might have required diets better than any we used to accomplish protection. These findings are completely in line with the nutritional principle [2, 7] that common food environments are consistently suboptimal, and hence are always subject to improvement. When, as suggested by van Heyningen's review [5], investigators have failed to prevent galactose-induced cataracts, it has been because they have failed to recognize this principle and have never tried seriously to improve to the limit the total environment of their experimental animals.

It is evident that from our study no one could derive a precise list of the nutrients involved in protecting against cataract, nor does our study rule out the possibility that for some or all individual animals, certain specific nutrients may be crucially limiting factors in the nutritional team. We have not proved by actual experiment that leaving out any one of the essentials would have resulted in failure to protect. Neither have we studied the possible effect of imbalance between nutrients. We have not ruled out the possibility that there is a glucose-galactose synergism involved in cataract production. Our simple experiment shows that when we attempted to furnish enough of all the essentials, success was attained. Many further experiments will be required to clear up numerous uncertainties.

If a physician were to treat an obscure malady by giving his patient several drugs at the same time, in the hope that one or another of the drugs might bring relief, this may be reprehensible, and would aptly be dubbed the "shotgun" approach. To extend this disapprobation to the administration of several nutrients simultaneously is to miss one of the most vital principles of nutritional science — the teamwork principle. Because of this teamwork principle, the administration of many nutrients at the same time is not only entirely logical but basically essential. When we do this we are following in the footsteps of nature. When human beings are fortunate enough to maintain health by consuming wholesome food, this is accomplished by reason of the fact that they consume regularly every one of the about 40 nutritional essentials. It is not following nature's strategy if we consume tryptophan on Monday, ascorbic acid on Tuesday, calcium on Wednesday, etc. We utilize in our bodies all nutritional elements simultaneously every day.

The careful discrimination between nutrient action and drug action is necessary if we are to avoid serious pitfalls. For example, the Food and Drug Administration is inclined to rule that drugs in order to be sold must be both "safe" and "efficacious." If we unfortunately and uncritically apply the same criteria to nutrients, we immediately condemn most nutrients as unsuitable for sale, because while they are usually safe, they are, generally speaking, not efficacious when administered singly. For example, there is probably no single nutrient that would be at all "efficacious" in preventing cataracts in rats; the entire team of nutrients, on the other hand, is extremely efficacious.

Attacking specific diseased conditions *seriatim* with the purpose of ascertaining what nutrition can do to prevent or alleviate them is certainly not fashionable today in the area of medical science. We can hope that our unqualified success in preventing galactose-induced cataracts in rats, once a "long-term aim," may help make the nutritional strategy more fashionable.

Immediately our success in preventing cataracts in rats leads to the questions: Can the cataracts associated with diabetes be prevented by a sophisticated nutritional teamwork approach? Can the cataracts often associated with human senility be prevented by regularly providing potential victims with an excellently proportioned set of nutritional elements?

It may be presumed that the rats in our experiments which were completely protected from galactose-induced cataracts were able, by having all their nutritional needs adequately satisfied, to build and adapt enzyme systems to metabolize galactose in such a way as to obviate its damaging effects. If the crucial agent concerned in cataract production in rats is galactitol [8], its formation was probably minimized when the metabolic operations flowed smoothly in a normal manner. If galactitol is involved in the production of senile cataracts, its effects in humans can probably be minimized by furnishing all the raw materials needed for promoting its normal metabolism. If sorbitol [9] (or another polyalcohol) is involved in the production of diabetic cataracts, then its deleterious action can probably be minimized in diabetics by providing the cells and tissues with a complete complement for building effective metabolic machinery.

The results obtained in the curative experiment were definitely positive, but the regressions were slow and incomplete presumably because of the slow rate of metabolism in the lens of the eye. It seems possible that if the dietary challenge offered these rats had been less severe or if the change in diet had been instituted at the very first sign of cataract instead of waiting until the cataracts were well formed, the responses might have been more favorable.

Cataracts in rats was chosen by us as a diseased condition to attack merely by "pulling it out of the hat," as something that could be studied objectively and conveniently. There is little evidence on which to predict in advance how many other diseased conditions in rats will respond similarly to the nutritional teamwork approach — other eye maladies, atherosclerosis, carious teeth, delayed bone healing after fracture, production of malformed young, etc. Substantial evidence is available to suggest that this approach will prevent the production of malformed young [10], but the other diseased conditions have not been explored with due consideration of the total food environment and the teamwork principle.

In the arena of human disease prevention, our unqualified success with galactose-induced cataracts in rats suggests that added emphasis on sophisticated nutritional teamwork be encouraged for the prevention not only of human cataracts and other eye maladies but also diseases of obscure etiology such as multiple sclerosis and muscular dystrophy, also mental retardation, ischemic heart disease, dental diseases, allergies, arthritis, premature senility, obesity, mental disease, alcoholism, and even cancer. To promise success in these numerous areas would be extravagant, but on the other hand, it can be stated that serious sophisticated trials of the teamwork approach — such as we have used to prevent cataracts in rats — have never been made in connection with any of the human diseases mentioned. Much of the nutritional exploration related to these areas can unfortunately be characterized as merely "dabbling," rather than dealing seriously with the total food environment.

REFERENCES

1. Williams, R.J. (1971) *Nutrition Against Disease* Pitman Publ. Co., New York), p. 212 *et seq*.
2. Williams, R.J., Heffley, J.D., Yew, M.L.S. & Bode, C.W. (1973) "A renaissance of nutritional science is imminent," *Perspect. Biol. Med.* 17, 1-15.
3. Mitchell, H.S. & Dodge, W.M. (1935) "Cataract in rats fed on high lactose rations," *J. Nutr.* 9, 37-49.
4. van Heyningen, R. (1971) "Galactose cataract: A review," *Exp. Eye Res.* 11, 415-426.
5. Lerman, S. (1965) "Metabolic pathways in experimental sugar and radiation cataracts," *Physiol. Rev.* 45, 98-122.
6. Williams, R.J., Heffley, J.D. & Bode, C.W. (1971) "The nutritive value of single foods," *Proc. Nat. Acad. Sci.* USA 68, 2361-2364.
7. Williams, R.J. (1974) *Physicians Handbook of Nutritional Science* (C.C Thomas, Springfield, Mo.), in press.
8. Kinoshita, J.H., Merola, L.O. & Dirkmak, E. (1962) "Osmotic changes in experimental galactose cataracts," *Exp. Eye Res.* 1, 405-410.
9. van Heyningen, R. (1959) "Formation of polyols by the lens of rats with 'sugar' cataracts," *Nature* 184, 194-195.
10. Williams, R.J. (1971) *Nutrition Against Disease* (Pitman Publ. Co., New York), chap. 4.
11. Fox, M.R.S. & Briggs, G.M. (1960) "Salt mixtures for purified-type diets: III. An improved salt mixture for chicks," *J. Nutr.* 72, 243.

7
Micronutrient Deficiencies in Major Sources of Calories*

"The elements (zinc, manganese, chromium, etc.) can not be synthesized by living things, as are the vitamins, but must be captured by plants from soil or sea to enter the food chain. Animals raised for profit are fed luxus amounts of essential trace metals; man gets minimal amounts"

HENRY A. SCHROEDER

PRECIS

The author claims that the refining, freezing, canning and other processing of foods robs them of vitamins (which are sometimes replaced or supplemented) and such trace elements as zinc, manganese, chromium, etc. (which are not replaced, though they can be). There is scattered evidence that these losses may be linked to certain metabolic disorders and chronic diseases such as hypertension and atherosclerosis. He notes that mammals other than man need, and get, more trace metals in their diets for optimal health and function, i.e., farm and laboratory animals.

The major sources of caloric energy in the American diet are starches, sugars and fats. In their raw or natural states, the micronutrients necessary for metabolism of these foods are present in adequate amounts.

When these foods are refined, processed, heated or stored, losses of micronutrients can occur, sometimes in relatively enormous quantities. Most Americans depend largely on refined and processed foods for their caloric intakes. The questions arise: are these foods nutritionally adequate? Can possible deficits in organic and inorganic micronutrients be met easily by other foods containing abundances of vitamins and trace minerals? Is it possible that, despite claims that the American diet is the best in the world, the diet is actually marginal or deficient in several trace nutrients, as others claim?

In order to evaluate the major sources of calories in this light, we can apply a simple yardstick to each source, based on the known daily requirement of the micronutrient [1], and its concentration in the food. The moist weight of the food consumed daily in an average diet is about 1.0 kg [2]. If 1.0 kg of a food daily were the sole source of energy, and the daily requirement of the vitamin or mineral were 1.0 mg, the food would contain 1.0 ppm of the micronutrient and the requirement would be met. If two foods made up the diet, one containing 2.0 ppm of the micronutrient and the other 0.5 ppm, it would be necessary to consume a diet of which 37.5 percent comprised the first food and 62.5 percent the second to meet the requirement. This diet would then be "balanced."

*Reprinted with permission: *Medical Counter-point*, Volume 3, #7, July 1971.

DEFICIENCIES OF VITAMINS

Wheat and its products supply a sizeable proportion of the energy in occidental food. Its principal product, bread, is usually made from refined white flour, from which the germ and bran are removed; patent flour comprises 68-72 percent of the whole wheat kernel. Losses of protein, carbohydrate and calories are negligible; half the fat is left in the flour. However, most of the vitamins and minerals, which are concentrated in germ and bran to supply the needs of the growing seed until its roots can be established in the soil, are removed from the flour [3]. Some 24 bulk and trace elements and vitamins are depleted to the extent of 40-96 percent of the amounts in whole wheat; four (thiamin, riboflavin, nicotinic acid and iron) are returned to the flour, which is then called "enriched." The residue, known as millfeeds, is truly enriched with all micronutrients [4]; it is fed to domestic animals.

There are four vitamins of concern which are depleted in white flour and not restored. Some 50 percent of the pantothenic acid, 66.7 percent of the folacin, 71.8 percent of the B_6 and 86.3 percent of the tocopherol are removed [3]. Applying our yardstick, flour contains one-fourth of the requirement of vitamin B_6 and folacin, the minimum requirement of pantothenic acid and 7.3 percent of the requirement for tocopherol. Tocopherol is further lost on storage of flour.

The vitamin B_6 contents of raw corn (4.7 ppm), brown rice (5.5 ppm), whole rye flour (3.0 ppm), whole bulgar (2.5 ppm), whole wheat flour (3.4 ppm) and whole wheat breakfast cereal (3.9 ppm) exceed the dietary requirement (2.0 ppm). Three of four corn products, all of 6 rice products, each of two rye products, oatmeal, all of 13 wheat products, bread and cake contained from 17 to 50 percent of the minimal requirement. As for pantothenic acid, 15 of 20 of these grain products had less than the minimal amount recommended, or 5 ppm [3, 5]. Furthermore, published data [6] show that there is less, and often considerably less, than the recommended amounts of biotin and folacin in corn, rice and wheat products — white bread, for example, having only 7.3 percent of the biotin and 37.5 percent of the folacin presumed needed.

Vitamin B_6 was depleted in all of 12 canned vegetables to levels less than half the minimal requirement and in seven of 10 canned fish and all of 19 frozen vegetables to less than the minimal requirement. Only fresh meats and fish supplied adequate amounts; processed meats did not, all of five analyzed being deficient. Rough calculations indicate that it would be almost impossible to construct a diet of frozen and canned vegetable foods, processed meats, canned fish, dairy products and refined grains containing 2 mg B_6 per day, unless large amounts of bran and germ products were added to each meal. There were similar but less extensive losses of pantothenic acid in canned foods, 25 of 33 failing to meet requirements [3].

Refined white sugar contains virtually no vitamins, although sugar cane juice and molasses have the water soluble-vitamins, including adequate amounts of B_6 and pantothenic acid. Refined fats may be low in tocopherol; lard has only 20 ppm, which is below requirements of 25-30 mg. Tocopherol deteriorates with storage and freezing. Fats have virtually no water-soluble vitamins. Therefore, two other major sources of calories are depleted of the organic micronutrients necessary for their metabolism.

The conclusion that the American diet is inadequate in vitamin B_6 is reinforced by the findings of Murphy et al. [7], who analyzed 300 Type A school lunches for vitamins and iron. These lunches included milk, meat, poultry, fish, egg or peanut butter, two vegetables, whole grain or enriched bread and butter or margarine. More than half, or 171 of the schools did not meet the nutritional goal for B_6, and 7 percent served lunches with less than a quarter of the goal.

Based on experiments in monkeys [8], vitamin B_6 deficiency has been proposed as a casual factor in human atherosclerosis [9].

The vitamin B_6 requirements have been set at 2.0 mg per day for adults, 2.5 mg per day for pregnant and lactating women, and 1.4-2.0 mg per day for adolescents [1]. Of 552 foods analyzed, 31.0 percent had concentrations of 2 ppm or more, many of them seeds, nuts, condiments, yeasts, or dried meats and fish. When dried legumes, seeds and nuts were excluded, only 77 foods, mainly raw fish and meats, had levels of B_6 over 2.5 ppm (13.9%), indicating the virtual impossibility of providing the requirements of pregnancy in a well-rounded diet. In 83 baby foods, only 28.9 percent had 2 ppm or more B_6 [3].

DEFICIENCIES OF TRACE ELEMENTS

The situation with the essential trace elements in refined foods is equally precarious, from the viewpoint of nutritional requirements. We have analyzed many foods and food fractions. Thirteen bulk and trace elements were depleted from wheat by refining of flour. The bulk minerals, sodium, potassium, magnesium, calcium, phosphorus were lost to the extent of 60-84.7 percent. Trace metals were lost to the extent of 40-88.5 percent [10, 17]. The most serious losses occurred in chromium, zinc and manganese, which are concentrated in germ and bran. Selenium was distributed throughout the grain, so that losses from the endosperm were minor. The resultant product, patent flour, is poor in minerals, and the residue, millfeeds, is rich.

Refined white sugar contains very small amounts of trace metals. Its ash content is about 0.15 percent, compared to 3-5 percent for raw sugar, which is rich in metals. From 87-100 percent of seven metals are removed in the refining; molasses, the residue, contains virtually all of them. Molasses is added to cattle feed as an excellent nutrient, but white sugar lacks the micronutrients necessary for its metabolism.

Polished rice, another staple carbohydrate, is depleted of six trace elements, in amounts ranging from 40-83 percent of those in unpolished rice. Copper is removed only to the extent of 25 percent. The final amounts are too low for good nutrition [3].

When foods are refined or fractionated and partitioned, as occurs when oils or fats are removed, some of the essential metals necessary for the metabolism of one fraction are largely found in the others. Thus, flour, polished rice, corn starch, corn oil, white sugar, butter, egg white, beef tallow and lard are deficient in zinc, and their residues adequate. Flour, gluten, corn starch, white sugar and skimmed milk are deficient in manganese. From this viewpoint, an heretical case can be made for the inadequacy of skimmed milk as a complete food, for it contains virtually no chromium, manganese or molybdenum, which are concentrated in butter. Butter itself has only 6 percent of the magnesium in raw milk, but contains most of the copper and cobalt of whole milk. Thus, neither fraction is as complete a food as whole milk [3].

Where the metal goes when foods are fractionated seems to depend upon its affinity for protein or fat. Magnesium, zinc and molybdenum are apparently bound to protein in foods, whereas chromium, manganese, cobalt and copper are lipotropic. Therefore, partitioned foods are likely to be in a state of unbalance in trace elements and magnesium, most of which are essential for the metabolism of glucose and fat. Applying our yardstick based on calculated requirements of magnesium and trace metals, of 200 ppm magnesium, 15 ppm zinc, 0.5 ppm chromium, 2.2 ppm manganese, 3 ppm copper, and 0.2 ppm molybdenum, flour, polished rice, corn starch, corn oil, white sugar, skimmed milk, beef fat and lard failed to meet the goals in all cases but for copper in rice.

THE "UNBALANCED" DIET

In an average diet of 2900 calories, fat probably contributes 1000 calories; sugar 400-500 calories (121 g per day is the national average); proteins 400 calories; and other carbohydrate 1000 calories, of which most comes from grains. Unless the grains are unrefined oats, rye, barley, millet or buckwheat, the major carbohydrates consumed are marginal in certain vitamins and trace minerals necessary for optimal health, sugar contributing "empty calories" and wheat contributing deficient calories. Similarly, processed protein foods contain significantly lesser amounts of micronutrients, both trace elements and vitamins, than they do in the natural state.

Partially "empty" calories are also provided by refined fats and oils. In some, but not all, cases a person can make up these deficiencies in vitamins and trace elements by the regular use of wheat germ, bran and other concentrated breakfast cereals, fresh meats, liver and fish. The average person probably does not. It would be most difficult to obtain adequate amounts of vitamin B_6 and chromium from frozen, processed and canned foods, hard to obtain adequate quantities of vitamin E and zinc, and difficult to obtain adequate zinc, even by changing dietary habits radically.

REQUIREMENTS OF OTHER MAMMALS
FOR TRACE ELEMENTS

Vitamins and trace elements are very basic factors in mammalian metabolism and that of other living things. The elements cannot be synthesized by living things, as are the vitamins, but must be captured by plants from soil or sea to enter the food chain. Animals raised for profit are fed luxus amounts of the essential trace metals: man gets minimal amounts. The recommended concentrations in swine feeds are as follows (ppm): zinc 34-50, manganese 40-50, copper 5-10; in ruminant feeds, zinc 30-100, manganese 20-40, copper 4-10 [18]. Calculated concentrations in human diets are (ppm): zinc 8-15, manganese 2-3, copper 2-3, in terms of solid food. Many diets have lesser concentrations. Laboratory animals (mice, rats, guinea pigs, rabbits, dogs) are fed in standard chows (ppm); zinc 18-178, manganese 40-121, copper 12-21. Monkey chow has (ppm) zinc 20, manganese 44, copper 12. It is not known why all mammals but man appear to require these relatively large amounts of trace metals for optimal health and function.

SUBTLE EFFECTS OF DEFICIENCIES OF TRACE ELEMENTS

What are the real or possible consequences of marginal intakes of trace elements? The most obvious results are basic metabolic alterations leading to chronic diseases. Several metabolic diseases common in older persons have been implicated. Just as the marginal intake of a vitamin results in poor function, so does a marginal intake of an essential element result in abnormal function. The abnormality is not necessarily directly lethal, but it may lead to a chronic disease with fatal consequences.

Chromium deficiency, which is prevalent in this country and is unusual in the Orient, Africa and the Middle East, is a causal factor in atherosclerosis [19]. The disorder, which involves glucose and lipid metabolic alterations, has been reproduced in rats by deficiency of chromium and prevented by feeding chromium or sugars containing chromium [20]. The human deficiency is the result of removing chromium by refining sugar, flour and fats. Chromium is essential for glucose and cholesterol homeostasis [20]. It is possible that concomitant vitamin B_6 deficiency causes sub-endothelial arterial lesions from alterations in the synthesis of mucopolysaccharides, which then fill with lipids; this process has been demonstrated in monkeys [8].

Plasma zinc levels were significantly low in pregnancy, in women taking oral contraceptives, in patients with chronic leg ulcers, alcoholic cirrhosis of the liver, other types of liver disease, active and inactive tuberculosis, pulmonary infections, myocardial infarction, and uremia. They were low in children with Down's syndrome, and with retarded growth [22]. Oral zinc therapy has resulted in enhanced growth and sexual development, healing of ulcers [23], improved liver function, and improved circulation to the legs of persons with atherosclerotic ischemia or intermittent claudication [24]. It is apparent that zinc deficiency is not uncommon in the general population and that low plasma levels can be restored by supplementation. Therefore, there is just as much reason to restore zinc to foods from which it has been removed as to restore iron.

One consequence of the depletion of zinc from flour concerns the failure of simultaneous depletion of cadmium. Excess cadmium is a factor in arterial hypertension [25]. Intestinal absorption of cadmium is increased with low intakes and suppressed by high intakes of zinc. Cadmium is distributed throughout the grain of wheat and rice; zinc is largely in the germ and bran [14]. Thus, removal of the zinc by refining results in effectively more cadmium being made available to the body; it accumulates in kidney and blood vessels, altering reactivity.

Manganese deficiency in man is conceivable only from indirect evidence. There is much less in human than in animal tissues, and less in American than in foreign human tissues. Intakes are low compared to the needs of domestic animals. Manganese is concerned in lipid and probably glucose metabolism. Results of marginal intakes in man have yet to be delineated.

Therefore, the average American diet, composed as it is of processed, frozen, stored, canned and refined foods, is probably marginal, and in some cases, partly deficient in several essential micronutrients, especially vitamin B_6, pantothenic acid, tocopherol, chromium, zinc and possibly manganese. The results of these inadequacies are several chronic diseases and conditions which are characterized by metabolic abnormalities. These abnormalities are not compatible with optimal function, or in other words, good health.

ADDENDUM

After this paper was submitted, Murphy et al., [26] reported analyses of 300 type A school lunches for five essential trace metals and four non-essential ones. According to accepted criteria, these diets were deficient in chromium, manganese and copper, low in strontium and adequate in zinc. They contained small amounts of cadmium and barium, and normal amounts of aluminum and boron. Although these standard diets for school children were adequate in most major nutrients, deficiencies in elemental micronutrients, as well as vitamins, were apparent.

REFERENCES

1. Food and Nutrition Board, National Research Council. "Recommended Dietary Allowances." 7th revised edition, National Academy of Sciences, Washington, D.C., 1968.
2. Household Food Consumption Survey, Report No. 6. "Food Consumption of Households in the United States, 1955," US dept. of Agriculture, Household Economics Research Division, Washington, D.C., 1957.
3. Schroeder, H.A.: Losses of vitamins and trace minerals resulting from processing and preservation of foods. Amer. J. Clin. Nutr. 25:562, 1971.
4. The Millers' National Federation, The Millfeed Manual, Chicago, Ill. 1967.
5. Orr, M.L.: Pantothenic acid, vitamin B_6 and vitamin B_{12} in foods. Home Economics Research Division, Agricultural Research Service, US Dept. of Agriculture, Washington, D.C., 1969.
6. Mitchell, H.A., Rynbergen, H.J., Anderson, L. and Dibble, M.V.: "Cooper's Nutrition in Health and Disease," 15th Ed. Lippencott Co. Philadelphia, 1968.
7. Murphy, E.W., Koons, P.C. and Page, L.: Vitamin content of Type A school lunches. J. Amer. Dietetic Assoc. 55:372, 1969.
8. a) Rinehart, J.F. and Greenberg, L.D.: Arteriosclerotic

lesions in pyridoxine deficient monkeys. Amer. J. Path. 25:481, 1949.

b) Rinehart, J.F. and Greenberg, L.D.: Pathogenesis of Experimental arteriosclerosis in pyridoxine deficiency, with notes on similarities to human arteriosclerosis. Arch. Path. 31:12, 1951.

9. Schroeder, H.A.: Is atherosclerosis a conditioned pyridoxal deficiency? J. Chron. Dis. 2:28, 1955.

10. Schroeder, H.A., Balassa, J.J. and Tipton, J.H.: Abnormal trace elements in man. Chromium. J. Chron. Dis. 15:941, 1962.

11. Schroeder, H.A., Balassa, J.J. and Tipton, I.H.: Essential trace metals in man: Manganese: A study in homeostasis. J. Chron. Dis. 19:545, 1966.

12. Schroeder, H.A., Nason, A.P. and Tipton, I.H.: Essential trace metals in man: Cobalt. J. Chron. Dis. 20:869, 1967.

13. Schroeder, H.A., Nason, A.P., Tipton, I.H. and Balassa, J.J.: Essential trace metals in man: Copper. J. Chron. Dis. 19:1007, 1966.

14. Schroeder, H.A., Nason, A.P., Tipton, I.H. and Balassa, J.J.: Essential trace metals in man: Zinc. Relation to environmental cadmium. J. Chron. Dis. 20:179, 1967.

15. Schroeder, H.A., Balassa, J.J. and Tipton, I.H.: Essential trace metals in man: Molybdenum. J. Chron. Dis. 25:562, 1971.

16. Schroeder, H.A., Balassa, J.J. and Tipton, I.H.: Essential trace metals in man: Molybdenum. J. Chron. Dis. 23: 227, 1970.

17. Schroeder, H.A., Nason, A.P. and Tipton, I.H.: Essential metals in man: Magnesium. J. Chron. Dis. 21:815, 1968.

18. Megown, J.W.: Trace mineral facts brought up to date. The Feed Bag, March, 1966.

19. Schroeder, H.A., Nason, A.P. and Tipton, I.H.: Chromium deficiency as a factor in atherosclerosis. J. Chron. Dis. 23:123, 1970.

20. Schroeder, H.A., Mitchener, M. and Nason, A.P.: Influence of various sugars, chromium and other trace metals on serum cholesterol and glucose of rats. J. Nutr. 101:247, 1971.

21. Mertz, A.: Chromium occurrence and function in biological systems. Physiol. Rev. 49:163, 1969.

22. Halsted, J.A. and Smith, J.C.: Plasma-zinc in health and disease. The Lancet 322 (Feb. 14), 1970.

23. Henzel, J.H., DeWeese, M.S. and Lichti, E.L.: Zinc concentrations within healing wounds. Arch. Surg. 100:349, 1970.

24. Henzel, J.H., Lichti, E.L., Keitzer, F.W. and DeWeese, M.S.: Efficacy of zinc medication as a therapeutic modality in atherosclerosis: Follow-up observations on patients medicated over prolonged periods. Proc. Fourth Ann. Conf. Trace Substances in Environmental Health, Univ. of Missouri, Columbia, 1970.

25. Schroeder, H.A.: Cadmium as a factor in hypertension. J. Chron. Dis. 18:647, 1965.

26. Murphy, E.W., Page, L. and Watt, B.K. Trace minerals in type A school lunches. J. Am. Dietetic Assoc. 58:115, 1971.

8
The Name of the Game is the Name*

E. CHERASKIN

The following is a statement delivered by Mr. Thomas J. Watson, Jr., Chairman of the Executive Committee of the International Business Machine Corporation at the Mayo Clinic in Rochester, Minnesota, on 19 November 1970 [1].

Let me start by asking a question that this great medical center brings to mind: How would you like to live in a country which, according to the figures available in the United States during the past two decades:

has dropped from seventh in the world to sixteenth in the prevention of infant mortality; has dropped in female life expectancy from sixth to eighth; has dropped in male life expectancy from tenth to twenty-fourth; and which has bought itself this unenviable trend by spending more of its gross national product for medical care ($1 out of every $14) than any other country on the face of the earth?

You know the country I am talking about: Our own U.S.A., the home of the free, the home of the brave, and the home of a decrepit, inefficient, high-priced system of medical care. Just look for a moment at what some of the figures mean. They mean that in infant mortality we have been overtaken by France, the U.K., and Japan, that in male life expectancy we have been overtaken by France, Japan, West Germany and Italy. I know experts can disagree over our precise international standing. And I realize that medical problems in the United States, Europe and Japan are not identical. But the evidence overwhelmingly indicates that we are falling down on the job, heading in the wrong direction, and becoming as a nation a massive medical disgrace.

The plethora of such pronouncements makes it now abundantly clear that health is the fastest growing failing business in these United States [20]. While the problem is without argument, there is no paucity of debate with regard to its causes and solutions. Some experts contend that the major, if not sole, cause is a lack of doctors; other equally-credentialled authorities claim that it is not the number but the uneven distribution on a rural-urban basis or specialty-general practice ratio which is the crux of the problem. There are students of the problem who plead for more fundamental research; others for more applied investigation; still others for better communication between basic and clinical research.

Quite probably, the health delivery disaster is a multifactorial problem and the explanations offered above and others play a role. However, it is the purpose of this report to bring into focus one item which has received practically no attention. More specifically, it will be the aim of this document to demonstrate that, in tradional medicine today, the name of the game is the name. Phrased another way, it is the thesis of this presentation that great strides toward a solution of the present health dilemma could come about if less attention were directed to diseases and more emphasis placed on mistakes of living.

To develop the theme of this report logically, attention will first be devoted to an experimental model which identifies the proper place for disease states and for mistakes in living. This will be followed by an analysis of the mechanism by which man becomes ill. Lastly, utilizing this seemingly new approach, illustrations will be cited to underline the kind of information which can then be generated and its impact upon the health delivery system.

THE SPHERE OF MAN

In one sense, man may be viewed as a multi-lamellated sphere [3]. Any way one turns a ball, it looks the same. However one inspects man peripherally, the conclusions are the same. True, viewed on one side, there may be a limp characteristic of a cerebrovascular accident; examined from a different angle, there are only pimples. But these and, in fact, all other peripheral stigmata possess a common denominator; they all reflect an index of the syndrome of sickness (Figure 1).

As successive layers of the lamellated sphere are unveiled, one reaches the core. Likewise in man, stripping away layer after layer brings into focus the central problems.

The outer, the most peripheral ring, is readily inspected in both a sphere and in man. At this level, one can make three clinical observations. First, it is possible to identify evidence of the ravages of classical disease such as the characteristic gait of a

*Reprinted with permission: *Proc. San Diego Biomed. Symposium*, 13:31-39, 1974.

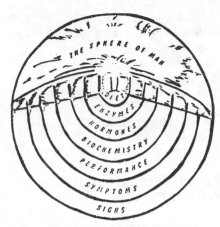

Fig. 1. Man may be likened to a lamellated sphere. The periphery of both is easily inspected. Layers can be progressively removed exposing the core.

stroke, the skin eruption of impetigo, a carious tooth. In actuality, this type of workup, though common and deemed worthy, is simply an accounting of the damage largely derived from a peripheral inspection of man. As Immanuel Kant has so aptly put it, "Physicians think they do a lot for a patient when they give his disease a name".

Second, signs and symptoms may be obtained at this peripheral level which provide a measure of pathosis referable to a particular system or site even though the clinical picture does not fit the textbook description of a particular syndrome.

Finally, it is possible to establish simply the number and kind of signs without regard to how or where they fit into systems, sites, or syndromes. In other words, one can simply use the total number of clinical findings as an index of incipient disease.

If one strips off the outer layer (Figure 1), into focus comes the zone of symptoms. Alterations of taste, smell, hearing, sight, and touch may be reported as symptoms. Where the outer layer ends and the next most peripheral one begins can be quite arbitrary. The decision as to whether a particular finding is a sign or symptom can be argued. For example, bleeding when observed by the doctor is a sign; when reported by the patient is a symptom.

Symptoms are not as measurable as signs and can only be derived through interrogation by means of classical interview or by questionnaire. In general, symptoms precede signs. Most significantly, symptoms, like signs, can be fitted into specific syndromes with specific names (the box on the right in Figure 2), viewed in systems and sites (the center box in Figure 2), or simply totalled as the sum of nonspecific clinical problems expressed as symptoms and signs (the box on the left in Figure 2).

As one continues the peeling process. (Figure 1), one eventually reaches the core illustrated here as diet. Since nutrients are the building blocks from which enzymes and hormones are made, it is obvious that all of the peripheral layers reflect the dietary imbalances, inadequacies, and excesses. Other core problems include physical activity, genetics, alcohol, tobacco, coffee and tea, smog, preservatives, insecticides, light, and still other known and unknown variables. What is important is that the name of the game does not truly reflect the importance of the core factors. For example, when one succumbs to pneumonia, does one die because of the pneumococcal invasion or the fact that a poor vitamin C state lowers resistance to the microbial invasion?

THE NATURAL HISTORY OF DISEASE

The usual pictorial portrayal of the natural history of the disease process in man shows that, with advancing age, there is a progressive increase in symptoms and signs (Figure 3). As a matter of fact, it is generally conceded that older people tend to have more clinical findings than younger people, that older people tend to die more readily, and that older persons with clinical problems die more readily than older persons without clinical symptoms and signs. What is usually not underlined is that, with time, there is an increase in variance (shown by the gray area in Figure 3). This then means that some older people are afflicted with fewer symptoms and signs than other younger subjects. Hence, this suggests that the common, so-called normal, increase in clinical symptoms and signs with time, meaning age, is not an inevitable ingredient of the aging process. Recognition of this fact is a critical point, namely that much of the clinical picture heretofore ascribed to the physiologic aging process is, in fact, simply an expression of pathosis. That the usual aging course of events is not physiologic allows that the process be slowed, stopped, reversed, or even completely prevented (Figure 4).

All disease is preceded by an incubation period. In the instance of acute mechanical trauma (e.g., an automobile accident), the incubation is brief and inconsequential from a diagnostic and therapeutic point of view. In the case of the acute

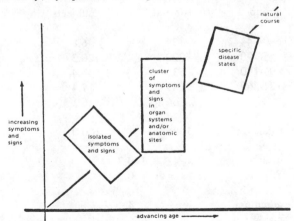

Fig. 2. The clinical sequence of events in chronic disease. At first, there are few and diverse symptoms and signs [box on the left]. With time, the findings become more numerous and localized in a system or site [center box]. Finally, the clinical evidence fits the textbook picture of a particular disease or syndrome [box on the right].

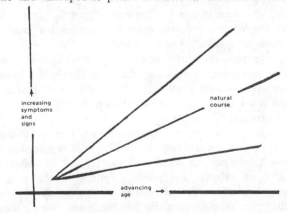

Fig. 3. The usual clinical sequence of events. With time, there is a progressive increase in symptoms and signs [shown by the rising center line]. However, with advancing age, there is also an increase in variance [pictured by the widening gray area]. This suggests that some elderly persons show fewer findings than other younger individuals.

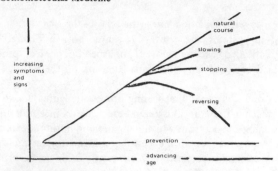

Fig. 4. The five possible clinical events are shown. First, the clinical course continues unchanged. Second, the progress may be slowed. Third, it is sometimes possible to halt the pattern. Fourth, there is a chance of reversing the state of affairs. Finally, the ideal is to subtend an angle of zero with real primary prevention [prevention of occurrence].

infectious disorders like the measles, the incubation period is somewhat longer, approximately ten days, and more significant from a diagnostic and treatment standpoint. With the chronic disorders (e.g., myocardial infarction, cerebrovascular accident, rheumatoid arthritis, periodontal disease), the incubation time extends over months and frequently years or decades. Clearly, the longer the incubation period, the greater the opportunity to anticipate the end-problem and, hopefully, abort the process.

Initially, the patient notes only few and seemingly unrelated findings. There may be irritability, for example, associated with leg cramps. Because these apparently independent symptoms and signs do not fit any textbook description of a particular disease, the complaints may either be ignored or assigned a meaningless label, or regarded as a minor emotional problem. In any case, because the clinical problem cannot be given a name, the treatment is purely symptomatic. At this stage, the clinical picture is shown by the box on the extreme left (Figure 2).

If the clinical situation just described continues, as is so often the case, then the number of symptoms and signs progressively multiplies. Sooner or later, the findings begin to crystallize in systems, organs, or in localized sites. For example, the patient earlier described now finds himself with several gastrointestinal complaints (e.g., indigestion, anorexia, constipation, and hemorrhoids). At this stage, the constellation is still not classifiable with textbook terminology. Hence, treatment is usually symptomatic or the patient is advised that the problem should be observed. If many organ systems or anatomic sites are involved, the syndrome might, by exclusion, be assigned a psychologic etiology. This is the story pictured in the middle box (Figure 2). In any case, because the clinical problem cannot be assigned a name, the treatment is symptomatic.

Finally, when the syndrome is clearly identifiable in terms of a classical textbook description, then the illness is assigned a label. In conventional medicine, it is only at this point that a diagnosis is justified. This is the situation pictorially portrayed on the extreme right (Figure 2).

In other words, in the traditional practice of medicine, disease does not really exist until a diagnosis is established. A diagnosis is only possible when a set number and constellation of findings ripen. Hence, for practical purposes, the long and tortuous incubation period clinically, biochemically, enzymatically goes frequently unlabelled or meaninglessly tagged. Clearly, the name of the game is the name!

The implications of this name-calling game are enormous. For example, the present concern with vitamin C is that, in its absence, it is possible to develop scurvy though it is granted that scurvy is rare and highly unlikely. Similarly, the concern with vitamin B_1 (thiamin) and vitamin B_3 (niacin) is because of beri-beri and pellagra, both rare and unlikely syndromes. Since the name of the game is the name, vitamin E is still under considerable question since it has not been identified with a particular disease even though it may be important in a host of vital metabolic processes.

THE PRACTICAL REVERBERATIONS OF A NEW PHILOSOPHY OF MEDICINE

We have now seen that the present health delivery system only recognizes a disease when a set of findings can be identified consistent with a textbook description. In other words, the name of the game is, in fact, the name. An attempt will now be made to show that, by switching the emphasis from classical syndromes to the earliest stages of pathosis in terms of mistakes of living, new and productive vistas open which could significantly alter the present health delivery system.

We have been conducting a study of the health of health professionals for a number of years. More precisely, we have been engaged in a multiphasic testing program of 832 doctors and their wives over an eight-year period.

It is safe to conclude that no scurvy was identified in this group. In other words, there is no evidence to suggest pathosis which would fit the box on the right in Figure 2. Since vitamin C deficiency is presumed the sole factor in scurvy, the assumption follows in traditional circles that the vitamin C intake in this group must therefore be optimal. Table 1 summarizes the distribution of reported daily vitamin C consumption in this group over the eight year period. Three points warrant particular mention. First, the average daily intake is 140 mgm. which is approximately threefold greater than the new recommendations of 45 mgm just recently announced by the Food and Nutrition Board of the National Research Council-National Academy of

Table 1. Distribution of daily vitamin C consumption (seven-day survey)

vitamin C group	number of subjects	percentage of subjects
0- 44	74	6.8
45- 90	220	20.3
91-180	537	49.4
181-269	189	17.4
270+	66	6.1
total	1086	100.0
mean	140.3	
S.D.	80.5	
minimum	4	
maximum	666	
range	662	

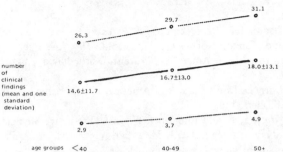

mean number of clinical findings (Cornell Medical Index Health Questionnaire) in terms of advancing age

Fig. 5. With advancing age [on the horizontal axis], there is an increase in clinical symptoms and signs [on the vertical axis].

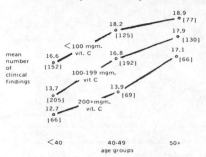

mean number of clinical findings (Cornell Medical Index Health Questionnaire) in terms of daily vitamin C consumption

Fig. 6. With advancing age, those consuming the largest amount of vitamin C [200+ mgs. daily] tend to report the fewest clinical findings.

Sciences [4]. Parenthetic mention should be made that the recommended daily intake has recently been lowered from 60 mgm. [5]. Second, it is noteworthy that the group range is considerable, of a magnitude of approximately 166-fold from 4 to 666 mgm. Finally, according to the cutoff point of 45 mgm. now set, approximately one in thirteen to one in fourteen subjects display suboptimal if not scorbutic intake.

Figure 5 is a pictorial portrayal of the total clinical symptoms and signs encountered in this presumably nonscorbutic group in terms of age. It is evident that, with advancing age (moving from left to right on the abscissa), there is a mean increase in clinical findings from 14.6 in the youngest group to 16.7 and 18.0 in the intermediate and advanced age groups respectively. This is quite in accord with the observations of a diagonal line earlier described (Figure 3). It is also noteworthy that the variance increases with advancing age from 11.7 to 13.0 to 13.1 respectively supporting the gray area of variance previously discussed (Figure 3). The question to be resolved is whether there is any parallelism between this nonspecific clinical picture and daily vitamin C consumption in nonscorbutic subjects.

Figure 6 depicts the relationship between clinical symptoms and signs as pictured on the ordinate in terms of age as described on the abscissa and in the light of daily vitamin C intake. It is clear that the group characterized by the lowest ascorbic acid consumption (less than 100 mgm. per day) shows, at all age groups, the greatest number of clinical symptoms and signs (16.6, 18.2, and 18.9). The group representing the highest vitamin C intake (200+ mgm. daily) is associated with the least clinical pathosis at all temporal points (12.7, 13.9, and 17.1). Finally, the group occupying an intermediate position in terms of daily vitamin C intake (100-199 mgm.) occupies an intermediate place in terms of clinical symptoms and signs (13.7, 16.8, and 17.9).

The point of the story, as underlined by this particular exercise, is that the present health-disease patterns become more meaningful when one discards the traditional disease classification (in this case, the syndrome of scurvy) for the earliest evidence of the syndrome of sickness (clinical symptoms and signs) and when one grants that small differences in vitamin C intake may be viewed as a mistake in living.

There are many other, and protean, implications of this philosophy. In fact, too many applications evolve to be included within the limits of these pages. One will be considered because of its singular importance.

There is no denying the heated debate generated by Professor Linus Pauling with the appearance of his paper on orthomolecular psychiatry [6], followed by his book, Vitamin C and the

Common Cold [7], and his most recent release, Orthomolecular Psychiatry [8]. One of the controversies stemming from his work is the dosage of vitamins which should be consumed under health and disease conditions.

For example, according to the Food and Nutrition Board, 45 mgm. vitamin C daily is adequate to maintain optimal health in the reference human [4]. Professor Pauling contends that the daily intake should range from a low of 250 mgm. (which is five-sixfold the traditional recommendation) to 10000 mgm. (which is 222 times the current recommendation). The burning question is how to develop an experimental model to resolve this dilemma.

Figure 7 is an attempt to resolve the question through a study of the daily vitamin C consumption in a progressively healthier sample. Ten hundred eight-six observations were made on the doctors and their wives. The mean number of clinical symptoms and signs was 16.2 (described on the horizontal axis). The daily vitamin C consumption was found to be 140 ± 81 mgm. (pictured on the ordinate).

As one moves from right to left, the group becomes progressively healthier by virtue of the fact that they manifest progressively fewer symptoms and signs. For example, 1061 of the 1086 reported less than 50 clinical findings. In other words, the 25 with more than 50 clinical findings have been excluded. The daily vitamin C consumption is 141 ± 81 in the group with a mean of 14.1 findings. As one proceeds from right to left on the abscissa, the mean daily ascorbic acid intake progressively increases. Hence, within the limits of this experiment, those subjects with no clinical findings consume about 167 mgm. vitamin C daily

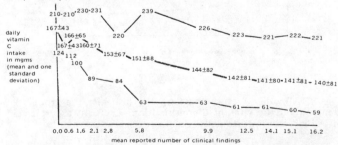

relationship of reported daily vitamin C consumption (seven-day dietary surveyland reported total clinical findings—Cornell Medical Index Health Questionnaire) in a presumably health male and female sample

Fig. 7. In a progressively healthier sample of subjects as judged by progressively fewer symptoms and signs [on the abscissa], the mean daily vitamin C consumption is progressively higher [on the ordinate].

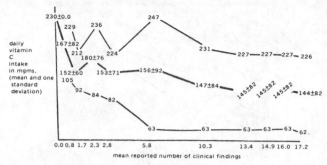

Fig. 8. The patterns described in Figure 7 is repeated in an older age group [40+ years] except that the reported daily vitamin C intake levels are higher.

which is about almost four times the present recommendation of 45 mgm.

Since time is a factor, meaning that vitamin C intake times time is a more reliable reflector of vitamin C needs, the story just described is repeated with those subjects 40+ years of age. The overall pattern is the same except that the vitamin C daily values are somewhat higher (Figure 8).

Thus, this approach indicates that the healthier the group, the greater the daily ascorbic acid intake. Additionally, the older the group the greater the daily vitamin C consumption. Hence, here is a model to develop the optimal and possibly ideal daily vitamin C consumption (Figure 9).

SUMMARY

There are a number of factors which contribute to the fact that the existing health delivery system is a national disaster. One, not mentioned, is the medical addiction to disease classification. If one diverts one's attention from diseases to mistakes in living, a new and refreshing approach to the solution of the national medical problem comes into focus.

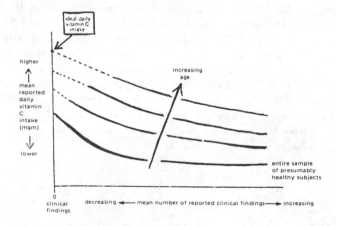

Fig. 9. All other factors constant, the healthier the group, the greater the daily vitamin C consumption. The daily ascorbic acid intake increases additionally, the older the studied sample.

REFERENCES

1. Watson, T.J. *Remarks on health care.* Presentation before Mayo Clinic, Rochester, Minnesota, 19 November 1970. Reprinted in J. Amer. Soc. Prevent. Dent., January-February 1973.

2. Schorr, D. Don't get sick in America. 1970. Nashville, Aurora Publishers, Inc.

3. Cheraskin, E. and Ringsdorf, W.M., Jr. Predictive Medicine: a study in strategy. 1973. Mountain View, California, Pacific Press Publishing Association.

4. National Academy of Sciences-National Research Council. Recommended daily dietary allowances. Revised 1973.

5. Food and Nutrition Board, National Research Council. Recommended dietary allowances. Publication #1964. Seventh edition. 1968. Washington, D.C., National Academy of Sciences.

6. Pauling, L. Orthomolecular psychiatry. Science 160: #3825, 265-271, 19 April 1968.

7. Pauling, L. Vitamin C and the common cold. 1970. San Francisco, W.H. Freeman and Company.

8. Hawkins, D. and Pauling, L. Orthomolecular psychiatry. 1973. San Francisco, W.H. Freeman and Company.

9
"Linus Pauling before Congress"*

LINUS PAULING

I am Linus Pauling, Director of the Linus Pauling Institute, Menlo Park, California, and, since 1 August 1974, Professor Emeritus in Stanford University. For many years I was Professor of Chemistry in the California Institute of Technology, Oxford University, University of California, and Stanford University. During the past forty-three years my work has covered many fields of physics, chemistry, biology, and medicine. In 1935 I began studying the properties of hemoglobin and other proteins and the nature of serological reactions in the natural process of immunity. In 1949 my students and I published a paper on the molecular basis of the disease sickle cell anemia and formulated for the first time the concept of molecular disease. Since 1954 my research has focused on the molecular basis of mental disease, the role of vitamins in relation to both mental disease and health in general, and the development of improved methods of chemical analysis of body fluids for diagnostic and therapeutic purposes. I have received the Nobel Prize for Chemistry in 1954, the Nobel Peace Prize for 1962, the Phillips Medal of the American College of Physicians for contributions to internal medicine, the Thomas Addis Medal of the American Nephrosis Society, the Modern Medicine Award, the U.S. Presidential Medal for Merit for contributions to the war effort during the Second World War, and additional awards in science, medicine, and other fields.

I first became aware of the value of an increased intake of vitamins in connection with my studies of schizophrenia. In 1968 I published papers entitled "Orthomolecular Psychiatric and Somatic Medicine" and "Orthomolecular Psychiatry," in which I discussed the significant role of vitamins and other natural substances in determining the mental and physical health of a person [1, 2]. In 1970 I published a book entitled "Vitamin C and the Common Cold," in which evidence was presented showing that an increased intake of vitamin C leads to improved health, as shown by a decrease in the amount of illness with the common cold [3]. As a result of my studies of vitamins during the past ten years I have reached the conclusion that the proposed FDA regulations restricting the sale of vitamins would do serious damage to the health of the American people if they were to go into effect. I believe that these proposed regulations

are based upon a misunderstanding and misinterpretation of the facts about the role of the vitamins in nutrition, on the part of the Food and Drug Administration. I recommend passage of the Proxmire bill, which would restrain the Food and Drug Administration from making such recommendations.

I advocate some controls over the sale and advertising of vitamins, but not through classifying them as drugs. For example, I advocate that labels should state the composition of preparations, giving, for example, the amount of rose-hip powder contained in a vitamin C tablet described as Rose-hip Vitamin C.

1. *The meaning of Recommended Dietary Allowance.* There is a serious misunderstanding by the FDA and most people of the meaning of the expression "Recommended Dietary Allowance (RDA)." The RDA, as formulated by the Food and Nutrition Board of the National Academy of Sciences — National Research Council, is described as being adequate for most people. This description is usually interpreted as meaning that it approximates the optimum intake for most people, that is, the intake that leads to the best of health. With this interpretation the proposed regulation classifying as drugs preparations that contain in a day's tablet more than the U.S. RDA (the U.S. RDA varies between 100 percent and 150 percent of the Food and Nutrition Board's RDA), and thus restricting their sale and use, would seem to be unobjectionable. This interpretation, however, is wrong.

The RDA for a vitamin is not the allowance that leads to the best of health for most people. It is, instead, only the estimated amount that for most people would prevent death or serious illness from overt vitamin deficiency. Values of the daily intake of the various vitamins that lead to the best of health for most people may well be several times as great, for the various vitamins, as the values of the RDA. The proposed regulation restricting the sale of vitamins, through classifying them as drugs, could lead to great damage to the health of the American people, by interfering with their obtaining vitamins in the optimum amounts, such as to lead to the best of health.

The FDA in making its proposed regulations about vitamins seems to have misunderstood the meaning of RDA, as formulated by the Food and Nutrition Board. The Food and Nutrition Board has stated in its reports that the RDA's are the amounts of vitamin C and other nutrients that protect against overt manifestations of scurvy and other deficiency diseases, and are not the amounts that lead to the best of health. This point has recently

*Presented before the Senate Subcommittee on Health, Sen. Edward Kennedy, Chairman. Reprinted with permission: *Healthline*, Volume I, #2.

been emphasized by Dr. Harper, the Chairman of the Committee on Recommended Dietary Allowances of the Food and Nutrition Board. Dr. Harper has recently [4] quoted the statement by the chairman of the first committee on RDA's that they "are not recommendations for the ideal diet," and also the statement of another nutritionist (Dr. Hegstedt) that the term "recommended allowance" was adopted "*to avoid* any implication of finality or . . . optimal requirements."

There is need for further research to determine reliably the values of the optimum daily intakes of the various vitamins. The presently existing evidence indicates that for several vitamins the optimum daily intake may be two to five times the RDA, and that for vitamin C, in particular, the optimum daily intake for different people probably lies between five and one hundred times the RDA. Since most vitamins are known to have very low toxicity and few side effects, even when taken in massive amounts, there is no justification for the proposed FDA regulation restricting their sale in the amounts that might include the daily intakes that lead to the best of health.

Some of the evidence about the optimum daily intake of various vitamins, especially vitamin C, is summarized in the following paragraphs.

2. *Vitamin C and the common cold.* There is overwhelming evidence that an increased intake of vitamin C, several times the RDA (which is now 45 mg per day for an adult) provides significant protection against the common cold [3]. For example, Cowan, Diehl, and Baker of the University of Michigan School of Medicine reported that students who received 200 mg per day in addition to that in their ordinary diet (probably approximately the RDA) had only about two thirds as much illness with the common cold (69 percent as much) as students who received an inactive placebo tablet [5]. The Swiss physician, Dr. G. Ritzel reported that school boys who received 1000 mg of vitamin C per day had only one third as much illness with the common cold (37 percent) as those who received a placebo [6]. Anderson, Reid, and Beaton of the University of Toronto reported a thirty percent decrease in respiratory illness for subjects receiving 1000 mg per day, [7] and Coulehan et al. reported thirty percent decrease for older children receiving 2000 mg per day, in comparison with those receiving a placebo [8]. Several other recent studies have given similar results. The evidence is overwhelming that a significant protective effect against this important disease, the common cold, the cause of more illness than all other diseases, is provided by an intake, daily, of vitamin C several times the RDA.

It is estimated that at the present time millions of people in the United States are providing themselves with some protection against the common cold by ingesting several hundred or a few thousand milligrams of vitamin C each day. Many of these people have verified the value of an increased intake of vitamin C through their own experiences. There is no sound scientific or medical justification for limiting the availability of vitamin C to these people, in the way that would be effected by the proposed FDA regulations.

3. *Vitamin C and the healing of wounds and burns.* It is well known that the intake of amounts of vitamin C greater than the RDA favors the healing of wounds and burns and the union of fractured bones. The concentration of vitamin C in the blood of a person who has been injured drops significantly below the normal value, unless he is given extra vitamin C. Many physicians and surgeons give vitamin C to patients who have been injured or are undergoing operations. The extensive literature about vitamin C in relation to the healing of wounds, burns, and fractures is surveyed in the book on vitamin C by Irwin Stone [9].

The mechanism of the effectiveness of vitamin C in wound healing is understood, at least in part. Vitamin C is required for the synthesis of collagen, the principal structural protein in the body, an important constituent of bone, skin, tendon, and the intercellular cement holding the cells of the body together.

It is a part of ordinary life for most people to suffer occasional minor cuts, abrasions, and burns. Their healing is expedited by an intake of vitamin C greater than the RDA. This effect can be considered a part of the justification for a daily intake greater than the RDA.

4. *Vitamin C and back trouble.* A troublesome and rather common complaint is back trouble, which may involve only the minor nuisance of pain in the lower back, or may develop into a serious disease, sometimes requiring operation. Ten years ago Dr. James Greenwood, Jr. of Houston, Texas, reported that he himself and many of his patients were able to alleviate and control their back trouble by an increased intake of vitamin C, usually about 1000 milligrams per day (twenty times the RDA). In his 1964 paper [10] he reported from a study of over 500 patients his conclusion that "a significant number of patients with disc lesions were able to avoid surgery by the use of large doses of vitamin C." He found that the back pain returned when the daily intake of vitamin C was decreased, and was again controlled by an increased intake. Dr. Greenwood has just informed me (in July 1974) that his extensive added observations over the last ten years provided additional substantiation for his earlier conclusion that an intake of about 1000 milligrams of vitamin C per day has significant value in preventing back trouble, as well as other manifestations of a poor state of health. His observations accordingly support the conclusion that an intake of several hundred or 1000 milligrams per day of vitamin C may approximate the optimum intake.

The effect of vitamin C in controlling back trouble can, of course, be attributed to its known effectiveness in strengthening connective tissue by favoring the synthesis of collagen. An increased strength of connective tissue should improve health in various respects, including providing protection against ordinary complaints other than back trouble. This effect of an increased intake of vitamin C accordingly provides another argument against the proposed FDA regulations and for the Proxmire bill.

5. *Vitamin C and heart disease.* The most common cause of death of American people is now cardiovascular disease, and its age-specific incidence has been increasing during recent decades. Many more young men and women die of disease of the heart and blood vessels now than fifty or one hundred years ago. The tendency to die of heart disease at an earlier age is an indication of poorer health. Evidence now exists strongly suggesting that an increased intake of vitamin C improves the health in such a way as to lead to a decreased incidence of heart disease.

The incidence of heart disease is higher for people with a high concentration of cholesterol in the blood than for those with a lower concentration. Several investigators have shown that an increase in intake of ascorbic acid leads to a decreased incidence of heart disease. The evidence has been reviewed recently by Krumdieck and Butterworth [11]. Ginter has obtained evidence that the mechanism of this effect is that an increased concentration of ascorbic acid leads to an increased rate of destruction of cholesterol by converting it to bile acids [12]. Knox has reported that people in England with a high intake of ascorbic acid have a significantly lower death rate from ischemic heart disease and cerebrovascular disease than those with a low intake of ascorbic acid [13]. Krumdieck and Butterworth in their discussion of the pathogenesis of atherosclerosis [11] conclude that "vitamin C seems to occupy a position of unique importance by virtue of its involvement in two systems: the maintenance of vascular integrity and the metabolism of cholesterol to bile acids," and suggest that it is pertinent to consider the adequacy of the present values of the RDA for vitamin C.

A beneficial effect of vitamin C in relation to heart disease and cerebrovascular disease may be attributed not only to the effect of the vitamin in increasing the rate of destruction of cholesterol but also to its known effect in strengthening the blood vessels through its participation in the synthesis of connective tissue. Dr. Constance Spittle in her study in England found that a significant decrease in cholesterol concentration in the blood is achieved by an intake of 1000 milligrams of vitamin C per day. This observation provides additional evidence that the optimum intake of vitamin C, leading to increased resistance to cardiovascular disease, may be in the neighborhood of 1000 milligrams per day.

6. *Vitamin C and cigarettes.* It is well known that people who smoke cigarettes are, on the average, in poorer health than those who do not smoke. This poorer health is evidenced by an increased incidence of heart disease, cancer, and other diseases. The incidence of disease in general is doubled for the average cigarette smoker, leading to a decrease by eight years in the length of the period of good health and of life. It is also known that the concentration of vitamin C in the blood of cigarette smokers is less than that in the blood of non-smokers. The destruction of vitamin C by the smoking of cigarettes at the rate of one pack a day is such that a normal concentration of the vitamin in the blood can be achieved only by the ingestion of 1000 to 3000 milligrams of the vitamin per day. This intake may be considered to approximate the optimum intake for cigarette smokers. Since half of the adults in the United States smoke cigarettes, an average of one pack per day, the people who smoke cigarettes have to be considered as ordinary people, rather than patients under treatment by a physician. The proposed FDA regulations would operate to interfere with the improvement of their health by cigarette smokers through the ingestion of the amount of vitamin C needed to counteract its destruction by the cigarettes that they smoke, and would thus operate to the detriment of the health of a significant fraction of the American people.

7. *Antiviral and antibacterial action of vitamin C.* Many investigators have reported that vitamin C inactivates viruses in vitro (references are given in the book by Irwin Stone [9]). The viruses that have been studied include poliomyelitis virus, vaccina virus, hoof-and-mouth virus, rabies virus, tobacco mosaic virus, and a number of bacterial viruses. Murata and Kitagawa [15] have recently reported that the inactivation results from the scission of the nucleic acid of the virus by free radicals formed during the oxidation of the vitamin C. The inactivation of viruses occurs at a significant rate for concentrations of vitamin C that can be reached in the blood with a high intake, 1000 milligrams per day, and is much less at a low intake, the RDA. Some

protection against viral diseases (poliomyelitis, hepatitis, fever blisters, shingles, virus pneumonia, measles, chickenpox, virus encephalitis, mumps, infectious mononucleosis) has been reported by several investigators. References are given by Stone [9].

Inactivation of bacterial toxins by vitamin C and bacteriostatic and bactericidal action of the vitamin against several bacteria have also been reported, and some success in controlling various bacterial infections in man by an increased intake of the vitamin has been reported (references in Stone [9]). The possibility that an increased intake of vitamin C has some general protective effect against both bacterial and viral diseases should not be rejected.

One of the most potent defense mechanisms of the body is the destruction of invading bacterial cells by the leukocytes of the blood (phagocytosis). It has been known for thirty years that vitamin C is needed for effective phagocytic activity of leukocytes. It is also known that wounds, infections, and other stresses lead to a decrease in the leukocyte concentration of the vitamin to below the phagocytically effective level, unless the intake of the vitamin is considerably greater than the RDA. Hume and Weyers in Scotland have recently reported that in subjects who receive the ordinary intake of vitamin C the concentration in the leukocytes drops and remains below the phagocytically effective value when the subject catches cold [16]. In consequence the resistance of the person against a secondary bacterial infection is low. An intake of 200 milligrams per day is not enough to keep the concentration in the leukocytes sufficiently high, but an intake of 1000 milligrams per day plus 6000 milligrams per day for three days when a cold is contracted suffices to keep the concentration high enough to provide protection against the secondary bacterial infections that often accompany the common cold, as well as against other bacterial infections, which often are incurred under conditions of stress.

8. *Animals that make their own vitamin C.* Most animals manufacture ascorbic acid in the cells of their body, and do not need to have this substance, which is vitamin C, in their foods. It is unlikely that animals would synthesize more ascorbic acid than the amount corresponding to optimum health. Hence the amounts that are made by animals, two to nineteen grams per day (calculated to 70 kilograms, 154 pounds, body weight, the weight of a man) suggest that similar amounts may be near the optimum for man. The mammals that have been studied range from the mouse, weighing about 20 grams (less than one ounce), to the goat, nearly as large as a man, and the amounts manufactured are approximately proportional to body weight for these various species. The mouse has been reported to manufacture 19 grams per day, calculated to 70 kilograms body weight, and the goat 13 grams per day, on the same basis.

These values provide additional evidence that the optimum intake for man is much larger than the RDA, perhaps one hundred times as large.

9. *The feed of laboratory animals.* The Food and Nutrition Board of the National Academy of Sciences — National Research Council formulates the values of the RDA of various vitamins for human beings. There is another committee, the Committee on Animal Nutrition of the National Academy of Sciences — National Research Council, that makes similar recommendations for domestic animals. It is my opinion that the recommendations of the Committee on Animal Nutrition are based on sounder

evidence than those of the Food and Nutrition Board on human nutrition, because of the well known difficulties of carrying out controlled experiments with human subjects.

Also, I believe that human beings are sufficiently similar in their nutritional requirements to other mammals as to justify the assumption that the optimum intakes of vitamins for animals may be applied also to human beings. Some evidence for this assumption is provided by the fact that the amounts of various vitamins (other than vitamin C) in the recommended feed of animals is not much different for different species of animals. By examining the report of the Committee on Animal Nutrition [17] I have found that the amount of vitamins contained in a day's ration of semi-purified feed (for a man, the amount with food energy 2500 kilocalories) for various vitamins other than vitamin C is usually between two and five times the corresponding RDA for man. The amounts in the recommended feed for these animals may well approximate the optimum amounts, in that many studies have been made of the composition of the feed of laboratory animals that leads to the best growth, proper reproductive capacity, and least loss through infectious disease. We might conclude that these facts indicate that the optimum intake of several vitamins (vitamin B_1, vitamin B_2, vitamin B_6, vitamin A) for man are in the range two to five times the respective RDA's.

The guinea pig and the monkey resemble man in requiring exogenous vitamin C. The recommended purified diets for the guinea pig and the monkey contain 1100 milligrams and 1250 milligrams, respectively, of vitamin C in the ration with 2500 kilocalories of food energy, corresponding to the intake of a 70-kilogram man. These animals, which are smaller than man, eat somewhat more food, per kilogram, than man, and the daily intakes are several times greater. The values 1100 milligrams and 1250 milligrams of vitamin C per day, per 2500 kilocalories of food energy, presumably approximate the optimum intake, and may well be pertinent to man.

Several studies have been made of the intake of vitamin C necessary for good health in the guinea pig. Calculated to body weight of 70 kilograms, the intake of 350 milligrams per day suffices to give good growth, 700 to prevent pathological lesions of the teeth, and 1400 milligrams per day to provide a high degree of phagocytic activity of the leukocytes to protect the animal against infection. A careful study, using several measures of good health, has been reported by Yew to indicate an optimum intake of 3500 milligrams per day (per 70 kilogram body weight) [18]. All of these studies of guinea pigs and other laboratory animals suggest that for man the optimum intake is in the range of a few grams per day, far larger than the RDA.

10. *Vitamin C, mental alertness, and general well-being.* Many people have referred to an increase in mental alertness and general feeling of well-being accompanying an increased intake of vitamin C. Some have reported a failure to observe such an effect. One carefully planned and executed study about vitamin C and mental alertness is that of Kubala and Katz [19]. The subjects were school children and college women, in four schools. It was found that the average IQ was higher for the subjects with a high concentration of vitamin C in the blood serum (about 1.10 milligrams per deciliter) than for those with a low concentration. There was an increase by 3.54 IQ units in the IQ for the low group after they had received a glass of orange juice containing 90 milligrams of vitamin C every day for four months, with very little change for the subjects with high concentration of vitamin

C. Kubala and Katz suggest that the increased values of the measured IQ result from an increase in "alertness" or "awareness" caused by the improved nutritional state, and that the subjects with a low level of vitamin C in the blood were functioning at less than maximum capacity. These observations accordingly indicate that an intake of vitamin C that does not provide a blood plasma concentration greater than 1.1 milligrams per deciliter is not adequate, in that it does not permit the person to function at maximum capacity. The intake required to achieve this high concentration of vitamin C in the plasma is about three times the recommended daily allowance.

A study of the general state of health of adults in relation to intake of vitamin C has been reported by Cheraskin [20]. The 1086 subjects were physicians or dentists and their wives, who were followed over a period of eight years. The number of clinical symptoms and signs of imperfect health was determined (Cornell Medical Index Health Questionnaire), and the intake of vitamin C was obtained through a seven-day survey. It was found that for each age group the number of clinical symptoms and signs decreased with increase in the intake of vitamin C. The indications of ill health were greatest for those receiving less than 100 milligrams per day, less for those receiving 100 to 200 milligrams per day, and least for those receiving 200 milligrams per day or more. There is clear indication that some improvement in health is associated with an increase in intake of vitamin C to more than 200 milligrams per day, which is more than four times the RDA.

This evidence, too, supports the conclusion that the optimum intake of vitamin C is much greater than the RDA for the vitamin.

11. *The low toxicity of vitamins.* Vitamin C has been described as one of the least toxic substances known. People have ingested 125 grams (over a quarter of a pound) at one time without harm, and an equal amount has been injected intravenously into a human being without harm. It is unlikely that ingestion in the amounts two grams to twenty grams per day, the amounts synthesized by animals, over long periods of time would lead to harm. It has been suggested that a high intake of vitamin C continued for a long time might lead to the formation of kidney stones, but in fact not a single case has been reported in the medical literature. Physicians who have supervised hundreds of subjects who ingested four grams per day of vitamin C or more for periods of a year or more have reported that there were no serious side effects.

Some ascorbic acid is converted in the body to oxalic acid, which could lead to the formation of kidney stones of the oxalate type. A careful study showed that the amount of oxalate was increased very little by an intake of four grams of vitamin C per day, and is only doubled for an intake of ten grams per day, for normal subjects. One man has been found who converts a large amount of ingested C into oxalic acid; this unusual person should, of course, refrain from ingesting large amounts of the vitamin. It is to be anticipated, of course, that because of individual variability an occasional person might not be able to tolerate a high intake of vitamin C. The number of people with such an idiosyncrasy is probably quite small.

The other water-soluble vitamins are reported to be similarly innocuous, with no known lethal dose for humans. The fat-soluble vitamins, vitamin A and vitamin D, are toxic in large doses, many times the RDA. It should be required that a statement about this toxicity be printed on labels.

The toxicity of vitamin A and vitamin D have, in my opinion, been overemphasized, especially when they are advanced as an argument against the ingestion of amounts of the other vitamins larger than the RDA's. A comparison with aspirin, which is generally considered to be a rather safe drug is interesting. The number of deaths from aspirin poisoning is estimated to more than 1000 times the number from overdoses of vitamin A and vitamin D. No deaths from overdoses of any other vitamins have ever been reported.

I conclude that the possible toxicity of vitamins provides no justification for the new FDA regulations.

12. *Conclusion.* I believe that the vitamins are important foods, and that the optimum daily intakes of vitamin C and other vitamins, leading to the best of health, are much larger than the present Recommended Dietary Allowances. I believe that the American people should not be hampered in their efforts to improve their health by an intake of vitamins approaching the optimum intake. The proposed FDA regulations would operate in a serious way to make it difficult for the American people to obtain these vitamins, by classifying them as drugs in daily amounts greater than the U.S. RDA's. I accordingly support legislation that will prevent the Food and Drug Administration from carrying out this unwise action.

The values of the RDA for various vitamins have been set by the Food and Nutrition Board by consideration only of the amounts needed to prevent death or serious illness from a dietary deficiency. No serious consideration whatever has been given to the question of the optimum daily intake, the amount that leads to the best of health.

In the foregoing paragraphs I have summarized the evidence for vitamin C. This evidence indicates that the optimum daily intake for human beings probably lies between about 250 milligrams per day and 10 grams per day, different for different people. It is accordingly probably between five and two hundred times the RDA for vitamin C. For other vitamins, for which less evidence is available, the optimum daily intake may be between two and five times the RDA.

For several years I have taken 6000 milligrams of vitamin C each day. I take it as pure crystalline L-ascorbic acid or as 1000 milligram tablets. If the FDA regulations were to go into effect, I would be put to added trouble and expense. I might be restricted to buying tablets containing the U.S. RDA of 100 milligrams, so that I would have to swallow sixty of these tablets each day. This would mean ingesting a large amount of filler and binder in the tablets, the filler and binder constituting a larger fraction of the 100-mg tablets than of the larger tablets. Also, the small tablets are more expensive, per gram of vitamin C, than the larger tablets. An alternative would be for me to go to the trouble of getting a physician to prescribe large doses of vitamin C for me. Aside from the trouble of getting the physician to do this, I would have to pay his fee, and would also have to pay the customary higher price for prescription items. I am sure that the new regulations, if they were to go into effect, would operate to the detriment of the health of the American people.

As a scientific investigator, I am interested in carrying on research on medical problems, including the problem of determining as reliably as possible the values of the optimum intakes of vitamins and other nutrients. Classification of vitamin C as a drug would in my opinion work a serious hardship on the research effort at a time when it should be most encouraged. The regulations about research on the effects of drugs on human subjects, which in my opinion are quite proper, would operate in an unnecessarily restrictive way to hamper research in the field of nutrition, especially research on the improvement in general health of people accompanying an increased intake of various vitamins.

As a consumer, I am concerned about the misrepresentations and over-pricing that have existed in connection with the sale of vitamin C and other vitamins. Even at the present time, some vitamin C preparations are being offered for sale at prices as much as one hundred times those of essentially equivalent preparations. Advertising is often misleading in suggesting a difference in vitamin C depending upon whether it contains wild rose hips or is a preparation of pure crystalline L-ascorbic acid. Preparations presently available under the name Rose-hip Vitamin C may contain less than one percent of rose-hip powder, with less than one hundredth of one percent of the vitamin C coming from rose hips. The proposed FDA regulations do not in my opinion establish an effective mechanism for protecting the consumer against the abuses of misrepresentation and over-pricing. A more direct approach, I believe, lies in implementation and enforcement of strict requirements about truth in advertising and initiation of a broad-based campaign of consumer education. It should be required, for example, that the actual amounts of the various components of each vitamin C preparation be stated on the label. Requirements of this sort about truth in advertising and labeling would be extremely helpful in eliminating some of the most serious consumer abuses.

I believe that the expression "Recommended Dietary Allowance" used by the Food and Nutrition Board and by the FDA is misleading, in that the RDA's are not the amounts that should be recommended as providing the best of health, but are only the amounts, probably much smaller, that prevent death or serious vitamin deficiency disease. I suggest that the name Recommended Dietary Allowance should be replaced by the name Minimum Dietary Allowance (MDA), which represents in a better way the actual significance of the amounts. I suggest also that the Food and Nutrition Board and the Food and Drug Administration should introduce a new range of quantities that might be called the Recommended Daily Intake (RDI). The RDI should be recommended as a range, corresponding to the known amount of individual variability. For vitamin C I suggest on the basis of the evidence summarized above that the RDI for an adult should be 250 milligrams to 4000 milligrams per day. Similar ranges of the RDI could be suggested for other vitamins, with values somewhat larger than the RDA's. I recommend also that the Federal government should support research to obtain more reliable information about the optimum daily intakes (RDI's) than is available at the present time.

I appreciate the opportunity to address the Committee on a matter of such significance to the health and well-being of the people of the United States. Thank you.

REFERENCES

1. Pauling, L. (1968) "Orthomolecular psychiatry," *Science 160*, 265-271.
2. Pauling, L. (1968) "Orthomolecular somatic and psychiatric medicine," *J. Diseases of Civilization 12*, 1-3.
3. Pauling, L. (1970) *Vitamin C and the Common Cold* (W.H. Freeman and Co., Inc., San Francisco).
4. Harper, A.E. (1974) "Official dietary allowances: those pesky RDAs," *Nutrition Today 9*, March-April 15-25.
5. Cowan, D.W., Diehl, H.S., and Baker, A.B. (1942) "Vitamins for the prevention of colds," *J. Amer. Med. Assn. 120*, 1268-1271.
6. Ritzel, G. (1961) "Kritische Beurteilung des Vitamins C als Prophylacticum und Therapeuticum der Erkaltungskrankheiten," *Helv. Med. Acta 28*, 63-68.
7. Anderson, T.W., Reid, D.B.W., and Beaton, G.H. (1972) "Vitamin C and the common cold: a double-blind trial," *J. Canadian Med. Assn. 107*, 503-508; correction 108, 133 (1973).
8. Coulehan, J.L., Reisinger, K.S., Rogers, K.D., and Bradley, D.W. (1974) "Vitamin C prophylaxis in a boarding school," *The New England J. of Medicine 290*, 6-10.
9. Stone, I. (1972) *The Healing Factor: Vitamin C Against Disease* (Grosset and Dunlap, New York, N.Y.).
10. Greenwood, J., Jr. (1964) "Optimum vitamin C intake as a factor in the preservation of disc integrity," *Med. Ann. Dist. of Columbia 33*, 274-276.
11. Krumdieck, C., and Butterworth, C.E., Jr. (1974) "Ascorbate-cholesterol- lechithin interactions: factors of potential importance in the pathogenesis of atherosclerosis," *Am. J. Clin. Nutr.* August.
12. Ginter, E. (1973) "Cholesterol: vitamin C controls its transformation to bile acids," *Science 179*, 702-704.
13. Knox, E.G. (1973) "Ischemic-heart-disease mortality and dietary intake of calcium," *Lancet i*, 1465-1468.
14. Spittle, C. (1971) "Atherosclerosis and vitamin C," *Lancet ii*, 1280-1281.
15. Murata, A., and Kitagawa, K. (1973) "Mechanism of inactivation of bacteriophage J_1 by ascorbic acid," *Agr. Biol. Chem. 37*, 1145-1151.
16. Hume, R., and Weyers, E. (1973) "Changes in leucocyte ascorbic acid during the common cold," *Scot. Med.J. 18*, 3-7.
17. Committee on Animal Nutrition, National Academy of Sciences - National Research Council (1962) "Nutrient requirements of domestic animals," *NAS-NRC* 990.
18. Yew, M.-L.S. (1973) "Recommended daily allowances for vitamin C," *Proc. Nat. Acad. Sci.* USA 70, 969-972.
19. Kubala, A.L., and Katz, M.M. (1960) "Nutritional factors in psychological test behavior," *J. Genet. Psychol. 96*, 343-352.
20. Cheraskin, E. and Ringsdorf, W.M. (1974) "Human vitamin C requirement: relation of daily intake to incidence of clinical signs and symptoms," *IRCS 2*, 1379.

10
Significance of High Daily Intake of Ascorbic Acid in Preventive Medicine*

FREDERICK ROBERT KLENNER

INTRODUCTION

The American Medical Association in its introduction to *Nostrums, Quackery and Pseudo-Medicine* states: "In from 80 to 85 percent of all cases of human ailment, it is probable that the individual will get well whether he does something for his indisposition or does nothing for it. The healing power of nature, fortunately for biologic perpetuity, works that way." These percentages are relative. Increased population and greater concentration in terms of living patterns, as well as other types of insult to the body, will frequently change this index. As physicians we have a duty to get the patient well, irrespective of his chance for self-healing with diet or herbs. Hippocrates once declared, "Of several remedies physicians should choose the least sensational." Vitamin C would seem to meet this requirement.

THE VIRUS STORY

The common cold has received renewed interest since publication of Pauling's book [1]. Brody, [2] in 1953, after studying vitamin C and its effect on colds in college students, advised that ascorbic acid be given early and often and in sufficient amounts. This confirmed what we had been experiencing and reporting over a period of several years. The response that we observed with massive and frequent doses of ascorbic acid in treating the common cold alerted us to the real significance of this treatment in preventive medicine. In February 1948, [3] I published my first paper on the use of massive doses of vitamin C in treating virus pathology. By February 1960, [4] some 25 scientific papers later, I realized that every head cold must be considered as a probable source of brain pathology. Many have died, especially children, following the sudden development of cerebral manifestations secondary to even a slight head and/or chest cold. These insidious cerebral happenings are responsible for the so-called crib deaths attributed to suffocation. They die by suffocation, but by way of a syndrome similar to that found in cephalic tetanus toxemia culminating in diaphragmatic spasm, with dyspnea and finally asphyxia. These infants and children who have been put to bed apparently well, except for an insignificant

nasal congestion, will demonstrate bilateral pneumonitis at autopsy. Adequate vitamin C, taken daily, will eliminate this syndrome. A similar pathology, dubbed Crib Syndrome, is less acute but unless recognized and treated heroically, the infant will also die. This condition is probably due to severe brain trauma received at time of delivery. Laryngismus stridulous will be present in this condition and the child will sound as if it has a cold. Calcium gluconate and massive, frequent injections of vitamin C will also reverse this pathology. The recognized treatment is daily oral dihydrotachysterol. Adequate ascorbic acid taken during the period of gestation will also prevent the occurrence of this syndrome. The information relative to crib syndrome is backed by case histories at Annie Penn Memorial Hospital, Reidsville, N.C. I have seen children dead in less than two hours after hospital admission, having received no treatment, simply because the attending physicians were not impressed with their illness. A few grams of ascorbic acid, given by needle, while they waited for laboratory procedures or examination to fit their schedule, could have saved their lives. I know this to be a fact because I have been in similar situations and by routinely employing ascorbic acid have seen death take a holiday. In a paper titled "An Insidious Virus," [5] I reasoned that it should be a *maxim* of medicine for large doses of vitamin C to be given in all pathological conditions while the physician ponders his diagnosis. The wisdom of this dictum is backed by many hundred cases under our supervision. I have seen critically ill chest patients well enough to go home after intravenous injection of 1 or 2 liters of 5 percent dextrose in water, each carrying 50 gm ascorbic acid. This procedure resulted in a dramatic transition from sickness to health.

Virus encephalitis can also be associated with the common cold as a result of the presence of herpes simplex in cold sores. Lerner [6] and associates believe that thousands of cases exist yearly from this route. Of this number, they estimate that one third die; and of the survivors, eight out of nine have residual brain damage. Their work suggests that passive hemaggluting antibodies in the cerebrospinal fluid are a better indicator of the presence of infectious virus than are circulating antibody titers in the serum. The simple herpes virus from the insignificant fever blister, but possessing the capability of producing encephalitis, can remain hidden for years in the neuron according to Drs. Stephens and Cook [7]. This confirms the thinking of Good-

*Reprinted with permission: *Journal of Preventive Medicine*, Spring, 1974.

pasture [8] given to us many years ago. Thus, a herpes simplex virus once present in a cold sore, although healed and leaving no evidence of lip pathology, could ignite later by simple exposure to ultraviolet light. How many mothers are endangering the lives of their children by sun-bathing, laboring under the belief that they are improving their health? Roizman [9] believes that all children are infected by age 5, but that only 1 percent experience true clinical illness. For many years investigators thought that each recurrence of fever blisters represented a new infection. Evidence is accumulating that shows the herpes simplex virus is harbored in dormant form until a physiologic or emotional event provokes the virus to produce the typical herpetic lesion. In one case with five repeats of herpes virus erupting at yearly intervals and at the same site, 7-10 gm ascorbic acid by mouth, daily, was found to eliminate this pathology.

Effecting a cure when a virus is the offending agent, and many times bringing about this change in the short space of 24 hours, is a rewarding moment in medicine. Vitamin C treatment must be intensive to be successful. Use veins when practical, otherwise give vitamin C intramuscularly. Never give less than 350 mg/kg body weight. This must be repeated every hour for 6 to 12 times, depending upon clinical improvement, then every two to four hours until the patient has recovered. Ice cubes held to the gluteal muscle before and after injection will reduce or eliminate pain and induration. When treatment continues for several days, the child can be placed on an ice cap between injections. When employing vitamin C intravenously, it is best to use sodium ascorbate and the solution free of all additives except sodium bisulfite. The dose of vitamin C using a syringe should range between 350 mg and 400 mg/kg body weight. In older patients or when very high doses are required the vitamin can be added to 5 percent dextrose in water, in saline solution or in Ringer's solution. The concentration should be approximately 1 gm to 18 cc fluid. Bottle injections will need 1 gm calcium gluconate one to two times each day to replace calcium ions removed by the high intravenous schedule. One quart of milk daily will suffice when using the vitamin intramuscularly. In place of milk one can substitute calcium gluconate tablets. Supplemental vitamin C is always given by mouth. As a guide in determining the amount and frequency of injections we recommend our Silver Nitrate-Urine test [10]. This is done by placing ten drops of 5 percent silver nitrate in a Wasserman tube and adding ten drops urine. A color pattern will develop showing white, beige, smoke gray or one that looks like fine grain charcoal. Charcoal is the color needed and the test is performed at least every four hours. The test itself is read in one minute.

These large doses of ascorbic acid will also bring all body tissue back to saturation which means that the white blood cells will now be capable of destroying other pathogens that might be clouding the picture. Unless the white blood cells are saturated with ascorbic acid they are like soldiers without bullets. Research on this is now under way at the Bowman Gray School of Medicine by McCall and Cooper [11]. White cells ingest bacteria and in the process produce hydrogen peroxide. Hydrogen peroxide will combine with ascorbic acid to produce a substance which is lethal to bacteria. I have seen diphtheria, hemolytic streptococcus and staphylococcus infections clear within hours following injections of ascorbic acid in a dose range of from 500 mg to 700 mg/kg body weight given intravenously and run in through a 20G needle as fast as the patient's cardiovascular system would allow.

Part of the white cells are lymphocytes. They, too, play an important role in survival from infection. We found in several cases of trichinosis [12] that the behavior of the lymphocytes was the real story of the changing blood picture and actually determined the course of the disease. Wintrobe [13] observed that the function of the lymphocytes was stimulation of antibody formation and that the lymphocytic response runs parallel with the recovery of the patient. This build-up of antibodies appears directly proportional to the concentration of ascorbic acid in all body tissue, and yet we give vaccines but pay no attention to the degree of tissue saturation of ascorbic acid. Dr. Nossal [14] of the Institute of Medical Research, Melbourne, Australia, wonders about the mechanism by which lymphocytes, on meeting antigens, decide to be turned on or off. He asks what physiological mechanism underlies the discrimination between immunization and the induction of immunological tolerance? We would suggest that it is controlled by vitamin C which in turn affects the negative charge which then influences the response of the lymphocyte. Ginter [15] of the Research Institute of Human Nutrition, Bratislava, offers some evidence to this effect in his statement: "that all reactions which are connected with vitamin C have oxidation-reduction features. It is therefore probable that the biological function of vitamin C can be located in the metabolic reactions which are connected with electron transfer."

The killing power of ascorbic acid is not limited to just herpes simplex and the adenovirus. When proper amounts are used it will destroy all virus organisms. We found measles to be a medical curiosity. Specifically we observe that vitamin C given prophylactically, by mouth, was not protective unless 1 gm was given every two hours around the clock. One gram every four hours would modify the attack. One gram given every four hours intramuscularly was also protective. With our own children we kept the measle syndrome going off and on for 30 days by giving 1 gm every two hours for two days, then off for two days. The disease was then stopped by continuing 1 gm every two hours, by mouth, for four days. By 1950 we learned that we could kill the measles virus in 24 hours by giving intramuscular injections in a dose range of 350 mg/kg body weight every 2 hours. We also found that we could dry up chicken pox in the same time, but more dramatic results were obtained by giving 400 mg/kg body weight intravenously. Two to three injections in 24 hours were all that was required. We published these results in 1951 [16]. Recently, we cured a man weighing 85 kg in four days taking 30 gm each day by mouth. In conclusion, the killing power of ascorbic acid on virus bodies has been demonstrated by me in hundreds of cases, many of which were treated in our hospital with nothing but vitamin C. We have published some 28 papers on this matter.

In certain individuals some virus conditions have a slower response. Herpes zoster and mumps belong to this group. We found that in these conditions equally rapid destruction of the virus could be effected through the use of adenosine-5-monophosphate. Adenosine was given according to age and weight, 25 mg in children and 50-100 mg intramuscularly in adults. This was given every 12 hours along with ascorbic acid. Adenosine will sometimes precipitate a mild reaction in that the patient will feel a fullness in his head with varying degrees of nausea. Inhalation of aromatic spirits of ammonia will quickly relieve and, if used before injection, will prevent this condition. Their response, when adenosine was administered, led us to theorize that when a cell has been invaded by a foreign substance, like virus nucleic acid, enzymic action fostered by ascorbic acid contributes to the breakdown of virus nucleic acid to adenosine deaminase which converts adenosine to inosine. Some individuals cannot manufacture sufficient adenosine to cope with this phase of purine metabolism under certain stress conditions associated with virus pathology. The net result from this chemical action is to catabolize purines rendering them unavailable for making additional virus nucleic acid. Ascorbic acid is further unique in that it possesses the capability of entering all cells. After entering a virus infected cell, ascorbic acid proceeds to take up the protein coats being manufactured by the virus nucleic acid, thus preventing the assembly of new virus units. These newly made macromolecules within the host cell soon create a situation where the tensile strength of the cell membrane is exceeded with resulting rupture and cell death. Ascorbic acid, when given in the massive amounts that accomplish full tissue saturation, will also enter those cells harboring the so-called dormant virus. Where the vitamin C removes the protective protein coat of the virus the micromolecule formed will act in the capacity of a repressor factor inhibiting further activity of the virus nucleic acid which is then destroyed by additional vitamin C. We offer as proof of this the instance of a patient having herpetic lesions for five years and being cured with continuous high daily intake of ascorbic acid. In acute virus infection, associated with a virusemia, ascorbic acid given intravenously will remove the protein protective coat from the virus body, leaving the denuded virus unit vulnerable to the leukocytes for destruction. Note that adrenal cortex extract and/or desoxycorticosterone acetate must also be considered for support of the adrenals in a debilitated patient.

THE CHOLESTEROL STORY

Next in importance to the virus is the story of cholesterol. One must understand, as noted by Ginter [17], that acute scurvy and chronic hypovitaminosis C are metabolically different conditions. On this point the Food and Life Yearbook, 1939, U.S. Department of Agriculture, had this to say: "Even when there is not a single outward symptom of trouble, a person may be in a state of vitamin C deficiency more dangerous than scurvy itself. When such a condition is not detected, and continues uncorrected, the teeth and bones will be damaged, and what may be even more serious, the blood stream is weakened to the point where it can no longer resist or fight infections not so easily cured as scurvy."

Working with guinea pigs many research groups have proved that acute avitaminosis C produces an increase in cholesterol concentration in the whole body. This increased concentration of whole body cholesterol in scorbutic guinea pigs can be caused either by increased biosynthesis or by slowed down cholesterol metabolism. The main pathway of cholesterol catabolism is in conversion to bile salts. The stimulating effect of ascorbic acid on the oxidation of polyunsaturated fatty acids and decreased oxidation of linolenic acid in the tissues of scorbutic guinea pigs has been well documented. Mjasnikova [18] found that intravenous injections of high doses of ascorbic acid to patients with high level blood cholesterol is followed by a distinct decrease of cholesterolemia. It must be remembered that the referred high doses of vitamin C employed by other scientists does not approach the dose schedule that we recommend. For example,

Tjapina [19] reported on the effect of intravenous doses of 500 mg ascorbic acid on cholesterolemia in patients suffering from atherosclerosis. The hypocholesterolemic effect from vitamin C was apparent within one hour. With continued daily injections of 500 mg there was continued drop in blood cholesterol. Spittle [20] showed that blood cholesterol levels, in humans, vary with the amount of vitamin C employed. In our own experiences we lowered the blood cholesterol in one patient 42 points in six weeks by increasing the vitamin C intake by mouth from 10 gm to 20 gm each day. Spittle advanced the theory that atherosclerosis is a long-term deficiency or negative balance of vitamin C, which permits cholesterol levels to build up in the arterial system and results in changes in other fractions of the fats. Ginter [21] also demonstrated that with a high cholesterol diet, guinea pigs used up all their dietary vitamin C while rats and rabbits who manufacture their own vitamin C showed a gain in ascorbic acid tissue levels. Ginter also showed that experimental animals given 50 mg vitamin C each day had cholesterol deposits 40 percent lower than animals fed the same diet but given only 5 mg of C daily. In a survey of 1000 school children Ginter et al showed that 97 percent suffered from vitamin C lack during winter months when C-rich fruits and vegetables were less abundant [22]. The children also showed corresponding rise in cholesterol. Czechoslovakian workers also reported that when guinea pigs are fed a diet deficient in vitamin C and rich in cholesterol, they frequently develop gallstones [23]. Small reported to the Society of University Surgeons in New Orleans in 1973 that when gallstones are removed from patients they are 60-70 percent cholesterol [24]. This suggests a causative factor in human gallstone formation. Reviewing the literature and summarizing his own studies, Ginter concluded that there is no doubt that the daily intake of ascorbic acid in the control of cholesterol will have a more pronounced effect in those persons who are already saturated with vitamin C. Tjapina and many others have reported that when amounts of ascorbic acid as low as 500 mg each day, by needle, were continued for 60 days, the clinical picture in the majority of the patients was dramatic, especially concerning the manifestations of coronary artery disease. Willis [25] reported that in scorbutic guinea pigs, fatty desposits on the aorta were formed very quickly, even without adding cholesterol to their diet. In 1957, Willis [26] found that when ascorbic acid was given to these scorbutic guinea pigs, the atherosclerotic lesions were quickly absorbed. Ascorbic acid is directly associated with the mechanism involved in the pathogenesis of human atherosclerosis. Duguid [27] found alterations of ground substance observed in atherosclerosis that produced experimentally to be morphologically similar. Electrocardiographic tracing by Shafer [28] on scorbutic animals showed that with prolonged vitamin C therapy, abnormalities disappeared entirely. Stamler [29], following the mortality rate for middle aged persons, found a significant drop with improved nutrition with supplemental C.

We must protect our heart from stress. Adequate vitamin C is one answer. Asahina and Asano [30] of the Toho University School of Medicine in Tokyo found that the larger the dose of ascorbic acid given to experimental rats, the longer they survived in decompression chambers in which the air was made to approximate that found at elevations of 33,000 feet. When ascorbic acid was given in amounts representing 14 gm in a human, only half their animals expired. In humans we have observed that 30 gm in 24 hours is critical in any acute situation.

Had the Japanese doubled their vitamin C dose they probably would have had no deaths.

THE HEAVY METAL STORY

Heavy metal poisoning is another morbid chapter in medicine. Lead poisoning comes from many sources. Auto exhaust, smelter furnaces and storage battery factories lead the list. Mercury takes second place. It is estimated that at least 1 million children in the U.S. have some degree of lead poisoning. In 1964 Mokranjac and Petrovic [31] studied the effect of mercury chloride in guinea pigs when ascorbic acid was administered in different ways. They first gave each animal 200 mg of vitamin C a day for one week (this roughly would represent 14 gm in a human) and then administered a dose of mercury proved beforehand to be 100 percent fatal. They then continued to give 0.2 gm of vitamin C daily. After 20 days the animals were all alive proving that vitamin C had protected them from certain death. If they gave vitamin C before and none after poisoning, two died. If vitamin C was given daily after poisoning, nine of 25 died; and if a single massive shot was given after poisoning, eight of 25 died. This again confirms that high daily intake of vitamin C will protect one from many of the ills seen today. The same can be said for lead poisoning. One of the more common types of lead poisoning is seen in long-term workers in lead storage battery plants. All have subclinical scurvy. Adequate ascorbic acid intake would eliminate the monthly blood examination for red cell stippling. The report by Dannenberg [32] that high doses of ascorbic acid were without effect in treating lead intoxication in a child must be ignored, since his extremely high dose was 25 mg by mouth four times a day and one single daily injection of 250 mg of C. Had he administered 350 mg/kg body weight every two hours, he would have the other side of the coin.

Monoxide poisoning is another killer or crippler. Persons living in most American cities are frequently exposed to 100 ppm (that is, 115 mg/cu mm) of carbon monoxide in the ambient air for varying periods of time and may attain carboxyhemoglobin blood levels up to 10 percent [33]. Carboxyhemoglobin blood levels up to 7 percent have been reported in cigarette smokers. These levels of carbon monoxide are quite capable of causing considerable interference with tissue oxygenation in man by displacing oxygen from the hemoglobin molecule and shifting the oxyhemoglobin dissociation curve to the left. Anderson [34] reports a definite link between carbon monoxide, both in the atmosphere and in cigarette smoke, with cardiac function. Normal coronary arteries can readily dilate and supply an increased demand; while diseased coronary arteries (e.g., angina pectoris) may not be able to meet this challenge. The hypoxic effect of carbon monoxide may act in a synergistic manner with other factors operative in ischemic heart disease, outstripping the limited coronary reserve and augmenting the production of stress-induced myocardial ischemia. Interesting is the report by Pelletier [35] who has shown experimentally that once you stop smoking, your ascorbic acid level approaches that of the non-smoker. Victims of house fires, especially children, succumb more often to monoxide poisoning, which is overlooked in the course of treating the burn. Mayers [36] warns physicians that symptoms of smoke poisoning might be delayed from 3 to 48 hours. In cases of this nature ascorbic acid serves a dual purpose.

A dose of 500 mg/kg body weight of vitamin C given intravenously will immediately neutralize the carbon monoxide or smoke poisoning while at the same time it will prevent blood sludging which is a major factor in the development of third degree burns.

OTHER APPLICATIONS

Other therapeutic effects of vitamin C include the following. Vitamin C will also destroy pseudamonis, locally as a 3 percent spray and systemically with massive frequent injections. This has been demonstrated in case histories on burns treated at Annie Penn Memorial Hospital, Reidsville, N.C. It is a demonstrated principle that the production of histamine and other end products from deaminized cell proteins, released by injury to cells, is a cause of shock. The clinical value of ascorbic acid in combating shock is explained when we realize that the deaminizing enzymes from the damaged cells are inhibited by vitamin C. Chambers and Pollock [37] have reported that mechanical damage to a cell results in pH changes which reverse the cell enzymes from constructive to destructive activity. The destructive activity releases histamine, a major shock-producing substance. Ascorbic acid, when present in sufficient amounts, inhibits this enzyme transition.

Ascorbic acid will reverse shock found in other areas of medicine. In one patient who had taken 2640 mg Lotusate (talbutal), the blood pressure was 60/0 when first seen in the emergency room. Twelve gm sodium ascorbate was administered with a 50 cc syringe. In ten minutes the blood pressure was recorded at 100/60. Over 100 additional grams were given intravenously over the following three hours, at which time the patient was awake. Shock from toxalbumin, neurotoxin, proteotoxin, muscarine and formic acid responds equally as well to high doses of vitamin C. Keeping the tissues saturated will prevent such experiences or make recovery by additional vitamin C a routine matter.

Blumberg, writing in *Medical World News,* noted that the discovery of the Australian antigen raises hopes for an effective hepatitis vaccine. Many controversial studies have been reported in the use of this antigen. Another controversial substance, vitamin C, will cure viral hepatitis in two to four days and allow the patient to immediately resume his usual activities. It should be given in a dose range of 500 to 700 mg/kg body weight every 8 to 12 hours. Our latest case was given 5 gm sodium ascorbate, as crystals dissolved in 200 cc water or fruit juice, every 4 hours — i.e., 30 grams per 24-hour period. All symptoms and signs were removed in 96 hours. By contrast treating virus hepatitis with an immunizing agent would possibly require several vaccines in a single hepatic epidemic. If you want results, use adequate ascorbic acid.

THE CANCER STORY

The question of virus and cancer association is still academic. Herpes simplex causing cervical cancer appears to be positive. We have cured many fever blisters by applying a 3 percent ointment of vitamin C to the lip 10-15 times a day. This is put in a water soluble base. I think that it is time for those women with a family history of cervical cancer to douche with a 3 percent solution of ascorbic acid at the first report of cervical erosion. Tamponing with a 3 percent solution should also be done by the physician. Twenty grams of vitamin C daily by mouth along with local application of vitamin C could erase this form of malignancy. Virus and breast cancer, which in the mouse has been established, seems likely to be confirmed in women on the basis of a hereditary factor along with a virus role. Paul Broca (1866) pointed out that ten of 24 women among his immediate forebearers had died of cancer of the breast. J.A. Murray (1911) demonstrated that mice with familial history of breast cancer developed breast cancer at an incidence three times that of mice with no familial history of tumor. Feller and associates found particles resembling type B and C viruses in eight of 16 human milk specimens from women with breast cancer but in only one of 43 apparently cancer-free women. These are stepping stones which serve to give warning that women from cancer-prone families should not breast feed their children. What will daily high intake of vitamin C do in altering the breast cancer picture? The answer is waiting for experimental work to be done with mice from knowledge gained from Bittner's classic cross-suckling experiment.

The role of ascorbic acid in treating virus cancer pathology can be seen with its action in mononucleosis. Large doses of vitamin C, given intravenously, will eliminate this virus in just a few days, the actual time being directly proportional to the amount of the vitamin employed in relation to the severity of the infection. A research team at Yale, after studying hundreds of college students, believe they have evidence that associates the Epstein-Burr virus with Burkett lymphoma [38, 39]. This has also been confirmed by researchers at Children's Hospital, Philadelphia, Pa. Many investigators have been working with immunological procedures for the treatment of malignant disease. As we noted earlier, unless the patient's tissues are saturated with vitamin C, the response in this area will be negated. Massive employment of vitamin C will make possible prolonged radiation therapy in late cases. It will also prevent radiation burns. Who can say what 100 gm or 300 gm given intravenously, daily, for several months might accomplish in cancer. The potential is so great and the employment so elementary that only the illiterate will continue to deny its use. Schlegel [40] has demonstrated that the use of ascorbic acid as low as 1.5 gm each day will prevent recurrence of bladder cancer. This is the so-called wasted vitamin C.

OTHER APPLICATIONS

Rous [41] has found that just 3 gm daily, by mouth, for four days will completely relieve all symptoms of urethritis. He believes that the urethral irritation is caused by phosphatic crystals formed in the urine because of insufficient acidity. Ascorbic acid, in this case, acidified the urine enough to force the crystals back into solution. The neglected chronic cystitis which is the rule with ammonical decomposition in the bladder, most always associated with marked alkalinity of the freshly voided urine, will cease to be a clinical entity once people take at least 10 gm vitamin C every day. This will also eliminate the backwash type pyelitis so debilitating, especially in women of childbearing age.

In over 300 consecutive obstetrical cases, we found that the simple stress of pregnancy increased the ascorbic acid demand up to 15 gm daily. This simple stress of pregnancy becomes meaningful when we review the work of Conney [42] on mammalian synthesis of vitamin C in the rat. Compared to a 70 kg individual the rat would make, under stress, 15.2 gm of C each day. Compare this to the 100 mg now recommended in pregnancy by the National Academy of Science and National Research Council and the disparity is shocking. Fred Stare's 40 mg/day is catastrophic. This must be changed. There are at least 16 categories [42], not including scurvy, that cry out against minimal daily requirements for vitamin C. There can never exist a situation where a set numerical unit of vitamin C will meet the needs of all men. This is true because people are different and these same people experience different situations at various times. Roger Williams, speaking before the National Academy of Science in 1967, reported that among guinea pigs living in his laboratory, some needed 20 times more vitamin C than others to maintain health. We must accept Ginter's conclusion that acute scurvy and chronic hypovitaminosis C are metabolically different conditions. Antonowicz and Kodicek (1969), working with guinea pigs, discovered an extremely complex chemical process existing in animals receiving ascorbic acid which did not occur in the animals with scurvy. They found that glucosamine synthesis with the formation of galactosamine was normal in those animals receiving vitamin C but did not take place in those with scurvy.

Under a grant from the National Institute of Mental Health, Hepler and associates, according to *Medical Tribune*, reported that marijuana smoking caused a significant decrease in intraocular pressure. This decrease was found 30 minutes after smoking. In fine print they conceded that the drop was not significant after three hours. Thus, one would need be a chainlink smoker to maintain worthwhile levels [43, 44]. No mention was made of the many deleterious effects smoking marijuana has on the human body. Virno and associates [45], working in G.B. Bietti's eye clinic observed a pronounced reduction in intraocular pressure in the glaucomatous eyes by giving high daily doses of vitamin C. Bietti states that these high doses of vitamin C are a very effective hypotonic agent for intraocular pressure and when an intravenous dose calculated at 1 gm/kg body weight is administered, the action is predominantly by osmotic dehydration of the eyeball. Virno employed 35 gm by mouth in divided doses each day. This gave marked reduction of pressure within four hours and this was maintained even in patients where Diamox and Philocarpone had failed. Linner in several symposiums using 0.5 gm twice daily reported no significant changes in eye pressure. Linner used 1 gm and Virno 35 gm each day 5,000-10,000 units penicillin every four to six hours. The same type pathology is cured today in 24 to 48 hours using 1-3 million units. The size of the dose does make a difference — a real difference.

Dr. Linus Pauling has written that "Biochemical and genetic arguments support the idea that orthomolecular therapy may be the preferred treatment for many ill patients." It is difficult to understand why megavitamin therapy remains so controversial when massive doses of vitamin B_{12} are universally used in pernicious anemia and niacinamide to correct the pathology of pellagra. I have used 150,000-200,000 units of vitamin A in a case of ichthyosis. The patient has been taking this dose for ten years. His skin is clear with no signs or symptoms of vitamin A toxicity.

During the same time he has taken 10 gm of vitamin C each day. Is vitamin C the answer?

Hoffer [46] and Osmond were probably the first to realize the value of ascorbic acid as an adjuvant with niacin in treating schizophrenics. They employed from 6 to 8 gm daily. One acute case was given 1 gm every hour for 48 hours at which time the patient was completely recovered and remained so for six months without further treatment. Hawkins [47] found that by adding megavitamin treatment he doubled the recovery rate, half the rehospitalization rate and virtually eliminated self-destruction in dealing with schizophrenics who have a suicide rate 22 times that of the general population. Dr. Pauling enabled his clinic to treat seriously ill schizophrenics for $200 per patient per year and to reduce the number of patient visits from 150 per year to 15. Hawkins' method gives schizophrenic patients four gm ascorbic acid and four gm niacin or the equivalent in niancinamide, in divided doses, each day. Vanderkamp (1966) demonstrated that schizophrenics burn up ascorbic acid ten times faster than normal people. On an intake of four gm vitamin C each day, almost 100 percent of normal people will spill some degree of ascorbic acid into the urine. In schizophrenics one can often go as high as 40 grams/day before spilling occurs. I have observed this same picture in severe virus infections where the patient did not spill over into the urine until the second or third day, when a clinical response was evident. Milmer in Great Britain and Lucksch in Germany have reported significant improvement in schizophrenics given vitamin C alone. Both investigators used the double blind approach.

Ascorbic acid has value as an adjuvant in other medical syndromes. With para-aminobenzoic acid (PABA), which is a fraction of the B vitamins, it will cure trichinosis in nine days [48]. Used with intravenous mephenesin or methocarbamol, it will cure tetanus in 96 hours.

Arthritis is not only a crippler but also a nagger. Aspirin is the favorite medication of many physicians because it will ease the arthritic pain. This makes aspirin a good guy and a bad guy. The bad side is that those who take high aspirin therapy will also have low platelet and plasma levels for vitamin C. With low plasma levels there will also be depletion in the white blood cells. We know what this will do. As to platelets, their main business is to keep people from bleeding to death. When a blood vessel ruptures, collagen tissue, which makes up the basement membrane of blood vessels, is exposed. The collagen affects the platelets so that they release a mineral substance called adenosine diphosphate. This substance makes the platelets very sticky so that they cling together. Aspirin can destroy this substance, but adequate vitamin C will prevent this action. As the platelets act to seal off the wound, a second mechanism for clot formation comes into play. This is a liquid protein called fibrinogen. In a recent case in which the platelet count was abnormally low and bleeding was a serious problem, 25 gm of ascorbic acid daily by mouth raised the platelet count back to normal with cessation of bleeding. Vitamin C is also the number one agent in collagen formation. A person who will take 10-20 gm of ascorbic acid a day along with other nutrients might very well never develop arthritis. Abrams and Sandson [49] have pointed out that synovial fluid becomes thinner, thus allowing easier movement, when serum levels of ascorbic acid are high. Drugs such as ACTH and cortisone are noted for their ability to drain ascorbic acid in prolonged usage. In our experience we found that the patient who took vitamin C to tolerance made more rapid progress in reversing arthritic joints.

The importance of daily high intake of ascorbic acid in preventive medicine has no limits. Crest and Colgate might limit tooth decay to one cavity every checkup, a relatively high index. Ten or more gm of ascorbic acid from age 10 up and at least 1 gm for each year of life, each day, through age 9 will record no cavities. Our son who is 20 has never had a tooth cavity. The same schedule could eliminate disc pathology. McCormick believes the problem is avitaminosis C [50]. Greenwood [51] believes that adequate amounts of ascorbic acid seem necessary to disc metabolism and maintenance. In surgery we found that plasma determinations taken before starting anesthesia, at the conclusion of surgery, and six hours later, were constant. At 12 hours postoperative, there was a significant drop in vitamin C levels and at 24 hours there was a dramatic loss of the vitamin. We have always required the surgeon to give 10 gm before surgery, 10 gm in each postoperative bottle of fluids and 10 gm by mouth after discontinuing fluids. Crandon et al state that postoperative disruption of abdominal wounds occurs eight times more often in patients with vitamin C deficiency. Not only surgery but any type of wound or fracture will heal slowly or not heal at all without the benefits of adequate vitamin C. Powdered vitamin C mixed with water to form a paste and applied to poison ivy or oak will usually effect a cure in 24 hours when adequate vitamin C is also taken by mouth. Ascorbic acid does have a definite influence on the rheumatic heart, especially in the acute stage [52]. I have seen children with the heart impulse so great that it raised the bed covers with each contraction recover so completely that later in life they were inducted into the armed services. Massive daily doses will also cure tuberculosis by removal of the organisms' polysaccharide coat. It does the same with pneumococci. I am convinced that ten or more grams a day will prevent cancer of the lung in tobacco smokers. It will relieve prickly heat and prevent heat stroke. Vitamin C will immediately reverse heat collapse, cramps or exhaustion if 12 to 40 gm are given intravenously. It will bring recovery to electric shock victims if sufficient amounts are administered soon after the accident. Lightning victims can also be saved. I have done it. Chronic myelocytic leukemia responds dramatically to 30 or more grams daily by mouth. Pancreatitis can be cured in less than three hours with 50 gm intravenously, and ten gm daily by mouth is positive insurance that it will never return. Virus pancarditis as a sequela of an adenovirus infection can be relieved in 36 hours giving 400 mg/kg body weight, intravenously, every four to six hours. I have never seen a patient that vitamin C would not benefit. And, too, never send a boy to do a man's job; meaning the dose level is very important.

In closing, I would like to quote Herbert Spencer, who summed up rather well a caution I would like all of us to take to heart: "There is a principle which is a bar against all information, which is proof against all argument, and which cannot fail to keep a man in everlasting ignorance. That principle is condemnation without investigation."

SUMMARY

The drug evaluation book of the American Medical Association (1971) gives information on the value of ascorbic acid which is at least 30 years behind present day knowledge. The 200-500 mg of ascorbic acid which is recommended as the 24-hour dose in burn cases is a typical example. From clinical experience we know that ascorbic acid must be given to burn victims in massive, frequent intravenous injections. Thirty to one hundred grams daily is the proper amount to employ and this is given until healing takes place – 7-30 days depending upon the degree of burn. We have found and reported that this massive vitamin C therapy will eliminate skin grafting by keeping the tissues oxygenated. Ample supply of oxygen to the tissues will prevent blood sludging and in place of the third degree burns that develop on the fourth or fifth day, the eschars will drop off leaving normal tissue. These high doses of ascorbic acid will also remove the smoke poisoning found in many fire victims and save many lives, especially children who expire from the effects of monoxide gas. The statement found in the A.M.S. book mentioned above – that controlled studies have shown no benefit from large doses of ascorbic acid in human subjects – must be ignored. The large doses referred to never exceeded 5 gm and in most cases not more than that found in a quart of orange juice, for a 24-hour period. It is unfortunate that the editorial staff of the AMA failed to check out the world literature. An example of their high doses was an article by Dannenberg [32] which was published in the JAMA in which the author found no value in lead poisoning by giving extremely high doses of ascorbic acid to a child. Dannenberg's extremely high dose was 25 mg four times a day, by mouth, and one single intramuscular injection of 250 mg. Had Dannenberg employed 350 mg/kg body weight and given it, intramuscularly, every two to four hours he would have had a recovered patient in less than 72 hours. The amount of ascorbic acid employed in any given case is the all important factor. In 28 years of research we have observed that 30 gm each day is critical in terms of response. This seems to be true regardless of age and weight. In certain pathological conditions like barbiturate intoxication, snake bite or virus encephalitis, higher doses are required in some individuals. We have observed from experience and from review of the literature that 15 percent - 20 percent of humans require much more ascorbic acid than do others. Approximately 15 percent is in evidence when giving vaccines, since they make no antibodies. Roughly 15 percent of pregnant humans were scheduled, in the past, to become paralyzed if hit with the polio virus. Fifteen percent of over 3000 cases in our files required more ascorbic acid to prevent colds or to relieve the cold once infected. This percentage difference is the reason why one patient would die with pneumonia while another lived, when all other factors were apparently equal. This dosage factor alone has misled many scientists to disregard the value of ascorbic acid in virus pathology because they would see dogs die with distemper when they knew that the dog could make his own vitamin C. What they did not appreciate was that even the animal could not make enough vitamin C under certain situations. I have cured many dogs suffering with distemper by giving several grams ascorbic acid, by needle, every two hours. We also found in over 300 obstetrical cases that roughly 15 percent require as much as 15 gm supplemental vitamin C each day just to remain within normal limits. Ten grams each day was the highest requirement of the other 85 percent.

Herpes simplex virus and the adenovirus can be destroyed with high doses of ascorbic acid. Many infections can be prevented by taking adequate vitamin C, daily, by mouth – 1 gm for each year of life up to age 10 and after 10 years of age at least 10 gm vitamin C daily. With these amounts the patient will spill varying amounts into the urine. The kidneys have a threshold for vitamin C much like the spillway of a dam. Spilling is necessary to assure adequate amounts for various body tissues. For example, white blood cells are useless unless they are full of ascorbic acid, since it is the ascorbic acid which makes their phagocytosis and/or destruction of pathogens possible. Although herpes simplex usually shows itself as a small lip sore and the adenoviruses as a mild but lingering cold, both can become killers through passage of the virus to the brain. Either one can cause crib deaths, which is truly the real cause. Again, we point out that high daily intake of vitamin C can prevent this tragic incident. For this reason, if for no other, the National Research Council and the National Academy of Science must remove the so-called minimal daily requirement for this substance. Williams has shown and reported to the National Academy that even guinea pigs living in his laboratory differ in their requirements for vitamin C and that they differ each day, sometimes 20 times a given unit. Guinea pigs, like man, cannot manufacture ascorbic acid due to genetic fault. Scurvy which accounts for the thinking on the amount of vitamin C needed is actually of no consequence in terms of avitaminosis C, which can determine one's future existence. Ginter, after ten years of research with vitamin C, concluded that actue scurvy and chronic hypovitaminosis C are metabolically different conditions. Antonowicz and Kodiçk confirmed this by finding that glucosamine synthesis in the guinea pig with the formation of galactosamine was normal in those animals receiving vitamin C but did not take place in the presence of acute scurvy.

Ascorbic acid when taken in sufficient quantities will relieve the intraocular pressure in the glaucomatous eyes, will relieve such things as prickly heat, and is a positive reversal for pemphigus. Vitamin C when given by needle will destroy all viruses and many can be destroyed by taking 25-30 gm each day by mouth. Lesser amounts will protect against these pathogens. I have cured diptheria, hemolytic streptococcus and staphylococcus infections by employing vitamin C intravenously in a dose range of 500 to 700 mg/kg body weight. Doses under 400 mg/kg body weight can be given with a syringe using the sodium salt. This will always produce thirst. Fluids taken just before or immediately after will eliminate this annoyance. Doses above 400 mg/kg body weight must be diluted to at least 1 gm to 18 cc solution, using 5 percent dextrose in water, saline in water or Ringer's solution. One gram calcium gluconate must be added to these bottle injections to replace Ca ions pulled from the calcium-prothrombin complex. There is no limit to the amount that can be administered by vein when honoring these two precautions. The use of vitamin C in cancer will prove to be a very beneficial agent. We recommend bottle doses containing 60 gm vitamin C and such fractions of the B complex as 500 mg thiamin HCl, pyridoxine 300 mg, calcium pantothenate 400 mg, riboflavin 100 mg and niacinamide 300 mg. This is to be given daily or even twice daily. Vitamin C is a positive neutralizing agent in snake bite [53], spider bite [54] and insect stings. Our use of ascorbic acid in snake bite has been limited to the Highland moccasin, a member of the copperhead family. Other poisonous snakes are more deadly but we can easily calculate from our experience what dose to employ. In a 4-year-old receiving a full strike from a mature Highland moccasin, 12 gm was required. Unlike a virus that will continue production until completely destroyed, the venom of the snake is constant in that there will exist no later increase in amount. I would suggest 40-60 gm, as a starter, in a large diamondback or cottonmouth. Additional vitamin C can be given if needed since the patient will be well on the road to recovery with the first injection.

Adenosine monophosphate given with ascorbic acid will increase the potential of the vitamin. This can be given in doses from 25 mg in children to as much as 200 mg in adults. Our use of this agent has been limited to mumps and herpes zoster but we are now of sufficient knowledge to believe that its use should be routine. The aqueous solution is more efficacious than the gel. Some patients experience a fullness in the head, a sickish feeling in the chest and a slowed pulse rate. Aromatic spirits of ammonia as a smelling agent relieves or prevents this syndrome. At present we are using 50 mg doses more frequently, until we can establish a reason for this type response.

Ascorbic acid can be lifesaving in shock. Twelve grams of the sodium salt given with a 50 cc syringe will reverse shock in minutes. In barbiturate poisoning and monoxide poisoning the results are so dramatic that it borders on malpractice to deny this therapy. Surgeons must learn to employ ascorbic acid more liberally. Ten to twenty grams in the preoperative solutions and 10 gm in each postoperative bottle will all but eliminate surgical deaths and will reduce hospital stay by 50 percent. The same can be said for obstetrical cases. We found that obstetrical cases needed 4 gm each day the first trimester, 6 gm the second trimester and 8-10 gm the third trimester. Fifteen percent of the patients required 15 gm each day just to stay within normal limits.

Ascorbic acid is the safest and the most valuable substance available to the physician. Many headaches and many heartaches will be avoided with its proper use.

REFERENCES

1. Pauling, L.: *Vitamin C and the Common Cold.* San Francisco: W.F. Freeman & Co., 1970.
2. Brody, H.D.: *J. Amer. Diet. Assn.,* 29:588, 1953.
3. Klenner, F.R.: Virus pneumonia and its treatment with vitamin C. *Southern Med. Surg.,* Feb. 1948.
4. Klenner, F.R.: Encephalitis as a sequelae of the pneumonias. *Tri-State Med. J.,* Feb. 1960.
5. Klenner, F.R.: An insidious virus. *Tri-State Med. J.,* June 1957.
6. Lerner, M. et al: Detecting herpes encephalitis earlier. *Med. World News,* May 26, 1972.
7. Stephens, J.C. and Cook, M. Cases of the hidden herpes virus. *Med. World News,* Feb. 25, 1972.
8. Goodpasture, E.W.: Case of the hidden herpes virus. *Med. World News,* Feb. 25, 1972.
9. Roizmen, B. et al: Tracing herpes viruses. *Med. World News,* Oct. 1, 1971.
10. Klenner, F.R.: A new office procedure for the determination of plasma levels for ascorbic acid. *Tri-State Med. J.,* 5, 1956.
11. McCall, C.E. and Copper, R.: Vitamin C shows promise as a bactericidal agent. Bowman Gray School Med. *Med. Alumni News,* 14:1, Feb., 1972.
12. Klenner, F.R.: The treatment of trichinosis with massive doses of vitamin C and para-aminobenzoic acid. *Tri-State Med. J.,* 1952.
13. Wintroble, M.M.: *Clinical Hematology. Text Book.* Lea and Febiger, 3rd Edition, 1952.
14. Nossal, G.: Most killed vaccines in use termed not fit for a mouse. *Medical Tribune,* April 5, 1972.
15. Ginter, E.: The Role of Ascorbic Acid In Cholesterol Metabolism. Research Institute of Human Nutrition, Bratislava, 1970.
16. Klenner, F.R.: Massive doses of vitamin C and the virus diseases. *Southern Med. Surg.,* 1951.
17. Ginter, E.: Cholesterol and vitamin C. *Amer. J. Clin. Nutr.,* 24:1238-1245, 1971.
18. Mjasnikove, I.A.: O vlijaniji vodorastvorimych vitaminov na nekororyje storony obmena vescesty. *Tr. Vojennomorskoj Medicinsk. akademiji Leningr.,* 8:140-148, 1947.
19. Tjapina, L.A.: Vlijanie askorbovoj kisloty na cholesterine-miju pri giper toniceskoj bolezni i ateroskleroze. Giperto-niceskaja bolezn. *Tr. AMN SSSR,* 2:108-113, 1952.
20. Spittle, C.: Atherosclerosis and vitamin C. *Lancet, II*:1280-1281. 1971.
21. Ginter, E.: Effects of dietary cholesterol on vitamin C metabolism in laboratory animals. *Acta med. Acad. Sci. Hung.,* 27:23-29, 1970.
22. Ginter, E., Kajabal, I. and Nizner, O.: The effects of ascorbic acid on cholesterolemia in healthy subjects with seasonal deficit of vitamin C. *Nutr. Metabol.,* 12:76-86, 1970.
23. Ginter, E., Bilisics, I. and Cerven, J.: Cholesterol metabolism under conditions of acute and chornic vitamin C deficiency in guinea pigs. *Physiol. Bohemoslov.,* 14:466-471, 1965.
24. Small, D.: *Med. World News,* March 30, 1971.
25. Willis, G.C.: An experimental study of the intimal ground substance in atherosclerosis. *Canad. Med. Assn. J.,* 69:17-22, 1953.
26. Willis, G.C.: The Reversibility of Atherosclerosis. *Canad. Med. Assn. J.,* 77:106-109, 1957.
27. Duguid, J.B.: Pathogenesis of atherosclerosis. *Lancet,* 2:925, 1957.
28. Shafer, C.F.: Ascorbic acid and atherosclerosis. *Amer. J. Clin. Nutr.,* 23:27, 1970.
29. Stamler, J.: *Comprehensive Treatment of Essential Hypertensive Diseases.* Monograph on Hypertension. Merck, Sharp and Dohme.
30. Asahina and Asano: *Prevention,* July 1972. pp. 81-82.
31. Mokranjac, M., Petrovic, C.: Report on mercury studies in guinea pigs in relation to amounts of vitamin C administered. *C. R. Acad. Sci.,* Paris.
32. Dannenburg, A.M. et al: Ascorbic acid in the treatment of chronic lead poisoning. *JAMA,* 114:1439-1440, 1940.
33. Klenner, F.R.: The role of ascorbic acid in therapeutics. *Tri-State Med. J.,* Nov. 1955.
34. Anderson, E.W. et al: Carbon monoxide linked to heart disease. *JAMA,* 22:5, July 1972.
35. Pelletier, O.: Experiments with smokers and non-smokers. *JAMA,* April 1969.
36. Mayers, B.W.: Where there's smoke there may be carbon monoxide. *Med. World News,* Jan. 21, 1972.
37. Chambers R. and Pollock, H.: *J. Gen Physiol.,* 10:739, 1927.
38. Hellne, G. and Helene, W.: EB virus in the etiology of infectious mononucleosis. *Hosp. Practice,* July 1970.
39. Niderman, J.C.: College finding tie mono to EB virus. *Med. World News.* Dec. 1968.

40. Schlegel, G.E. et al: The role of ascorbic acid in the prevention of bladder tumor formation. *Trans. Amer. Assn. Genitourin. Surg.,* 61, 1969.

41. Rous, S.: Urethritis in men. *N.Y. Soc. Med.,* Dec. 15, 1971.

42. Klenner, F.R.: Observations on the dose and administration of ascorbic acid when employed beyond the range of a vitamin in human pathology. *J. Appl. Nutr.,* 23:3-4, 1971.

43. Leuchtenberger, C. and Leuchtenberger, R.: New dangers seen in marijuana. *Nature,* Nov. 1971.

44. Campbell, A.M.G. et al: Significant brain damage caused by smoking marijuana. *Lancet,* Dec. 1971.

45. Virno, M. et al: *Eye, Ear, Nose, Throat Monthly,* 64 Dec. 1967.

46. Hoffer, A.: Use of ascorbic acid with niacin in schizophrenia. *Canad. Med. J.,* Nov. 6, 1971.

47. Hawkins, D.: Back to reality the megavitamin way. *Med. World News,* September 24, 1971.

48. Klenner, F.R.: Recent discoveries in the treatment of lockjaw with vitamin C and Tolserol. *Tri-State Med. J.,* July 1954.

49. Abrams, E. and Sandson, J.: *Ann. Rheum. Dis.,* 27, 1964.

50. McCormick, W.J.: Intervertable Disc Pathology: A new etiologic concept. *Arch. Pre.,* 71:29, 1954.

51. Greenwood, J.: Optimum vitamin C intake as a factor in the preservation of disc integrity. *Med. Ann. D.C.,* 33:6, June 1964.

52. Massell, B.F., Warren, J.E. Patterson, P.R. et al: Antirheumatic activity of ascorbic acid in large doses. *New Eng. J. Med.,* 1950.

53. Klenner, F.R.: Case history: cure of a 4 year old child bitten by a mature Hiland moccasin with vitamin C. *Tri-State Med. J.,* July, 1954.

54. Klenner, F.R.: Case history: The black widow spider. *Tri-State Med. J.,* Dec. 1957.

11
A Review of Vitamin B₆

JOHN M. ELLIS

A fabulous nutrient — Vitamin B₆ — since its discovery in 1934 has stirred the minds of brilliant biochemists in laboratories of many countries. Necessary for protein metabolism in millions of human body cells, it may well be the link toward prevention of diseases only vaguely comprehended. These diseases include rheumatism, diabetes, arteriosclerosis, and associated heart attacks of the coronary occlusion type.

Tribute must be paid to biochemists, bless them, who have bit by bit added to understanding of Vitamin B₆. It is now known that this nutrient enters into more than 30 enzymatic reactions involving cells in the brain, liver, nerves, blood vessels, kidney, muscle, and ductless glands which produce certain hormones.

First evidence that Vitamin B₆ was essential to man came in 1952 when an excessively heated commercial milk formula caused convulsions in infants. It was thus proven that naturally occuring Vitamin B₆ was destroyed by heat to a point that — resulting deficiency in the diet caused serious impairment of brain function.

Further investigations in other clinics and laboratories revealed that there is a relationship between increased need for Vitamin B₆ and mental retardation. Convulsive seizures occurred in children who were mentally retarded, and these convulsions could be eliminated by using increased amounts of Vitamin B₆.

It was proven in other hospitals and clinics that patients with tuberculosis who were given certain drugs for treatment of tuberculosis developed neuritis in their arms and legs, hands and feet, and it was learned that Vitamin B₆ would relieve this neuritis. For this reason tuberculosis sanitariums began using large amounts of Vitamin B₆ which apparently was being destroyed by drug antagonists used in treatment of tuberculosis.

Radiologists began using Vitamin B₆ to some extent in an effort to relieve nausea associated with deep x-ray therapy in treatment of cancer. Obstetricians also claimed some success in treating nausea of pregnancy with Vitamin B₆.

Vitamin B₆ was found useful in relieving a rare type of anemia in which red blood cells were too small. This was not the usual iron deficiency anemia, but apparently resulted from a defective hereditary factor that was responsive to Vitamin B₆.

A peculiar type of photosensitivity has been treated successfully with Vitamin B₆. This rare disease condition is characterized by intolerance to sunlight and severe sunburn with very little exposure.

Briefly, it might be said that prior to 1961, clinical Vitamin B₆ deficiency had not been recognized except in infants who convulsed following use of a defective milk formula, and in patients with tuberculosis who developed neuritis as a result of treatment with drugs antagonistic to Vitamin B₆. There was a prevalent concept that Vitamin B₆ deficiency did not exist in the United States and that people who responded to Vitamin B₆ had rare and unusual disease conditions.

Between the years of 1961 and 1970, I conducted clinical studies in use of Vitamin B₆ in private practice of medicine in Northeast Texas and found that certain objective and subjective symptomatology common to many hundreds of people was responsive to Vitamin B₆.

The most frequent beginning symptom of increased need for or deficiency of Vitamin B₆ is a "numbness" or "tingling" sensation in the hands and fingers. More often the little finger is involved first. Particularly is this noticeable while driving an automobile. Usually a patient experiencing this paresthesia will state that his hands "go to sleep" when he lies in bed at night. As the disease condition progresses, the fingers become stiffened and there is a loss of flexion at the finger joints. Although a fist can be made to a fashion, tips of the fingers can not be pressed against the metacarpo — phalangeal crease of the palm. There is an associated weakness of handgrip accompanied by pain in the finger joints. Eventually there is a varying degree of swelling or edema of fingers and hands, and with progression of the disease condition, there is disturbance or loss of sensation and perception in finger tips.

As objective swelling or edema appears in the hands, wedding rings become tight and can only be removed forceably if at all. Sometimes a patient might exhibit very little swelling and yet be unable to perform usual chores that require normal handgrip. Such a patient may complain that at night a transitory paralysis of an entire arm is troublesome. Upon awakening, an arm may be found paralyzed until it is shaken by the opposite and unaffected hand.

Range of finger flexion is reduced and there is impairment of coordination of finger movement. Dishes and water glasses are apt to be dropped and broken on the kitchen floor while elderly women can no longer control their thimbles and needles in sewing. Carpenters and mechanics complain that they drop their tools if they are able to grip them at all.

Sensation in the tips of fingers of more severely affected

patients may be disturbed to a degree that glass, for example, feels the same as wood, or a seamstress may state that she can no longer distinguish the texture of cloth made either of wool or satin.

Patients in need of Vitamin B$_6$ often complain bitterly of night time "Charley horses," or leg cramps. They bolt from their beds and have excruciating pains in their legs and feet as they desperately try to massage the cramps or spasms from their feet and legs.

Symptomatology is the same in hands and fingers of both men and women. However, women are more severely affected near the age of menopause. They develop what has been called "menopausal arthritis." In addition to the disturbance of sensation and perception in fingers, women at time of menopause will develop painful and reddened little burs or knots on the sides of finger joints. These little burs were described by William Heberden in London in 1802. A hundred and sixty years later, I found that Vitamin B$_6$ given daily for 6 weeks will relieve pain in these little burs and reduce them in size to some degree.

Along with painful hand symptoms, there occurs varying degrees of painful arm and shoulder symptoms. There may be pain in the shoulder, beneath the shoulder blade, or in the arm between the shoulder and the elbow.

If a person with this symptomatology is asked about his condition, he will respond, "I have rheumatism."

The people studied in Northeast Texas, and there were hundreds, perhaps thousands that I saw, did have rheumatism, and they exhibited spectacular response to Vitamin B$_6$ given 50 milligrams daily by mouth.

At this point, it might be well to identify Vitamin B$_6$ to some extent. In small amounts it occurs free in nature as pyridoxine, pyridoxal, and pyridoxamine. Once taken into the human body, the natural forms combine with phosphate to form the reacting coenzyme, pyridoxal phosphate. In my clinical investigations of Vitamin B$_6$, I used pyridoxine tablets and in most cases gave pyridoxine 50 milligrams daily by mouth. There are dozens of patients in Northeast Texas who have taken pyriodoxine 50 milligrams daily for 8 years, and there are thousands who have taken pyridoxine 50 milligrams daily for the last 4 years. There have been no ill effects or side effects except in people who have stomach ulcers. It is believed that Vitamin B$_6$ has something to do with histamine production and very likely Vitamin B$_6$ increases production or action of stomach secretions. At any rate, people who have stomach ulcers should be under treatment before beginning use of Vitamin B$_6$.

Motion pictures taken before and after treatment with pyridoxine gave objective proof that Vitamin B$_6$ reduced swelling in hands and fingers, improved range of finger flexion, improved speed of finger flexion, improved coordination of finger movement, prevented transitory nocturnal arm paralysis, and halted night time leg cramps and muscle spasms. Subjectively, after 6 weeks of therapy, there was improvement of sensation and perception in finger tips, and there was elimination of numbness and tingling in hands and fingers. Shoulder pain was reduced or eliminated, and shoulder and arm function was improved. Finger joints that had been tender and painful before treatment were substantially improved after 6 weeks of therapy with pyridoxine.

An important relation to body fluid retention was established by these studies in Northeast Texas. When a patient with painful and swollen hands and fingers was given pyridoxine,

within 2 weeks there would be a loss of body weight amounting to as much as 5-7 pounds. Wedding rings could be slipped off and on fingers much more easily, and there was increased wrinkling of skin on the dorsum of hands, whereas before treatment the hands were "puffy" and "fat" in appearance. There was edema of hands and fingers in many patients long before there was experience of pain in arms and shoulders. Younger women noticed this edema most during the premenstrual period. Pyridoxine was given with considerable success in prevention and relief of premenstrual edema.

Since initiation of my studies with Vitamin B$_6$ in 1961, I have delivered about 175 newborn infants of mothers who were given pyridoxine 50-300 milligrams daily during pregnancy. There have been only two infants who showed evidence of increased need for Vitamin B$_6$ after birth. Both infants were born of mothers who had marked edema of pregnancy, and one had toxemia of pregnancy. At eight months of age, one of the infants, mentally retarded and troubled by convulsive seizures, would not move about the cradle and would not clutch a rattle. When pyridoxine was given 25 milligrams daily, this infant became much more active, more coordinated, and within one week would clutch and vigorously shake a rattle. The second infant which required an increased amount of Vitamin B$_6$ was born premature and had convulsions in an incubator until given 25 milligrams of pyridoxine by injection. At 3 years of age, this child began having light convulsive seizures, and a Ft. Worth pediatrician determined that there was an abnormally elevated blood sugar level after a sugar tolerance test. After receiving pyridoxine 50 milligrams daily, this child after more than a year has had no additional convulsive seizures.

After having delivered 175 infants to mothers who received large doses of pyridoxine, it should be reported that the infants grew normally, showed no dependency on Vitamin B$_6$ and are now doing successful work in grade school or kindergarten. Newborn infant mortality was less than 1 percent. None of the children born of these mothers who received large doses of pyridoxine has had behavioral problems. Several of the mothers stated that their children heard and remembered words easily, could say nursery rhymes at an early age, and could count at an early age. No controlled studies were done along this line, however. One observation seemed significant. These children were very active as determined by the mothers. They seemed well coordinated and agile in exercise and play. Future investigations should be done to determine if Vitamin B$_6$ is in some way related to prevention of obesity by enhancing physical activity at an early age. At any rate, let it be said that children now in grade school, born of mothers who received 50-300 milligrams daily of pyridoxine during pregnancy, are intelligent, very active, and apparently normal with no evidence of dependency on Vitamin B$_6$.

In attendance of expectant mothers during pregnancy, it was learned that this same syndrome of increased need for Vitamin B$_6$ appeared even more frequently among those pregnant than the rest of the population in Northeast Texas. There was "numbness" and "tingling" of fingers and hands, there was swelling of hands and feet, there was painful flexion finger joints, and there was a tendency toward incoordination of hand movements as indicated by frequent dropping and breaking of water glasses and dishes. Following treatment with pyridoxine 50-300 milligrams daily, it was my opinion that during pregnancy pyridoxine should be given in an increased amount as soon as pregnancy is diagnosed. Since pyridoxine is water soluble, any excess is within 8 hours excreted through the urine. For this reason, during pregnancy pyridoxine should be given one dose in the morning and a second dose at night.

Pyridoxine was specific for relief of edema of pregnancy. As much as 13 lbs. weight loss in 14 days was observed in one pregnant patient who received as little as 50 milligrams daily. During the last year, I have given pyridoxine 50 milligrams in the morning and 50 milligrams at night, along with a general vitamin-mineral capsule that contained 25 milligrams of pyridoxine, and I have seen no edema in hands and feet of pregnant women. No diuretics were used, and no attention was paid to salt in the diet.

It was proven during these studies that pyridoxine prevented and relieved the neuopathies of hands and fingers previously described in this paper. For this reason, it can be asserted that pyridoxine served not simply as a diuretic, but as a nutrient that was in support of the nervous system while at the same time it relieved edema of pregnancy.

It remains to be proven if pyridoxine will prevent eclampsia. In 8 years and 175 deliveries, I have had only one case in which there was appearance of convulsions during pregnancy. The patient had all signs of toxemia of pregnancy, and I reported the case. However, after 2½ years this patient began convulsing and although the convulsions were partially responsive to intravenous use of pyridoxine, it must be assumed that this patient was suffering with epilepsey. It might be said in passing that epilepsey can not be cured with pyridoxine. There has been some evidence that in treatment of epilepsey, pyridoxine reduced frequency and severity of seizures, and that it should be given as adjunctive therapy.

Motion pictures were taken of 3 infants born of mothers who had marked edema of pregnancy and who had received no therapy with pyridoxine until the last month of pregnancy. These infants less than 24 hours after birth exhibited remarkable wrinkling of skin. In my opinion this was an objective sign that the mothers had been edematous before birth of the infants, that the infants as fetuses had been edematous prior to use of pyridoxine, and that when pyridoxine was given the mothers during the last month of pregnancy, edema subsided in the mother and edema subsided in the fetus. One of these infants did not urinate for 24 hours after birth, and there was very little weight loss after birth. In fact, all three infants had less than usual loss in weight during the 72 hours following birth. In light of this evidence, it seems certain that in association with edema of pregnancy both mother and fetus are in dire need of greatly increased amounts of Vitamin B₆.

Some general comments might be offered relative to the studies in Northeast Texas which dealt with clinical use of Vitamin B₆. Onset of the disease syndrome known as rheumatism was gradual. There was edema of hands and fingers long before there was experience of pain and stiffness in shoulders. Occasionally there was a rather sudden onset of signs and symptoms that has been alluded to as the "shoulder-hand syndrome". The long standing cases were more difficult to relieve, and ordinarily the older aged people had less response to pyridoxine. There was no doubt, however, that patients with the "shoulder-hand syndrome" exhibited improvement of hand function, reduction of edema, and moderate relief of pain in shoulders when pyridoxine was given 50-100 milligrams daily for 6 weeks. Reduction of edema and improvement in hand function could be observed within one week of initiation of treatment.

A number of patients with diabetes mellitus had disturbed tactile sensation in fingers that responded to pyridoxine. It seemed that most elderly diabetics had edema in their hands and fingers, neuritis and neuropathies in their hands and fingers, and that these conditions responded to pyridoxine given 50 milligrams daily.

A more astute scientist would conclude his paper at this point and allow established facts to support this magnificent nutrient in making its own way toward a marvelous rendezvous in human destiny. After 9 years of working with diets and Vitamin B₆, one can not avoid the lure of suggestion. It has been proven by brilliant scientists in well recognized laboratories and accepted by the scientific community that on Vitamin B₆ deficient diets monkeys, dogs, and chickens develop arterial changes in keeping with that of arteriosclerosis in the human. It is well established that most people who have coronary artery thrombosis also have arteriosclerosis in the coronary artery. It also has been accepted that rheumatism and the shoulder-hand syndrome frequently appear at the same time or in company with coronary thrombosis, and their accomplice in the mystery of coronary thrombosis is diabetes with its notorious associate, advanced arteriosclerosis. One has only to know that rheumatism and the shoulder-hand syndrome are responsible to Vitamin B₆ to conclude that somewhere between early life of the fetus and terminal gasps of the coronary thrombosis victim, increased need for Vitamin B₆ stands paramount as the cause of the deadly heart attack and coronary occlusion. Very certainly one can conclude that increased amounts of Vitamin B₆ should be given those pregnant, those with rheumatism, those with diabetes, and those with heart disease.

Without approaching further the precipice of speculation, suffice it to say that in Northeast Texas between the years of 1961 and 1970 there was established by use of photographs and motion pictures conclusive objective evidence that numbers of people responded to Vitamin B₆; and included in the group were pregnant women, newborn infants, and those who had rheumatism, those who had heart disease, and those who had diabetes.

One would not intimate that Vitamin B₆ is the only nutrient necessary for prevention of any disease condition. There are other vitamins and other minerals that act and interact with Vitamin B₆, and all are important. There is a delicate balance of quantitative amounts so essential for proper function and utilization of each nutrient. Establishment of the optimum amount of nature's nutrients for human health is a fascinating challenge that makes a study of food so important and interesting.

A question arises as to why literally hundreds of people in one county in Northeast Texas were found to present so much evidence of disease that was responsive to Vitamin B₆. It must be assumed that either literally hundreds had an abnormal trait that required increased amounts of Vitamin B₆, or else there was frank deficiency among the population in Titus County. When as many as four families on the same street, and when repeatedly it was found that both a man and his wife had paresthesia of hands, along with other symptomatology just described, one can only state that there was extensive Vitamin B₆ deficiency in the population of Northeast Texas.

In the near future if our governement is going to seriously attempt to relieve malnutrition in the United States, monitoring stations manned by trained and talented technicians will have to take into account Vitamin B$_6$ deficiency. Biochemists now face the additional challenge of finding new and simple methods of determining Vitamin B$_6$ deficiency among the population.

A question arises as to whether or not there are chemical antagonists that are nullifying action of Vitamin B$_6$ in the human body, there is question of the amount that individuals are eating, and there is a question as to what effect cooking and food preparation has on Vitamin B$_6$ when it has been proven that there is destruction of the nutrient in cooking.

According to reports made by government scientists and others who have confirmed these reports, the leaves of plants contain more Vitamin B$_6$ than the stems. An example would be celery. There is more Vitamin B$_6$ in leaves than the tubers. An example would be potatoes. With this in mind, if one were considering onions for lunch, he would choose the little green ones and eat the blades first. Perhaps the blades of little green onions would add color to a nice salad prepared of other leafy vegatables and raw fruits. If we are talking about massive Vitamin B$_6$ deficiency in the United States, these little points are important.

Among foods that can be eaten raw, yeast is one of the best foods for man. It is rich in the B vitamins, B$_6$ included. Wheat germ is also a good source of Vitamin B$_6$. In general, it has been found that leafy vegetables contain more Vitamin B$_6$ than the fruits except avocados and bananas, both of which are rich in Vitamin B$_6$ and can be eaten without cooking. Bananas are a wonderful food, children like them, and because they are also rich in potassium, bananas supply a mineral which is very necessary in the daily diet.

In short, if one were to try to list foods rich in Vitamin B$_6$ and which could be eaten raw, he would think of yeast, wheat germ, avocados, bananas, green peppers, cabbage, carrots, pecans, and peanuts.

Fish, beef, and pork must be cooked because of fear of diseases caused by parasites. Lean beef has 2-3 times more Vitamin B$_6$ than vegetables. However, it has been reported that there is considerable loss of Vitamin B$_6$ during cooking of meat. Meat, fowl, and fish are eaten for their protein content. However, and fortunately, the amino acids are rather stable to heat. Amino acids in protein are not stored in the human body and must be eaten daily.

There may be a biochemical paradox, however, in consideration of protein and Vitamin B$_6$ in the U.S. national diet. It had been established by different scientists that addition of certain amino acids to the diets of B$_6$ deficient animals would aggravate the deficiency state. Some distinguished nutritionists at the U.S. Army Medical Research and Nutrition Laboratory in Denver, Colorado have confirmed this and proven further that young soldiers on high protein diets need more Vitamin B$_6$ than those on low protein diets. This can only mean that the affluent American with a marginal or submarginal intake of Vitamin B$_6$ is in further jeopardy when he subjects himself to a high protein diet. Clinical studies in Northeast Texas seemed to substantiate this because some of the most evident symptomatology appeared among dairymen and cattlemen who had access to farm products that were very high in animal protein.

In the United States of America, biochemists have determined that the average citizen eats daily 1.5 milligrams of Vitamin B$_6$ plus or minus .5 milligrams. In the best judgment after considered opinion, most scientists agree that the optimum intake of Vitamin B$_6$ for an adult should be 2.5-3 milligrams daily. If a person were to deliberately and intentionally eat as much Vitamin B$_6$ as his food, appetite, and stomach would allow, he would or could eat a maximum of 5 milligrams of Vitamin B$_6$ daily. It is to be remembered that in Northeast Texas pyridoxine 50 milligrams daily was the usual dose of Vitamin B$_6$ given to patients with evidence of increased need for Vitamin B$_6$. The intention was to safely relieve signs and symptoms of diseases found responsive to Vitamin B$_6$.

Much work lies ahead for those who are interested and want to work in the field of nutrition. Any knowledge gained is that much ahead. The final answers are not in, but many facts are now apparent. The person who finds the study of nutrition interesting, fascinating, and challenging will most likely enjoy better health, very likely live longer, and might enjoy the mission of helping his neighbors do the same.

REFERENCES

1. Brain, W.R., Wright, A.D., and Wilkinson, M. Spontaneous compression of both median nerves in carpal tunnel. *Lancet,* 1:277-282, 1947.

2. Cannon, B.W., and Love, J.G. Tardy median palsy; median neurities; median thenarneuritis amenable to surgery. *Surgery,* 20:210-216, 1946.

3. Ellis, J.M. *The Doctor Who Looked at Hands,* Vantage Press, 1966.

4. Gyorgy, P. Vitamin B$_2$ and pellagra-like dermatities in rats. *Nature,* 133:498, 1934.

5. Gyorgy, P. Developments leading to the metabolic role of vitamin B$_6$. *Am. J. Clin. Nutr.* 24:1250-1256, 1971.

6. Kotake, Y., Jr., Inada, Studies on xanthurenic acid. II. Preliminary report on xanthurenic acid diabetes. *J. Biochem.* (Tokyo) 40:291, 1953.

7. Kotake, Y., Jr., Inoto, Y. Studies on xanthurenic acid. X. Progressive depletion in the reduced gluthathionine content of the blood following xanthurenic acid injection. *J. Biochem.* (Tokyo) 41:627, 1954.

8. Kotake, Y., Jr. Experiments of chronic diabetes symptoms caused by xanthurenic acid, an abnormal metobolite of tryptophan. *Clin. Chem.* 3, 432, 1957.

9. Luhby, A.L., Davis, P., Murphy, M., Gordon, M., Brin, M., and Spiegel, H. Pyridoxine and oral contraceptives. *Lancet,* 2:1083.1970.

10. Luhby A.L., Brin, M., Gordon, P., Davis, P., Murphy, M., Spiegel, H., Vitamin B$_6$ metabolism in users of oral contraceptive agents. I. Abnormal urinary xanthurenic acid excretion and its correction by pyridoxine. *Am. J. Clin. Nutr.* 24:684, 1971.

12
What About Vitamin E?*
Eminent investigators now suspect it may be one of the key factors to help resist disease and slow the aging process

LINUS PAULING

"It is amazing that a substance such as vitamin E, on which many hundreds of papers have been written and to which four international symposiums have been devoted, has been the subject of calumny rather than investigation . . ." — Erwin Di Cyan, Ph.D., in *Vitamin E & Aging*

Vitamin E was discovered in 1922 by Herbert M. Evans, Professor of Biochemistry in the University of California, and his co-worker Katherine Scott Bishop. They showed that it is necessary for full health of rats, but the question of whether or not it is needed for man was not settled until recently. Only in 1968 did the U.S. Food and Nutrition Board finally decide that it is essential to human nutrition, and set the recommended daily allowance for an adult at 30 IU (international units).

During the intervening years a keen controversy developed about the possible value of vitamin E in far larger amounts than 30 IU per day for controlling or curing many serious diseases, including coronary heart disease and peripheral vascular disease. The controversy centered around the Canadian physician Dr. R. James Shute and his two sons, Dr. Evan V. Shute and Dr. Wilfrid E. Shute, who had begun using vitamin E in the treatment of disease in 1933. Their claims of success were contradicted by many other physicians, especially in the years around 1948, and for a quarter of a century the stand taken by nearly all medical authorities has been that vitamin E in amounts greater than the recommended daily allowance of 30 IU per day has no value in improving health or in preventing or controlling disease.

It is my opinion that the authorities are wrong about vitamin E, as they were about vitamin C.

SOME FACTS ABOUT VITAMIN E

When vitamin E was isolated from wheat germ oil in 1936 it was found to be a mixture of several similar substances, which are called alpha-tocopherol, beta-tocopherol, gamma-tocopherol, delta-tocopherol, and so on. Each of these can occur as the D form or the L form. They all have biological activity and antioxidant power, but in different amounts. Vitamin E capsules often contain pure alpha-DL-tocopheryl acetate, for which 1 milligrams equals 1 IU (international unit). They may, however, contain a mixture of tocopherols or their esters, in amounts such as to give the biological effect corresponding to the number of IU stated on the label. The biological and antioxidant effects do not change in quite the same way from one tocopherol to another, so that the number of IU is only a rough measure of the activity of vitamin E. Dr. Wilfrid Shute recommends that alpha-tocopherol (or alpha-tocopheryl acetate) be used in controlling heart disease.

Pure vitamin E is an oil, practically insoluble in water but soluble in oils and fats. It is found in many foods (butter, vegetable oils, margarine, eggs, fruits and vegetables) in amounts such that an average diet is estimated to provide about 10 or 15 IU perday. In 1968 the Food and Nutrition Board of the U.S. National Academy of Sciences National Research Council recommended a daily intake of 30 IU. The Board, until this time, had not accepted vitamin E as essential to human health. But in 1956 M.K. Horwitt and his collaborators (Horwitt et al, *American Journal of Clinical Nutrition*, 1956; 10,4:408) reported the results of a study of nineteen subjects (in a state hospital) who for several years received a diet containing only 3 IU of vitamin E and of nine subjects who received the same diet but with 18 IU. After about six months the subjects depleted of vitamin E began to show a pronounced increase in the fragility of the red blood cells. The concentration of the vitamin in the blood plasma changed only slowly, decreasing by about 5 percent per month. Other investigators showed that a diet high in unsaturated fatty acids causes manifestations of disease (muscular lesions, brain lesions) unless there is an increased intake of vitamin E. Horwitt mentions an infant who died, showing severe cerebellar damage, after receiving 23 grams of the unsaturated fat linoleic acid, with no added vitamin E, by intravenous feeding for nineteen days.

Much of the effectiveness of vitamin E may be ascribed to its function of preventing the oxidation of unsaturated molecules in the tissues and membranes of the body. Vitamin E is the principal fat-soluble antioxidant, and vitamin C (ascorbic acid) is the principal water-soluble antioxidant. They probably cooperated in providing protection for our bodies and slowing the aging process.

ON VITAMIN E AND AGING . . .

As Roger Williams, discoverer of the important B vitamin, pantothenic acid, puts it [1]:

Ascorbic acid (vitamin C) may delay old age because

*Reprinted with permission: *Executive Health*, Volume X, #1.

it has strong antioxidant properties (prevents un-wanted oxidations). This possibility is related to the action of other agents, particularly vitamin E, which function in a similar manner. Vitamin E deficiency has often been observed to cause biochemical and physiological changes similar to those that occur in old age. Like ascorbic acid, the most prominent known characteristic of vitamin E is its ability to act as an antioxidant.

Lipid peroxidation, the formation of harmful peroxides, from the interaction between oxygen and highly unsaturated fats (polyunsaturates) needs to be controlled in the body. Both oxygen and the poly-unsaturated lipids (fats) are essential to our existence, but if the protection against peroxidation is inade-quate, serious damage to various body proteins may result.

Vitamin E is thought to be the leading agent for the prevention of peroxidation and the free radical production which is associated both with it and with radiation. Vitamin E, along with a relatively large number of other antioxidants — ascorbic acid, ubi-quinones, sulfhydryl compounds, and the trace element selenium — do their jobs in a complicated manner. They protect the body against the damaging products formed when oxygen reacts directly with the highly unsaturated fatty substances which are essential parts of our metabolic machinery.

We do not know all the details of how these antioxidants do their work in practical situations, and the information probably would not be of interest to laymen anyway. As a practical matter, providing plenty of vitamin E and ascorbic acid — both harm-less antioxidants — is indicated as a possible means of preventing premature aging, especially if one's diet is rich in polyunsaturated acids.

A visible result of the harmful effects of peroxi-dation is the production of brown (lipofuscin-like ceroid) pigments which are deposited in various tissues, including the brain and heart. In one study, it was found that in vitamin E-deficient rats three to three and a half months old, the accumulation of these brown pigments in the adrenal glands approach that present in twelve-month-old animals fed an ordinary diet.

While no one seriously entertains the idea of a philosopher's stone which will prolong life indefi-nitely, the evidence at hand indicates that well-rounded nutrition, including generous amounts of vitamin C and vitamin E can contribute materially to extending the healthy life span of those who are already middle aged. The greatest hops for increasing life spans can be offered if nutrition — from the time of prenatal development to old age — is continuously of the highest quality.

ON THE SAFETY OF VITAMIN E . . .

Harmful side effects from very large doses of E have not been reported. In this respect it differs from the various drugs, such as aspirin (to mention one of the less dangerous), that are widely used in treating the diseases for which the Shutes claim that vitamin E is valuable. The fact that vitamin E is safe and the fact that the Shutes claim that it has value in treating coronary heart disease and several other diseases should have caused the skeptical medical authorities to carry out a thorough investigation by means of a number of large double-blind trials, in which patients in one group, selected at random, receive the vitamin, and those in another group receive a placebo (a harmless oil resembling the vitamin). But in fact these thorough investigations have not been carried out, 27 years after the original claims were made.

It has been argued that it was the duty of the Shutes to carry out these double-blind studies themselves. But the basic principles of medical ethics have made it impossible for them to do so. They themselves were convinced of the great value of vitamin E in 1946. A physician has the moral duty to give to each patient the treatment that he believes to have the greatest chance of healing the patient. Hence it was the duty of the Shutes to continue to use vitamin E for all their patients with the diseases that they had found vitamin E to control. To have kept this beneficial treat-ment from half of their patients would have been immoral.

But it would not be immoral for a skeptic, a physician who believes that vitamin E has no value, to carry out a double-blind study of this sort. It is not the Shutes, but rather the other members of the medical profession who have failed in their duty, by not having made extensive studies of vitamin E, when there was strongly suggestive evidence that this non-toxic, safe, natural substance has some value, probably even great value, in con-trolling diseases that each year cause about 200,000,000 patient-days of bed disability and 1,000,000 deaths in the United States.

HOW THE SHUTES USE VITAMIN E

In addition to many papers published in medical journals since 1946, the Shutes have described their methods and results in a book, *Vitamin E for Ailing and Healthy Hearts*, by Wilfrid E. Shute, M.D., with Harold J. Taub (Pyramid House, New York, 1969). The diseases discussed in separate chapters include coro-nary and ischemic heart disease and the accompanying angina, rheumatic fever, acute and chronic rheumatic heart disease, high blood pressure, congenital heart disease, peripheral vascular disease, varicose veins, thrombophlebitis, arterial thrombi, indolent ulcer, diabetes, kidney disease, and burns. They believe that vitamin E in doses between 50 IU and 2500 IU per day has value in treating all of these diseases. The vitamin E is given by mouth. An ointment (3 percent vitamin E in petroleum jelly) is also used for burns and ulcers and some forms of pain.

Wilfrid Shute states that in the 22 years before 1969 he had treated 30,000 cardiovascular patients. The records of hundreds of them have been published. For the most part, the only "control cases" have been provided by the record of the patient himself before he began vitamin E. For example, one patient, an elderly physician with diabetes, had severe ulceration and impair-ment of the circulation in one leg, so serious as to indicate that amputation was necessary. The leg was amputated. Ulceration and impairment of the circulation developed in the other leg. He then learned of the Shutes. Vitamin E was administered. After some months the other leg was healed, and amputation was avoided (Nelson George, *Summary*, 1951, 3:74).

Another patient, age 58 in 1951, had a coronary occlusion with posterior infarction. After two weeks in the hospital he was sent home, but was not able to work. After six months he was seen by Wilfrid Shute, who placed him on 800 IU of vitamin E per day. Within ten weeks he was free of symptoms and had returned to work. Seventeen years later he had an attack of auricular fibrillation, which was soon controlled with oxygen. He was in good condition in 1968, at age 76.

There are scores of such case histories in the book. They do not constitute proof, but there is no doubt that Wilfrid Shute is convinced that vitamin E is the most important substance in the world.

ON THE DANGERS OF AN UNBALANCED DIET

Some very important arguments about human heart disease have been advanced recently by Dr. T.W. Anderson, of the Department of Epidemiology and Biometrics, School of Hygiene, University of Toronto, Canada.

Dr. Anderson has now pointed out (the *Lancet*, ii, 298; 1973) that the nutritional muscular dystrophy that develops in animals that are given dietary unsaturated fatty acids without the protective antioxidants (vitamin E), making the animals liable to die suddenly of "heart attacks," especially when stressed, may occur in a subclinical form in human beings, especially males. The heart muscles would thus be rendered especially vulnerable to damage from a decreased blood supply, increasing the incidence of myocardial infarction. He suggested that there came a time, about 1920, when, as a result of changing practices in food processing, there occurred a dangerous decrease in the ratio of antioxidants to unsaturated fats in the available foods. (Cigarette smoking may of course also be in part responsible.) He mentions that "even such an apparently innocuous procedure as heating corn oil in air results in such a serious loss of antioxidants that if the oil is then fed to pigs the animals develop an acute and fatal myocardial degeneration" (B. Thafvelin, *Nature* 186-1169 (1960). Dr. Anderson has proposed and provided support for the hypothesis that coronary heart disease is a combination of diseases of the coronary artery and a disorder of the heart muscle caused by a dietary imbalance, essentially a deficiency of vitamin E (and perhaps also vitamin C) in relation to the amount of unsaturated fat that is ingested.

The ordinary modern diet, with bread made from flour from which the wheat germ is excluded, may provide only about 10 IU of vitamin E per day. An average diet in the old days may have provided 100 IU.

I believe that physicians should consider seriously the possibility that an increased intake of vitamin E (also vitamin C and other vitamins), in addition to their customary therapeutic measures, would benefit their patients.

Vitamin E differs from the other two fat-soluble vitamins (A and D) in that it seems to be completely non-toxic. No serious side effects of large doses of vitamin E have been reported. This fact suggests that persons who are not suffering from any illness may safely ingest an increased amount of vitamin E as a prophylactic measure, to decrease the chance of developing damaged blood vessels, a damaged heart, or some other serious condition. A younger person might do well on 100 IU per day, an older one on 400 IU or 800 IU.

REFERENCES

1. Williams, Roger J., Ph.D., D.Sc. Nutrition Against Disease: Environmental Prevention. (Copyright 1971, Pitman Publishing Corporation, New York/Toronto/London/Tel Aviv).

13
Tailoring the Dose*

WILFRID E. SHUTE

It is now nearly 24 years since we treated the first ten cardiac patients with alpha tocopherol. During these years we have personally cared for or supervised the treatment of more than 30,000 cardiovascular patients. Because much has been learned from this large experience and because of the appearance of some new and useful adjuncts to alpha tocopherol therapy, it now seems a good idea to specify the dosage schedule for the different cardiovascular conditions commonly met in such a practice.

It is noteworthy that time has shown alpha tocopherol to be unique in its ability to prevent coronary thrombosis, to dissolve fresh venous thromboses, and to decrease or abolish the symptoms that usually follow such disasters. Since these symptoms are chiefly limitation of exercise tolerance due to dyspnea, or angina pectoris, or both, the important action of alpha tocopherol here is its oxygen conservation. As shown in the experiments of air-force investigators, the administration of alpha tocopherol to normal animals decreases the oxygen requirements of muscle, cardiac and skeletal. Houchin and Mattill have also demonstrated this action of alpha tocopherol. In cardiac cases the oxygen needs are reduced, so anoxia to the degree that initiates angina pectoris or dsypnea is not reached as readily or at all. It should be noted that there are no safe rival drugs available to contest its powers and usefulness. The other fibrinolysins are still in the cautious, experimental stage.

Although it is about 110 years since Vogel first discovered cholesterol in the aorta, there is still no satisfactory evidence that coronary attacks can be prevented by controlling cholesterol values in the blood stream. Indeed it has been stated that cholesterol is not the major constituent in plaques in the coronary artery, yielding precedence to triglycerides. Talbott's article on cholesterol is refreshingly sane.

The almost universal use of the anticoagulants by cardiologists in treating coronary thrombosis, in both the acute phase and as long-term treatment, followed the paper published in 1948 by Irving S. Wright and his group. Why it took 12 more years for several thousand cardiologists and clinicians to discover that these drugs were of dubious value and also highly dangerous is hard to explain, just as it is hard to explain why these drugs are still in common use in 1969, some nine or ten years after they should

have been widely discarded, at least for chronic patients.

Similarly, bed rest for six weeks after an acute coronary episode is apparently more dangerous than useful, as discovered and reported by Samuel Levine in 1952. In this year, 1969, Levine's armchair treatment (with a reduction of the death rate to ten percent) is just beginning to be used in some parts of Canada by more than the author. As recently as 1964, one great Ontario hospital was reported to be disturbed by its 40 percent coronary death rate. The conclusion is inescapable that, for 11 years, this hospital had permitted four times as many patients with coronary occlusion to die as in a similar hospital in Boston! Early ambulation was the obvious major difference in the two centers.

Not only is alpha tocopherol the drug of choice in treating coronary artery narrowing and/or occlusion, but it is also effective in treating all other forms of heart disease with or without the help of other old and new drugs, such as digitalis, the chlorothiazides, Rauwolfia, diuretics, and such.

However, as is true for any useful drug, one must know how to use alpha tocopherol and must have a reliable preparation, properly assayed and labeled and one with which the physician is thoroughly familiar. Indeed, general acceptance of alpha tocopherol in treating cardiovascular disease might have been achieved long since had the earliest workers in the field used the same dosage schedule and product that we had used and upon which our original findings were released to the medical profession. For example, *only the alpha fraction* of the tocopherols is really effective. For this reason, it is essential to use a product in which the alpha fraction is assayed. So many of the tocopherol preparations are a combination of the tocopherols, and, unless the alpha fraction is potent and its potency known by assay, one is likely to earn a poor result.

Primarily it is because of its value as fibrinolysin and its oxygen conservation powers that alpha tocopherol is so useful in cardiovascular disease, although in acute rheumatic fever and acute glomerulonephritis its ability to decrease capillary permeability in a very short time may be what allows it to dispel signs and symptoms.

This note is, therefore, intended to serve as a guide to its intelligent therapeutic use. The key to success depends upon fitting the dosage to the individual patient's peculiar requirements. Different forms of cardiovascular disease require different

*Excerpted from *Vitamin E for Ailing and Healthy Hearts*, Copyright © 1969 by Wilfred E. Shute with Harold J. Taub. Reprinted by permission of Pyramid Publications (Harçourt Brace Jovanovich).

ranges of effective dosage. For example, coronary artery insufficiency, whatever the underlying pathology, responds usually to 800 to 1,200 I.U. of alpha tocopherol daily. However, individual patients may need much more. Starting a victim of chronic rheumatic heart disease on such a dose can lead to rapid deterioration or death. Intermittent claudication may be relieved on 800 I.U. a day, but this rarely. Sixteen hundred I.U. a day seems to be a wiser dose, and 2,400 I.U. can be needed.

CORONARY HEART DISEASE

Angina

Those patients who have a normal blood pressure, i.e., 120/80 or very nearly that, who have angina pectoris on effort or excitement, but no evidence of congestive failure, and whose electrocardiograms do not show evidence of myocardial infarction in the standard or five precordial leads.

These should be checked out very carefully to rule out intercostal tenderness in the left chest, a very frequent finding in right-handed people and a lesion which can simulate angina pectoris due to coronary sclerosis. We treat this intercostal neuralgia intensively in all patients, since it may either complicate a true case of angina pectoris or simulate it in cardiologically normal people.

We give these coronary patients 800 I.U. alpha tocopherol daily for six weeks. Since alpha tocopherol in cardiac patients takes five to ten days to begin to take effect and four to six weeks to diminish or relieve symptoms to the point where the results are obvious to patient and physician alike, we check all such patients after six weeks of treatment and often carry out a practical exercise tolerance test at the end of five or six weeks to establish the approximate degree of improvement.

If all or nearly all symptoms have disappeared, we maintain the patient on that dose indefinitely. He must take the full dose every day, since he can lose all relief from the treatment within three to seven days after cessation of therapy. A diminution of dosage will, of course, lead to a slower but certain return of symptoms. Very rarely a dosage of this degree may lead to gastric distress, but this will nearly always respond to the addition of three teaspoonsful of skim milk powder in a little milk or water after each meal with the added precaution of taking the alpha tocopherol half way through each meal.

If the patient is not improved on the original dosage level we raise it by 200 I.U. per day at six-week intervals until he is relieved or until we must admit defeat. Even then, mindful of our own experience and of Zierler's and Ochsner's work, we maintain a dosage of 800 I.U. a day to prevent intravascular clotting — aware that such patients stand a very real danger of coronary thrombosis.

Formerly we had to be very careful of patients in this category who had an elevated blood pressure, since large doses of alpha tocopherol, by increasing the tone of cardiac muscle, could elevate the blood pressure still more. However, we now start such patients on 800 I.U. a day, and proceed just as above, except that we place them on a suitable dose of hydrochlorothiazide. On their return visit in six weeks the blood pressure is usually lowered and can be satisfactorily controlled. Occasionally, we must add Rauwolfia or other such drugs. Rarely is the blood pressure reading higher than on the original examination.

Coronary Occlusion

Acute phase. The only correct time to begin the treatment of a case of coronary occlusion with alpha tocopherol is immediately upon establishment of the probable diagnosis! In such cases the full value of the oxygen-conserving power of alpha tocopherol and of its ability as a capillary dilator has a chance to salvage the heart. The infarct can be greatly reduced in size, and adjacent tissue death may be largely prevented. Later it is too late to prevent extensive tissue necrosis. Then all that can be done is to promote healing in the damaged myocardium surrounding the infarct, the areas commonly known as the zones of injury and ischemia; to increase the rate and extent of the opening up and establishment of collateral circulation and to ensure a firm scar tissue repair of the infarcted area. Of course, decreasing the oxygen need of the rest of the laboring heart is of real value and usually insures an added chance of survival.

These cases are ideal test problems, since in them all the powers of alpha tocopherol have their chance to demonstrate themselves. Indeed, one of the most dramatic proofs of the value of alpha tocopherol in coronary occlusion is demonstrable here, since in such fresh cases the electrocardiogram will show the change typical of the lesion, but to a diminished degree; thenceforward, the recovery of the electrocardiogram is more rapid and complete than it is without alpha tocopherol. We now have an interesting collection of such electrocardiograms.

The well-known drop in blood pressure that occurs in acute myocardial infarction allows full and immediate dosage in every case. Previously elevated pressures often remain within a normal range after recovery. Some will need antihypertensive drugs later, however.

We now start all acute cases on 1,600 I.U. of alpha tocopherol per day. A smaller dose is certainly adequate in the majority of cases, but it is better to make sure that maximum help is being given.

Postocclusion Status of Coronary Cases

We are seeing more and more fresh occlusions in consultation or in our own practice, but, of course, the majority of post-occlusal cases seen by us during the last twenty years have come weeks, months, or years after their accident. If cardiologists really believe that a majority of patients regain good or near-normal health following an occlusion, they are mistaken. Such patients are not deceived by the usual reassurance and six-monthly vists. The majority of those we have seen have had a definite and usually marked abnormality of the electrocardiogram. In the evaluation of treatment in these patients, the pulse rate and electrocardiographic changes become the best objective evidence of adequate dosage and, therefore, of adequate protection.

Here is one place where the clinician unaccustomed to tocopherol therapy must learn something entirely new. The myocardial infarct itself, the "zone of injury" next to it, and the "zone of ischemia" just outside that again form a total area affecting the electrocardiogram. As time goes on this area either is slightly decreased by the slowly forming anastomoses, or it remains constant, or it gradually spreads as the basic disease process worsens accordingly. The electrocardiogram either shows spontaneous improvement, or reaches a static state for months or years, or gradually shows an increase of abnormality, depending upon whatever variation just described has developed. However, when such a patient responds to adequate alpha tocopherol therapy we believe that the zone of injury may lessen, the zone of ischemia may perhaps become physiologically normal, and the total area can thereby be greatly reduced. At least such improvement is reflected by corresponding changes in the T wave of the electrocardiogram. This sequence, may we repeat, is scarcely known to the older cardiologists because it so rarely occurred in their experience before the day of alpha tocopherol.

For some reason patients with coronary occlusions often respond more rapidly and completely to alpha tocopherol therapy than do those having coronary sclerosis and angina pectoris, but without definite electrocardiographic evidence of infarction. Morris has shown convincingly that coronary thrombosis may be quite independent of atherosclerosis, although angina pectoris presupposes atheromatous changes.

Patients in this category are started also on 800 I.U. a day, with increases of 200 to 400 I.U. a day at six-week intervals, until improvement is obtained.

RHEUMATIC HEART DISEASE

(a) *Acute Rheumatic Fever.* The first attack: Here, as with acute coronary occlusion, the proper time to treat the patient is the moment the probable diagnosis is made. Under such circumstances all evidences of disease may disappear in as little as three to seven days — at least by three to four weeks. Fever, joint symptoms and signs, tachycardia, and elevated sedimentation rate will in many a case disappear entirely. Here also, irrespective of age, the full dosage of 600 units daily should be given by mouth.

(b) *Continuing Rheumatic Fever,* with marked damage to the heart, and with or without congestive failure, as long as there is no auricular fibrillation present.

Herein the ideal treatment is still as in (a) above. However, there are many cases in which the damage from earlier attacks is so great that the full dosage cannot be given immediately without precipitating congestive failure. If the heart size is nearly normal and heart damage moderate or relatively slight, we try full dosages as in (a). If we can send the patient to hospital and have full laboratory and other such facilities for treatment, we give a trial of full dosage, since here we are able to detect adverse responses as soon as they occur. In the majority of cases, however, we must treat these patients cautiously, giving 90 I.U. per day for the first four weeks, 120 I.U. daily for the second four weeks, and 150 I.U. for the third four weeks. Usually 150 I.U. is the maximum safe level of dosage.

(c) *Patients with beginning failure, after years of normal or comparatively normal health following recovery from an attack of acute rheumatic fever.*

This group is ideal to demonstrate the value of alpha tocopherol therapy. Compensation can be restored in most of them within a few weeks, and they seem to continue to improve steadily thereafter. It is in this group that diminution, and even the very occasional disappearance, of murmurs has been demonstrated by Dowd; even diminution of a moderate degree of cardiac enlargement can develop after two to three years of therapy. This is not too hard to understand if one thinks of the properties of alpha tocopherol, especially its effect on scar tissue

— and mitral stenosis, of course, is a scar process involving the angles of the cups of the mitral valve.

Many of these patients are first seen early in pregnancy and in these compensation is more difficult to achieve, requiring usually a larger dosage of alpha tocopherol and longer treatment.

Such patients should be started very gradually on alpha tocopherol. It will be 12 to 15 weeks before they notice real improvement. Meanwhile, if they show early congestive failure, it can now be easily and successfully treated with the newer diuretics until the end of this period of three and one-half months, after which such adjuncts to treatment can usually be safely stopped. We start such patients on 90 I.U. a day for one month, then give 120 I.U. for one month and then 150 I.U. permanently. 150 I.U. is usually an effective dose, and there is no need to increase it. Indeed, it may be several years before the maximum safe dose in such cases (300 I.U. a day) can be reached. Any attempt to increase beyond 150 I.U. can precipitate fresh congestive failure or palpitation. Strangely enough, a patient living a normal life on 300 I.U. for years (10 to 15) can sometimes be precipitated into failure by a mere 75 I.U. more.

A few cases require months to show satisfactory improvement, but persistence should turn virtually every case in this category into a satisfied patient.

(d) **Chronic Rheumatic Heart Disease.** These end states show congestive failure, auricular fibrillation, and very little or no exercise tolerance.

These cases which are so very common illustrate the failure of all conventional methods of treatment in rheumatic heart disease. This stage of partial to complete invalidism lasts for five to ten years, and its effect upon the patient and his relatives is sad to watch.

It is difficult to treat such cases even with alpha tocopherol, because it, of course, requires a miracle to make a heart so badly damaged function well enough to restore the patient even to a limited degree of normal living. A 50 percent improvement in a patient confined to bed still leaves him an invalid. Yet we have had patients in this category who had spent six to 19 months in bed under classical therapy, who were able to resume full activity and to maintain normal living with increasing strength. This has occurred in as little as a month of tocopherol treatment. Apparently the factors determining the extent of improvement are many and complex, although many of these are obvious to anyone understanding the basic pathology and the pharmacological effect of alpha tocopherol. We could mention just one here — alpha tocopherol has been shown to reduce the oxygen requirement of heart muscle by a great deal.

This type of case is still worth attempting to treat, since the results can be so valuable occasionally. Need we stress the fact that every aid in the pharmacopoeia must be used, especially at first, until the effect of alpha tocopherol has had a chance to show itself? Then gradually these older agents may be dispensed with, or used less often or in smaller dosage.

The most important point in treating these patients is to bring the congestive failure under control as quickly as possible by the use of the right amount of digitalis and diuretics, given as often as is necessary to relieve the failure completely. At the same time alpha tocopherol is begun. If the patient is under *close* supervision he should be given 300 I.U. of alpha tocopherol daily from the beginning, provided the physician is sufficiently experienced in using alpha tocopherol to know when his patient is showing evidence of excessive dosage. Since alpha tocopherol will not show much effect for about ten days and since intensive treatment of the congestive failure should show a steady improvement by the first ten days of treatment, this overdosage is being reached if the patient begins to show signs of increasing failure at about the ten- to 14-day period. If, however, the patient begins to improve more rapidly at this phase, full dosage is maintained thereafter until the fourth week, when the other accessory medications can often be reduced or stopped entirely. Some digitalis, usually much less than before treatment and much less than is necessary during the first two weeks, may be continued. That is a matter for professional experience and judgment.

If, however, the patient is one of those who cannot tolerate so large an initial dose, then alpha tocopherol should be stopped for two full days and the slower schedule adopted — 90 I.U. for four weeks, 120 I.U. for four weeks, and then 150 I.U. a day thereafter.

Curiously, patients in this group often do best on 150 I.U. a day — even better, indeed, than on the large dosage. One must find out by trial. For example, one patient was told by a very competent cardiologist that she would never do another bit of work of any kind, but has done her own housework for the last four years, taking 150 I.U. a day and nothing else, except for two short periods — once when she reduced her dose to 120 I.U. a day — with the recurrence of complete failure. So narrow a dosage tolerance is fairly common in this type of patient. In no other type is it so necessary to tailor the dose to the individual patient's requirement.

Most of our patients come from many miles away, and so we usually follow the slow dosage procedure. By the end of six months on any given dosage one can usually tell if it is the dose that will give the optimum results. Once improvement begins it will usually continue slowly for many months or years. While the improvement is so slow as to be very discouraging for three months or more on this slow schedule, it is really the most accurate way of arriving at the individual's correct dosage.

When too large a dose is given in any type of heart disease, the patient often shows an unusually rapid and encouraging response and then becomes worse again. When this happens, it is evidence that the optimum dosage level was reached and then exceeded. Since alpha tocopherol is rapidly excreted, stop the dosage for three days — no more — and begin again at approximately the right level, or just less.

In tailoring the dose to the individual's requirement, remember the general rule: a patient with a normal or low blood pressure and with no evidence of congestive failure can nearly, but not quite always, tolerate any quantity of alpha tocopherol. "It can do him no harm." So give him enough to do the job. Like digitalis and insulin and thyroid extract, the right dose is the dose that begins to show definite improvement, in four to six weeks in this case. The maintenance dose is the same. However, in the presence of hypertension or congestive failure, in advanced rheumatic heart disease, or both, be careful. Probably you can kill the patient if you are overzealous.

However, an exception to the presence of congestive failure, as a contraindication to high dosage of alpha tocopherol, is coronary heart disease following occlusion. In such a case we give full dosage, and the failure tends to clear up with the disappearance of myocardial anoxia. In rare cases where the patient is obviously dying of congestive failure in hypertensive heart disease the same applies. Tailor your dose to the patient's needs. Maintaining full dosage in the post-occlusive patient maintains better myocardial oxygenation.

SUMMARY

1. Alpha tocopherol has its own mechanics of action on damaged hearts, and its dosage levels, speed of ingestion, rate of excretion, potentialities for harm and toxicity must be understood if it is to be used successfully.

2. There is a dose appropriate to every patient. More or less may harm the patient. It may require weeks or months to determine what his dose should be.

3. Patience and skill are demanded by this type of treatment. There is no simple rule-of-thumb.

14
A New Brand of Nutritional Science*

ROGER J. WILLIAMS

INTRODUCTION

Senator Schweiker of Pennsylvania has introduced a bill into the U.S. Senate providing 5 million dollars yearly to ensure the teaching of nutrition in our medical schools. Regardless of the outcome of this unusual move to improve the curriculum of medical schools by outside influence, it is highly significant that many intelligent laymen see a desperate need for change. Historically this sentiment has been provoked by decades of neglect of nutrition by medical institutions. This neglect is freely admitted by many prominent leaders in the medical profession (Williams, 1971; Butterworth, 1974).

Without attempting to assess the elements of blame, it appears an undeniable fact that the opinion makers in medical education have for decades practically unanimously regarded the only type of nutrition they know as not worthy of the serious attention of medical scientists.

Certainly there are many highly competent investigators in this field; specialists who are carrying out highly commendable studies. Yet the material available for presentation in medical schools is largely descriptive, detailed but disjointed. Nutritional science has too long been lacking in fundamental guiding principles and its raw material has often remained a poorly digested mass.

What is needed is a newly developed type of nutritional science which will command respect and be regarded as eminently worthy of the attention of all medical scientists.

In this article I will attempt to outline the salient features of such a comprehensive nutritional science. We will seek to answer the questions, "What needs to be taught in medical schools about nutrition?" "What can adequately fill the evident gap in medical education?" The answers can best be outlined by presenting and discussing very briefly 12 propositions, the majority of which present truths that have been neglected in the past. The broad impact of the following 12 propositions seems inescapable.

*Reprinted with permission: *New Dynamics of Preventive Medicine*, Vol. 4, Leon R. Pomeroy, Editor (Selected papers from the 8th meeting of the International Academy of Preventive Medicine.)

1. Nutrients are essential parts of the human environment; human environments are by nature suboptimal.

Nutrients are essentially in the same category as oxygen and water and just as indispensable to life and health. There are approximately 40 chemical items which are the ABC's of nutritional science — amino acids, minerals, vitamins, etc. We do not know with certainty the precise number or identity of all these essential chemicals, let alone our quantitative needs for each, their quantitative distribution in foods and their interrelationships.

The fact that nutrients are part of our environment needs to be correlated with another fact: human environments as commonly encountered are suboptimal and always subject to improvement. With respect to climate we never encounter temperatures, humidity, wind and sunshine that are perfect at all times. Socially we do not encounter families and friends that are perfect specimens nor do we have perfect books and magazines to read. In the realm of nutrition there is no tree that bears a perfect food. Nutrition is always subject to improvement. "Normal nutrition" is some indefinite level of suboptimal nutrition. Food choices can yield every possible level of inferiority and excellence.

On the basis of present inadequate information it is impossible to know with certainty, how far removed from optimal any particular diet is. "Balanced diets" possess varying degrees of balance. Human environments and diets are always imperfect.

2. Nutrients as such always act as a team.

Comprehensive nutritional science must rise above the traditional piecemeal approach. Following this approach one might regard the subject of nutritional deficiencies fully exposed to view when deficiencies of each and every nutrient is separately considered. This would leave out, of course, myriads of real deficiencies (encountered by real people) — those involving simultaneous deficiencies (of varying degrees) of numerous combinations of nutrients.

The nature of the teamwork among nutrients appears when we reflect that thiamin cures beriberi not as a single acting agent, but because it happens to complete (imperfectly) the nutritional team furnished by polished rice. When niacinamide cures pellagra it is not a medicinal agent acting by itself; it happens to complete the nutritional team furnished by a diet consisting largely of corn bread and sow belly. Nutrients, unlike drugs, always act constructively. To function constructively they must act in co-operation with all other members of the nutrient team.

Vitamins and other nutrients have often been judged to be of dubious medical value because they do not cure specific diseases. These judgments involve acceptance of the piecemeal approach to nutrition and uninformed use of nutrient agents. When nutrients are used under conditions such that they might scientifically be expected to act, that is, recognizing the teamwork principle, they may bring dramatic results. The nutrients acting as a team make life possible; if any essential nutrient is lacking or is in short supply life and health cannot continue.

The teamwork of the nutrients is complicated by the numerous chemicals which are added to foods for other than nutritional reasons viz. as preservatives, texturizers, emulsifiers, stabilizers, etc. Modern nutritional science must approach such problems realistically (Hall, 1975).

3. Nutrition concerns real people; not hypothetical "man."

Neither medicine nor nutrition are "pure" sciences. If the findings of nutrition or medicine apply only to hypothetical "man" they are almost worthless.

Since everyone grants the applied nature of nutrition and of medical practice, the crucial question is: How different are real people from hypothetical "man?" This question can be partially answered by two sets of illustrations. Figure 1 shows the partial composition of the blood of "man" in contrast to levels of the same constituents in the bloods of 11 real people as shown in Figure 2. Figure 3 shows first the taste sensations, salivary composition and urinary constituents of hypothetical average "man;" in contrast there are shown 12 corresponding patterns of 12 real individuals including a pair of monozygous twins.

As some of my readers know, I have been at least mildly interested in biochemical individuality for approximately 30 years. On the basis of my extensive study of this subject, it is my opinion that a study of nutrition is a subterfuge when it is geared to the supposition that the general population is made up mostly of "normal healthy people" who correspond approximately to hypothetical man with about average nutritional needs.

Yet one can pick up book after book on nutrition to find in the index no citations under the headings of "individuality," "variations" or "normal variations." Books on nutrition are often written as though these phenomena did not exist. There are some notable exceptions to this rule. One is *Heinz Handbook of Nutrition* which discusses this problem briefly but ably in two pages, and then, unfortunately, lets the problem drop out of sight (Burton, 1959).

A really practical nutritional science must have as one of its cornerstones a grasp of the elementary facts of biochemical individuality. The value of nutritional study will be immeasurably enhanced by considering these facts. This aspect of nutrition is one which when developed will demand and get the attention of all health-minded medical scientists.

4. Body nutrition entails complete cellular nutrition including intercellular (cell to cell) nutrition and many other complexities.

This aspect of nutrition which gets down to the basic fundamentals has been neglected. This is unfortunate because in a real sense cellular nutrition is what nutrition is all about. If we can keep the cells of our body well nourished certainly our whole body will fare well. If some cells in our bodies are poorly nourished this can play havoc with the entire body mechanism.

I called attention several years ago to the potential importance of intercellular nutrition — the fact that some essential cellular nutrients are produced by other cells within the body. These ordinarily may not be body nutrients, but under some circumstances they may be. Such cell nutrients may include gluta-mine, inositol, lipoic acid and perhaps many other substances currently regarded as non-essential for the body as a whole. The failure to explore these possibilities points to the inadequacies of nutritional science so far as cellular nutrition is concerned. The neglect of cellular nutrition in the area of cancer research has recently been discussed (Williams, 1974).

Another complexity encountered in the field of cellular nutrition is the presence of foreign organisms in the intestinal tract and elsewhere. This itself constitutes a large field for explorations.

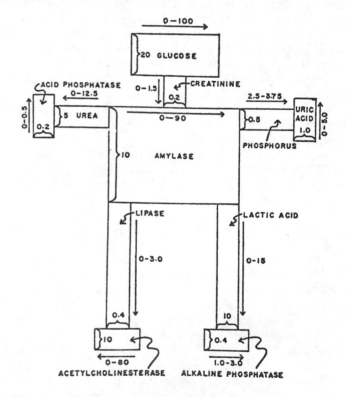

Figure 1.   "Normal" Blood. This diagramatic representation depicts partially the characteristics of "normal" blood. The average amount and "normal" variation of each of 11 blood constituents is represented by a rectangle. The longer dimension, indicated by an arrow, represents the average level, and the shorter dimension, indicated by a brace, represents the "normal" extent of variation. The scales are so adjusted as to present a reasonably proportioned diagrammatic picture of a man. From "Individual Patterns in Normal Humans: Organic Blood Constituents" by W. Duane Brown, Doctoral Dissertation, The University of Texas, 1955.

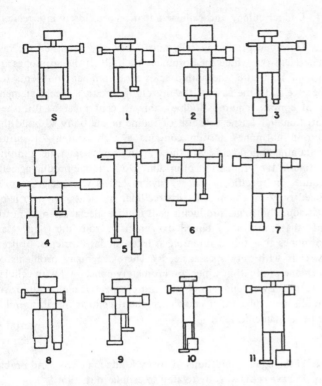

Figure 2. "Normal" Blood Variations. These diagramatic representations depict certain compositional levels in the fasting bloods of 11 healthy young men, in comparison with the "normal" or standard blood depicted in Figure 1. The levels and variations depicted for these 11 individuals were determined experimentally from 5 to 6 fasting blood samples from each, collected at about weekly intervals. These diagrams are reduced versions; the originals were drawn on exactly the same scale as that picturing "normal" blood. These representations appeared with permission in *You Are Extraordinary* by Roger J. Williams (Random House, New York, 1967) p. 22. They originated in "Individual Patterns in Normal Humans: Organic Blood Constituents" by W. Duane Brown, Doctoral Dissertation, The University of Texas, 1955.

Several of the 8 succeeding propositions yet to be discussed strongly implicate further consideration of cellular nutrition.

5. Digestion, absorption and circulation phenomena and derangements are vital parts of cellular nutrition.

Since cellular nutrition has in general been neglected, it has been common to under-emphasize the role of circulation in feeding the various cells and tissues of the body. Too often it has been assumed that once proper food is consumed, no further problems exist. The whole problem of "normal" individuality with respect to digestion, absorption and blood circulation has been largely unexplored. This is most unfortunate because nutritional problems arising in these areas are probably relatively common.

6. Prenatal nutrition is an important phase of internal cellular nutrition.

Prenatal nutrition has been of concern to nutritionists generally, but its findings have not influenced adequately the medical community. There has been a tendency on the part of physicians to ignore completely or to look upon prenatal nutrition as a last resort, in attempting to understand and/or explain miscarriages, premature births, deformities, discordancies, mental retardation and birth defects in general. Mediocre prenatal nutrition may be responsible for many of these difficulties.

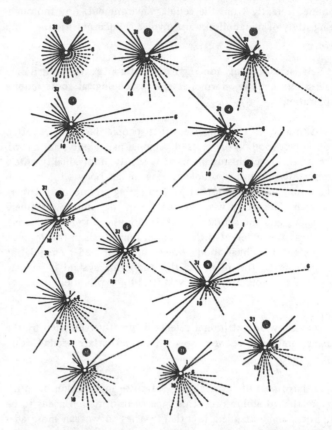

Figure 3. Individual Biochemical Patterns. Each radial line in these diagrams represents a separate type of measurement: (1-5) Taste sensitivities; creatinine, sucrose, KCl, NaCl, HCL (6-17) Salivary constituents; uric acid, glucose, leucine, valine, citrulline, alanine, lysine, taurine, glycine, serine, glutamic acid, aspartic acid (18-31) Urinary constituents; citrate, base R_F .28, acid R_F .32, gonadotropin, pH, pigment/creatinine, chloride/creatinine, hippuric acid/creatinine, creatinine, taurine, glycine, serine, citrulline, alanine. Each line represents the average of a series of determinations on each individual. Figures 1-12 represent different healthy individuals, including one pair of monozygous twins (11, 12). Figure 0 is the patternless hypothetical "average" or "normal." University of Texas Publication No. 5109 (1951) pp. 10-12.

Particularly if we accept the facts of individuality in nutrition and the concept that human environments are commonly suboptimal, we see that prenatal nutrition may be of phenomenal importance. Realistically we must grant that when a reasonably healthy woman becomes pregnant, the environment she provides for the growing fetus is probably more nearly ideal than other environments human beings usually encounter. This does not mean, however, that prenatal environments are uniformly optimal or that their excellence can be taken for granted.

It has been found in nutritional studies over several decades that in numerous diverse species, food that is adequate for ordinary maintenance of adult specimens may be quite inadequate to support good reproductive records.

7. Intracellular metabolism at the molecular level is made possible by, and is integrated with, cellular nutrition.

Two outstanding factors involved in intracellular metabolism are the enzymes and their substrates. The enzymes are built within the cells from cellular nutrients from the outside. The substrates of the enzymes are often exogenous in origin and are obtained directly from the cellular environment. Any thoroughgoing study of metabolism must involve cellular nutrition.

8. Self selection of food greatly influences the nutritional process; its cellular, hormonal and psychological roots require exploration.

Although it is recognized that people individually often choose their food on the basis of personal palatability, our knowledge of the mechanisms involved is scanty. Individuality enters prominently into this problem. How much body wisdom individuals may have with respect to their eating preferences is largely unknown. This body wisdom may be or may not be extremely important, and the sources of the wisdom need to be elucidated, as well as the inherent differences in individuals in this respect. The extent to which food choices are governed by regulating mechanisms in the brain or the endocrine system is vaguely known. The whole subject is a vast field for exploration.

9. The study of nutritional science is greatly facilitated by the close resemblance between species; this advantage needs further exploration.

A large part of the available definitive information on nutrition relates to albino rats. This type of information needs to be amplified and extended to other species so we can more adequately answer the questions, "To what degree can we trust the transfer of nutritional information from another species to human beings?" "Since rats and humans both show wide individual variability in nutritional needs, are the ranges such that much overlapping exists, with the result that requirements found for rats, as a group, may be adapted for humans, as a group?"

Complete assessment of the nutritional needs of several species would be valuable because it would throw light on questions such as the ones just considered.

10. Genetics, inheritance and molecular biology are permeated with nutritional problems and these disciplines cannot be studied adequately while disregarding cellular nutrition.

It is by no means enough for nutrition to be taught in medical schools to those few who may wish to specialize in nutrition. A substantial amount of nutrition should be taught to every health professional.

Those members of research teams which delve deeply into molecular biology and inheritance phenomena must have some expertise with respect to cellular nutrition. Every essential chemical item involved must either be produced within the cell or obtained nutritionally from the cellular environment. No adequate picture of such processes can be gained without considerations involving cellular nutrition.

11. Endocrinology and cellular nutrition are closely interrelated.

Hormone producing cells must always be furnished the raw materials from which the hormones are built. If the hormones are protein in nature, the amino acids are prominent nutrients for these cells. In the case of the thyroid hormone, a special element is, of course, required (iodine); this element must be furnished nutritionally. Is the sole use of iodine in the body to build the thyroid hormone? Insulin contains a high content of sulfur-containing amino acids. Are those amino acids sometimes limiting factors in the production of insulin? Do hormone producing cells require, in specific instances, raw materials which can be produced only by other cells (intercellular nutrients) or may it be that some hormone producing cells require special essential nutrients that must be obtained exogenously from the food? May hormones themselves function as intercellular nutrients, utilized by cells with very special needs? There are many problems of hormone production which are intimately concerned with cellular nutrition. Every endocrinologist and prospective endocrinologists should have substantial knowledge about cellular nutrition in his or her armamentarium.

12. Pathological conditions of many kinds may have, and probably do have roots directly related to cellular nutrition.

This last proposition has extremely wide scope and is discussed in part in my book, *Nutrition Against Disease* (Williams, 1971).

Some of the types of pathology included as having roots related to cellular nutrition are the following: birth deformities, blood vessel and other anatomical discordancies, mental retardation, infectious diseases, allergies, immunities, unusual drug response, arthritis, atherosclerosis, heart disease, mental disease, emotional stress, nervous tension, sleep aberrances, alcoholism, peridontal disease.

Elsewhere I have discussed a type of pathology which has not hitherto been recognized — generalized cytopathy (Williams, 1975). Pathology is often thought of as being localized in some particular organ or tissue. This pathology is different.

If, for example, an essential nutrient is in short supply in the body, every cell and tissue in the entire body may have its functions impaired. This type of general cell sickness unquestionably exists in different degrees whenever even mild nutritional deficiencies exist. Since cellular environments like human environments are commonly not optimal or perfect, this type of illness is probably the most prevalent of all. We are fortunate when its effects are minimal or better yet negligible. It is inconceivable to me that anyone could claim to have a comprehensive view of the subject of pathology and at the same time neglect cellular nutrition.

The development of a nutritional science such as we envisage will require time — there is much catching up to be done — and the efforts of many thousands of scientists will be involved. In the past decades there have been far too few medical scientists who have been interested in nutrition. Often nutrition is completely outside their scientific world.

We have presented 12 propositions in outline and have not attempted to discuss them in detail. There are three key phrases which can be used to call attention to the principal deficiencies of current nutritional science which has not been accepted as an integral part of medical science. These three phrases are: *Suboptimal nutritional environment, biochemical individuality,* and *cellular nutrition.* When the subject matter suggested by the discussion of these three topics is included in comprehensive nutritional science, this discipline will compel attention. Medical schools will be forced by student and popular demand to include such teaching in their curricula. Its relevance to health and medical practice cannot be doubted, because it paves the way for disease prevention.

REFERENCES

Burton, B.T., Ed., *The Heinz Handbook of Nutrition,* New York, New York, McGraw-Hill, 1959.

Butterworth, C.E., Jr., The Skeleton in the Hospital Closet, *Nutrition Today,* 9:4, 1974.

Hall, R., Is Nutrition a Stagnating Science? *New Scientist,* 2:9, 1975.

Williams, R.J., How Can the Climate in Medical Education be Changed? *Persp. in Biol. and Med.,* 14:608, 1971.

Williams, R.J., The Neglect of Nutritional Science in Cancer Research, *Congressional Record,* 120: October 16, 1974.

Williams, R.J., *Nutrition Against Disease,* New York, New York, Pitman, 1971.

Williams, R.J., The Range of Potential Benefits to be Derived from the Improvement of Nutritional Environments: A New Concept in Pathology: Generalized Cytopathy, *Physicians' Handbook of Nutritional Science,* Springfield, IL, Charles C. Thomas, 1975.

15
On the Orthomolecular Environment of the Mind: Orthomolecular Theory*

LINUS PAULING

"Varying the concentrations of substances normally present in the human body may control mental disease." – Linus Pauling

"The methods principally used now for treating patients with mental disease are psychotherapy (psychoanalysis and related efforts to provide insight and to decrease environmental stress), chemotherapy (mainly with the use of powerful synthetic drugs, such as chlorpromazine, or powerful natural products from plants, such as reserpine), and convulsive shock therapy (electroconvulsive therapy, insulin coma therapy, pentylenetetrazol shock therapy). I have reached the conclusion that another general method of treatment, which may be called orthomolecular therapy, may be found to be of great value, and may turn out to be the best method of treatment for many patients." – Linus Pauling, *Science*, April 19, 1968, p. 265

The author defines orthomolecular psychiatry as the achievement and preservation of good mental health by the provision of the optimum molecular environment for the mind, especially the optimum concentrations of substances normally present in the human body, such as the vitamins. He states that there is sound evidence for the theory that increased intake of such vitamins as ascorbic acid, niacin, pyridoxine, and cyanocobalamin is useful in treating schizophrenia. The negative conclusions of APA Task Force Report 7, *Megavitamin and Orthomolecular Therapy in Psychiatry*, he says, result not only from faulty arguments and from a bias against megavitamin therapy but also from a failure to deal fully with orthomolecular therapy in psychiatry. Three psychiatrists comment on Dr. Pauling's presentation.

Orthomolecular psychiatry is the achievement and preservation of mental health by varying the concentrations in the human

*Based on a lecture given at a meeting of the American College of Neuropsychopharmacology, Palm Springs, Calif., Dec. 4-7, 1973. Reprinted with permission: *Am. J. Psychiatry*, 131:11, November 1974.© Copyright 1974 American Psychiatric Association.

body of substances that are normally present, such as the vitamins. It is part of a broader subject, orthomolecular medicine, an important part because the functioning of the brain is probably more sensitively dependent on its molecular composition and structure than is the functioning of other organs [1].

After having worked for a decade on the hereditary hemolytic anemias, I decided in 1954 to work on the molecular basis of mental disease. I read the papers and books dealing with megavitamin therapy of schizophrenia by Hoffer and Osmond [2, 4] as well as the reports on studies of vitamins in relation to mental disease by Cleckley and Sydenstricker [5, 6] and others. In the course of time I formulated a general theory of the dependence of function on molecular structure of the brain and other parts of the body and coined the adjective "orthomolecular" to describe it [1].

There is no doubt that the mind is affected by its molecular environment. The presence in the brain of molecules of LSD, mescaline, or some other schizophrenogenic substance is associated with profound psychic effects. Mental manifestations of avitaminosis have been reported for several vitamins. A correlation of behavior of school children with concentration of ascorbic acid in the blood (increase in "alertness" or "sharpness" with increase in concentration) has been reported by Kubala and Katz [7]. A striking abnormality in the urinary excretion of ascorbic acid after an oral loading dose was reported for chronic schizophrenics by VanderKamp [8] and by Herjanic and Moss-Herjanic [9]. My associates and I [10] carried out loading tests for three vitamins on schizophrenic patients who had recently been hospitalized and on control subjects. The percentage of schizophrenic patients who showed low urinary excretion of each vitamin was about twice as great as that of the controls: for ascorbic acid, 74 percent of the schizophrenic patients showed low urinary excretion versus 32 percent of the controls; for niacinamide, 81 percent versus 46 percent; and for pyridoxine, 52 percent versus 24 percent. The possibility that the low values in urinary excretion of these vitamins for schizophrenic patients resulted from poor nutrition is made unlikely by the observation that the numbers of subjects low in one, two, or all three vitamins corresponded well with the numbers calculated for independent incidence.

There are a number of plausible mechanisms by which the concentration of a vitamin may affect the functioning of the brain. One mechanism, effective for vitamins that serve as coenzymes, is that of shifting the equilibrium for the reaction of apoenzyme and coenzyme to give the active enzyme. An example is the effectiveness of cyanocobalamin (vitamin B_{12}) given in amounts 1,000 times greater than normal to control the disease methylmalonic aciduria [11-14]. About half of the patients with this disease are successfully treated with megadoses of vitamin B_{12}. In these patients a genetic mutation has occurred and an altered apoenzyme that has a greatly reduced affinity for the coenzyme has been produced. Increase in concentration of the coenzyme can counteract the effect of the decrease in the value of the combining constant and lead to the formation of enough of the active enzyme to catalyze effectively the reaction of conversion of methylmalonic acid to succinic acid.

In the human population there may be several alleles of the gene controlling the manufacture of each apoenzyme; in consequence the concentration of coenzyme needed to produce the amount of active enzyme required for optimum health may well be somewhat different for different individuals. In particular, many individuals may require a considerably higher concentration of one or more coenzymes than other people do for optimum health, especially for optimum mental health. It is difficult to obtain experimental evidence for gene mutations that lead to only small changes in the properties of enzymes. The fact that genes that lead to large and more easily detectable changes in the properties of enzymes occur, as in individuals with methylmalonic aciduria, for example, suggests that mutations that lead to small changes also occur.

Significant differences in enzyme activity in different individuals have been reported by many investigators, especially by Williams [15], who has made many studies of biochemical individuality. It is likely that thorough studies of enzymes would show them to be similar to the human hemoglobins. A few of the abnormal human hemoglobins, most of which involve only the substitution of one amino-acid residu for another in either the alpha chain or the beta chain of the molecule, differ greatly in properties from normal adult hemoglobin, leading to serious manifestations of disease.

It was in the course of the study of one of these diseases, sickle cell anemia, that the first abnormal hemoglobin was discovered [16]. Most of the abnormal human hemoglobins, however, differ from normal hemoglobin in their properties to only a small extent, so that there is no overt manifestation of disease. There is, nevertheless, the possibility that even the small changes in properties of an abnormal hemoglobin associated with a mild hemoglobinopathy will have deleterious consequences. An example is the intolerance to sulfa drugs associated with the substitution of arginine for histidine in the locus 58 in the alpha chain or 63 in the beta chain. It is likely that individual differences in enzyme activity will in the course of time be shown to be the result of differences in the amino-acid sequences of the polypeptide chains of the apoenzymes.

More than 100 abnormal human hemoglobins are now known, and the human population may be expected to be similarly complex with respect to many enzymes, including those involved in the functioning of the brain. A tendency to schizophrenia is probably polygenic in origin. I have suggested [1] that the genes primarily involved in this tendency may well be those which regulate the metabolism of vital substances such as the vitamins.

Some vitamins are known to serve as coenzymes for several enzyme systems. We might ask if the high concentration of coenzyme required to produce the optimum amount of one active enzyme might not lead to the production of far too great an amount of another active enzyme. The answer to this question is that the danger is not very great. For most enzymes the concentration of coenzyme and the value of the combination constant are such that most (90 percent or more) of the protein is converted to active enzyme. Accordingly, a great increase in concentration would increase the amount of most active enzymes by only a few percentage points, whereas it might cause a great increase for a mutated enzyme.

THE ORTHOMOLECULAR TREATMENT OF SCHIZOPHRENIA

In the book *Orthomolecular Psychiatry: Treatment of Schizophrenia* [17] my colleagues and I pointed out that the orthomolecular treatment of schizophrenia involves the use of vitamins (megavitamin therapy) and minerals; the control of diet, especially the intake of sucrose; and, during the initial acute phase, the use of conventional methods of controlling the crisis, such as the phenothiazines. The phenothiazines are not, of course, normally present in the human body and are not orthomolecular. However, they are so valuable in controlling the crisis that their use is justified in spite of their undesirable side effects.

Hawkins [18, p. 640] stated that his initial combination of vitamins for the treatment of schizophrenia was 1 gm. of ascorbic acid, 1 gm. of niacinamide, 50 mg. of pyridoxine, and 400 I.U. of vitamin E four times a day. Other vitamins may also be given. A larger intake, especially of niacinamide or niacin, may be prescribed; the usual amount seems to be about 8 gm. a day after an initial period on 4 gm. a day.

The vitamins, as nutrients or medicaments, pose an interesting question. The question is not, Do we need them? We know that we do need them, in small amounts, to stay alive. The real question is, What daily amounts of the various vitamins will lead to the best of health, both physical and mental? This question has been largely ignored by medical and nutritional authorities.

Let us consider schizophrenia. Osmond [19, p. 200] stated that about 40 percent of schizophrenics hospitalized for the first time are treated successfully by conventional methods in that they are released and not hospitalized a second time. The conventional treatment fails for about 60 percent in that the patient is not released or is hospitalized again. Conventional treatment includes a decision about vitamin intake. Usually it is decided that the vitamins in the food will suffice or that a multivitamin tablet will also be given. The amounts of ascorbic acid, niacin, pyridoxine, and vitamin E may be approximately the daily allowances recommended by the Food and Nutrition Board of the U.S. National Academy of Sciences-National Research Council: 60 mg of ascorbic acid, 20 mg of niacin, 2 mg. of pyridoxine, and 15 I.U. of vitamin E. Is this amount of vitamins correct? Would many schizophrenic patients respond to their treatment better if the decision were made that they should receive 10 or 100 or 500 times as much of some vitamins? What is the optimum intake for these patients? I believe there is much evidence that the optimum intake for schizophrenic patients is much larger than the recommended daily allowances. By the use of orthomolecular methods in addition to the conventional treatment of schizophrenia, the fraction of patients hospitalized for the first time in whom the disease is controlled may be increased from about 40 percent to about 80 percent [19].

Ascorbic Acid

It was reported by Horwitt in 1942 [20] and by later investigators that schizophrenic patients receiving the usual dietary amounts of ascorbic acid had lower concentrations of ascorbic acid in the blood than people in good health. The loading-test results of VanderKamp [8], Herjanic and Moss-Herjanic [9], and Pauling and associates [10] have been mentioned above. In his discussion of ascorbic acid and schizophrenia Herjanic [21] concluded:

> The individual variation of the need for ascorbic acid may turn out to be one of the contributing factors in the development of the illness. Ascorbic acid is an important substance necessary for optimum functioning of many organs. If we desire, in the treatment of mental illness, to provide the "optimum molecular environment," especially the optimum concentration of substances normally present in the human body (Pauling, 1968 [1]), ascorbic acid should certainly be included [21, p. 314].

There is, moreover, a special reason for an increased intake of ascorbic acid by patients with schizophrenia or any other disease for which there is only partial control. About 60 mg. of ascorbic acid a day is enough to prevent overt manifestations of avitaminosis C (scurvy) in most people. However, there are several significant arguments to support the thesis that the optimum intake for most people is 10 to 100 times more than 60 mg. These arguments are summarized in the papers and books of Irwin Stone [22] and myself [23, 24]. They constitute the theoretical basis for the customary use of about 4 gm. of ascorbic acid a day in the orthomolecular therapeutic and prophylactic treatment of schizophrenia.

A significant controlled trial of ascorbic acid in chronic psychiatric patients was reported in 1963 by Milner [25]. The study, which was double-blind, was made with 40 chronic male patients: 34 had schizophrenia, 4 had manic-depressive psychosis, and 2 had general paresis. Twenty of the patients, selected at random, received 1 gm. of ascorbic acid a day for three weeks; the rest received a placebo. The patients were checked with the Minnesota Multiphasic Personality Inventory (MMPI) and the Wittenborn Psychiatric Rating Scales (WPRS) before and after the trial. Milner concluded that "statistically significant improvement in the depressive, manic, and paranoid symptoms-complexes, together with an improvement in overall personality functioning, was obtained following saturation with ascorbic acid" [25]. He suggested that chronic psychiatric patients would benefit from the administration of ascorbic acid.

We found [10] that of 106 of the schizophrenic patients we studied who had recently been hospitalized in a private hospital, a county-university hospital, or a state hospital, 81 (76 percent) were deficient in ascorbic acid, as shown by the six-hour excretion of less than 17 percent of an orally administered dose. Only 27 of 89 control subjects (30 percent) showed this deficiency.

Great deficiency (less than 4 percent excreted) was shown by 24 (22 percent) of the schizophrenic subjects and by only 1 (1 percent) of the controls. I have no doubt that many schizophrenic patients would benefit from an increased intake of ascorbic acid. My estimate is that 4 gm. of ascorbic acid a day, in addition to the conventional treatment, would increase the fraction of acute schizophrenics in whom the disease is permanently controlled by about 25 percent. Except for that of Milner [25], no controlled trial of ascorbic acid in relation to schizophrenia has been made, so far as I know.

Niacin and Niacinamide

The requirement of niacin (nicotinic acid) for proper functioning of the brain is well known. The psychosis of pellagra, as well as the other manifestations of this deficiency disease, is prevented by the intake of a small amount of niacin, about 20 mg. a day. In 1939 Cleckley, Sydenstricker, and Geeslin [5] reported the successful treatment of 19 patients with severe psychiatric symptoms with niacin, and in 1941 Sydenstricker and Cleckley [6] reported similarly successful treatment of 29 patients with niacin. In both studies, moderately large doses of niacin, 0.3 to 1.5 gm. a day, were given. None of the patients in these studies had physical symptoms of pellagra or any other avitaminosis. A decade later, Hoffer and Osmond [2, 3] initiated two double-blind studies of niacin or niacinamide in the treatment of schizophrenia. Another double-blind study was reported by Denson in 1962 [26]. In 1964 Hoffer and Osmond [4] reported that a 10-year follow-up evaluation of the patients in their initial studies showed that 75 percent had not required hospitalization, compared with 36 percent of the comparison group, who had not received niacin. Similar estimates have been made by Hawkins [18, p. 585]. There are, however, contradictory statements by other investigators. The question of the weight of the evidence is discussed below in the section on the APA task force report.

Pyridoxine

Pyridoxine, vitamin B_6, is used in the treatment of schizophrenia in amounts of 200 to 800 mg. a day by many orthomolecular psychiatrists. Derivatives of this vitamin are known to be the coenzymes for over 50 enzymes, and the chance of a genotype with need for a large intake of the vitamin is accordingly great. There is evidence that pyridoxine is involved in tryptophan-niacin metabolism.

A double-blind placebo-controlled study has been made of pyridoxine and niacin by Ananth, Ban, and Lehmann [27]. Their experimental population consisted of 30 schizophrenic patients: 15 were men, 15 were women, their mean age was 41.7 years, and their mean duration of hospitalization was 10.9 years. They were randomly assigned to three treatment groups: 1) the combined treatment group, which received 3 gm. of nicotinic acid a day for 48 weeks and 75 mg. of pyridoxine a day during three 4-week periods; 2) the nicotinic acid group, which received 3 gm. of nicotinic acid a day for 48 weeks and a pyridoxine placebo; and 3) the pyridoxine group, which received 75 mg. of pyridoxine a day during three 4-week periods and a nicotinic acid placebo. In addition, neuroleptic preparations were administered according to clinical requirements for the control of psychopathology. The investigators reported that "of the ten patients in each treatment group, seven improved and three deteriorated in the nicotinic acid group, nine improved and one deteriorated in both the combined treatment group and in the pyridoxine group" [27]. They also stated:

> Of the three indices of therapeutic effects, global improvement in psychopathology (Brief Psychiatric Rating Scale and Nurses Observation Scale for In-patient .Evaluation) scores was seen in all three groups: the number of days of hospitalization during the period of the clinical study was lower in both the nicotinic acid and the combined treatment group; and only in the combined treatment group was the daily average dosage of phenothiazine medication decreased. Thus, improvement in all three indices was noted in the combined treatment group.
>
> However, several side effects were observed during the therapeutic trials, indicating that the vitamins used are not completely safe [27, p. 381].

The investigators reached the conclusion that "on balance, these results suggest that the addition of pyridoxine may potentiate the action of nicotinic acid. Thus pyridoxine seems to be a useful adjunct to nicotinic acid therapy" [27, p. 381]. Hawkins [18] commented on this work in the following way:

> The therapeutic effect was demonstrable even though the patients had been hospitalized for an average of 10.9 years, were not on hypoglycemic diets, and the doses of both pyridoxine (75 mg. daily) and vitamin B_3 (3 gm. a day) were considerably below the dosages we routinely prescribe [18, p. 638].

Cyanocobalamin

A deficiency in cyanocobalamin (vitamin B_{12}), whatever its cause, leads to mental illness as well as to such physical manifestations as anemia. The anemia can be controlled by a large intake of folic acid, but the mental illness and neurological damage cannot. A pathologically low concentration of cyanocobalamin in the blood serum has been reported to occur in a much larger percentage of patients with mental illness than in the general population. Edwin and associates [28] determined the amount of vitamin B_{12} in the serum of every patient over 30 years old admitted to a mental hospital in Norway during a period of one year. Of the 396 patients, 61 (15.4 percent) had a subnormal or pathologically low concentration of vitamin B_{12}, less than 150 pg. per ml. (the normal range is 150 to 1,300 pg. per ml.). This incidence is 30 times as great as that estimated for the population as a whole. Other investigators have reported similar results and have suggested that a low serum concentration of vitamin B_{12}, whatever its origin, may cause mental illness. In addition, of course, mental illness may accompany some genetic diseases, such as methylmalonic aciduria, which can be controlled only by achieving a serum concentration of cyanocobalamin far greater than normal.

Minerals and Other Vitamins

There is some evidence that mental illness may result from deprivation of or abnormal need for minerals and other vitamins. (See, for example, Pfeiffer, Iliev, and Goldstein [29]). Further work in this field by psychiatrists and biochemists is needed.

THE APA TASK FORCE REPORT

In July 1973 an APA task force of five physicians and one consultant issued a 54-page report titled *Megavitamin and Orthomolecular Therapy in Psychiatry* [30]. In this report the Task Force on Vitamin Therapy in Psychiatry purports to present both theoretical and empirical reasons for completely rejecting the basic concept of orthomolecular psychiatry, which is the achievement and preservation of good mental health by the provision of the optimum molecular environment for the mind, especially the optimum concentrations of substances normally present in the human body.

Some Errors in the Report

It is mentioned in the report that in the treatment program of the orthomolecular psychiatrists "each patient may receive as many as six vitamins in large doses individually determined by the treating physician as well as other psychotropic drugs and hormones whose doses are also individually determined for each patient" (p. 46). The assumption is made by the task force that the optimum intake of vitamins for mental health is the conventional average daily nutritional requirement, with growth and development as the criteria: "In schizophrenia there is apparently an adequate vitamin intake for growth and development until the illness becomes manifest in the teens or early adult life" (p. 40). Mention is made in the report of the well-known genetic diseases with both psychic and somatic manifestations that can be controlled by an intake of a vitamin 100 or 1,000 times the usually recommended daily allowance, but the possibility that less obvious genetic differences could result in an increased individual need for a larger intake of vitamins in order to achieve good mental health, as discussed in my 1968 publication [1] and in the earlier sections of this paper, is rejected on the basis of arguments that have little value or pertinence.

One such argument is the following:

> The two theoretical bases adduced by megavitamin proponents for the effectiveness of NA therapy (nicotinic acid as a methyl acceptor and NAD deficiency) are in fact generally incompatible, because NAA [nicotinamide], when functioning as a vitamin, is bound to the remainder of the coenzyme molecule by the nitrogen of its pyridine ring and hence can no longer accept methyl groups. . . .
>
> Essentially, then, the two views of NA as a vitamin precursor of NAD and as a methyl acceptor are incompatible, except for the possibility that there is in schizophrenia double deficit — both a vitamin deficiency and a transmethylation defect and that nicotinic acid has the happy fortune to serve two purposes simultaneously (pp. 40-42).

There is an obvious error in this task force argument. There is no incompatibility between two functions of nicotinic acid; some molecules may engage in one function and others in the other. A defect in either function might be controlled by increasing the intake of the vital substance. A "double deficit" is not needed. The authors of the report would have seen the fallacy in their argument if they had set up some equilibrium and reaction rate equations, as was done in my 1968 paper [1].

The task force expresses an interesting misunderstanding of the nature of vitamins, in the following words: "By common definition a vitamin is not only an essential nutrient, but it is essential because it is transformed into a coenzyme vital for metabolic reactions" (p. 41). In fact, this is not the common definition of a vitamin; it is wrong. Some vitamins, including vitamin C, are not known to be transformed into a coenzyme. This misunderstanding by the task force may have contributed to the misinterpretation of the evidence for and the theoretical basis of orthomolecular psychiatry.

Nicotinic acid as a methyl acceptor is referred to in the report: "From Study No. 12: nicotinic acid in the dosage of 3000 mg. per day can neither prevent nor counteract the psychopathology induced by the combined administration of a monoamine oxidase inhibitor (tranylcypromine) and methionine" (p. 16). In fact, the molecular weights of nicotinic acid and methionine (a methyl donor) are nearly the same, 123 and 149, respectively. Instead of 3 gm., 16.5 gm. of nicotinic acid would have had to be given each day to accept the methyl groups donated by the 20 gm. of methionine that was given each day. The study referred to as number 12 [31], which resulted in an exacerbation of the illness of 30 schizophrenic patients who participated in it, has no value as a test of the methyl acceptor theory of nicotinic acid. Consideration of ethical principles may have kept the investigators from repeating the study with use of the proper equimolar amounts of nicotinic acid and methionine.

The Failure To Discuss Ascorbic Acid and Pyridoxine

In several places the APA task force report mentions the use of 1 to 30 gm. of ascorbic acid a day by orthomolecular psychiatrists. There are, however, no references to the literature. Milner's double-blind study [25] is not mentioned, nor is there any discussion of the many papers in which a low level of ascorbic acid in the blood of schizophrenics was reported. Neither the general theory of orthomolecular psychiatry, as presented in my 1968 paper [1], nor any of the special arguments about the value of ascorbic acid is presented or discussed in any significant way. There is, moreover, no discussion in the report of pyridoxine and no reference to the 1973 work by Ananth, Ban, and Lehmann [27] on the potentiation by pyridoxine of the effectiveness of niacin in controlling chronic schizophrenia. The title of the report, *Megavitamin and Orthomolecular Therapy in Psychiatry*, is completely inappropriate, and the general condemnation of megavitamin and orthomolecular therapy is unjustified.

Niacin

The report does say that it is possible that the other water-soluble vitamins will prove to be more effective than niacin, but it adds:

Nonetheless, the massive use of niacin has always been the cornerstone of the theory and practice of megavitamin advocates. Since this has proved to have no value when is it employed as the sole variable along with conventional treatments of schizophrenia, the burden of proof for the complex and highly individualized programs now advocated would appear to be on the proponents of such treatment (p. 46).

I shall point out below that the principles of medical ethics prevent orthomolecular psychiatrists from withholding from half of their patients a treatment that they consider to be valuable. Controlled tests can be carried out only by skeptics. I now ask whether the task force is justified in saying that the massive use of niacin has been proved to have no value when it is employed as the sole variable along with conventional treatments of schizophrenia. My answer to this question, from a study of the evidence quoted in the report, is that it is not justified.

The evidence that niacin has no value is far from conclusive. A beneficial effect of niacin or niacinamide was reported for three double-blind studies (two by Hoffer and Osmond and their collaborators [2, 3, 32] and one by Denson [26]) and in 12 open clinical trials by other investigators referred to in the report. On the other hand, the report mentions 7 double-blind studies in which a statistically significant difference between the niacinamide subjects and the controls was not observed.

A failure to reject with statistical significance the null hypothesis that the treatment and the placebo have equal value is not proof that the treatment has no value. The explicit statistical analysis of an alternative hypothesis should be carried out: for example, the hypothesis that there is a 10-percent or 20-percent greater improvement in the treated subjects than in the placebo subjects. No such analysis has been published.

In fact, some of the "negative" studies indicate that the treatment has value. The report states that "Greenbaum [33] reported a double-blind study of 57 schizophrenic children who received nicotinamide 1 gm. per 50 lbs. of body weight or placebo for six months. No statistically significant differences were seen in the two groups as a result of the treatment" (p. 11). It is true that no statistically significant differences were seen, but that is not the whole truth. The principal criterion of improvement in this study was the increase in the score on a clinical scale of observable behavior categories. The average improvement in the score of the 17 children receiving niacinamide was 4.0 units and that of the 24 controls was 2.6 units (there was a third group of 16 children who were given a tranquilizer and niacinamide). The children who were given niacinamide showed a 54-percent greater improvement than the children who were given placebo. The groups were too small, however, for the difference to be significant at the 95-percent level of confidence. This study does not prove that niacinamide has no value. Rather, it indicates that niacinamide has greater value than the placebo, even though it fails to show this at the customary level of statistical significance.

The Hoffer-Osmond Diagnostic Test

Two-thirds of the report relates to niacin, and one-third to the Hoffer-Osmond Diagnostic Test (HOD) [34], which has no special connection with megavitamin or orthomolecular psychiatry except that it was devised by the originators of niacin therapy. The report should have been given the title *Niacin Therapy and the HOD Test,* or published as two reports, one on niacin and one on the HOD test. It would have been still better for the task force to have discussed megavitamin and ortho-molecular therapy in psychiatry fully.

The Question of Controlled Experiments

The report refers to the low credibility of the megavitamin proponents, whose published results were not duplicated in studies carried out by one of the task force members (p. 48). The penultimate sentence of the report is, "Their credibility is further diminished by the consistent refusal over the past decade to perform controlled experiments and to report their new results in a scientifically acceptable fashion" (p. 48).

I have talked with the leading orthomolecular psychiatrists and have found that they feel the principles of medical ethics prevent them from carrying out controlled clinical tests, with half of their patients receiving orthomolecular therapy in addition to the conventional treatment and the other half receiving only the conventional treatment. It is the duty of the physician to give to every one of his patients the treatment that in his best judgment will be of the greatest value. Some psychiatrists, including Hoffer and Osmond, carried out controlled trials 20 years ago. They became convinced that orthomolecular therapy, along with con-ventional treatment, was beneficial to almost every patient. From that time on their ethical principles have required that they give this treatment and not withhold it from half of their patients. The task force is wrong in criticizing the orthomolecular psychia-trists for not having carried out controlled clinical trials during the last few years. Instead, it is the critics, who doubt the value of orthomolecular methods, who are at fault in not having carried out well-designed clinical tests.

It is also the duty of a physician to give to a patient a treatment that may benefit him and is known not to be harmful. The incidences of toxicity and other serious side effects of the doses of vitamins used in orthomolecular medicine are low. There is significant evidence that an increased intake of certain vitamins may benefit the patient. It is accordingly the duty of the psy-chiatrist to prescribe these vitamins for him.

The Bias of the Task Force

The last sentence of the report reads as follows:

> Under these circumstances this Task Force considers the massive publicity which they promulgate via radio, the lay press and popular books, using catch phrases which are really misnomers like "megavitamin therapy" and "orthomolecular treatment," to be deplorable (p. 48).

This sentence, like others in the report, shows the pre-sumably unconscious bias of the task force. "Promulgate" (mis-used here) is a pejorative word, and "catch phrases" is a pejora-tive expression. I do not understand why megavitamin therapy and orthomolecular treatment should be called misnomers. This concluding sentence, like many others in the book, seems to me

to have been written in order to exert an unjustifiably un-favorable influence on the readers of the report.

I have written two popular books, *No More War!* [35] and *Vitamin C and the Common Cold* [24]. I feel that each of them was worthwhile and that neither would have been easily replaced by a more technical book. The second book [24] was written because I had discovered in reading the medical literature that there was much evidence there about the value of ascorbic acid in decreasing both the incidence and the severity of the common cold and that this evidence had been suppressed or misrepre-sented by the medical and nutritional authorities. Since publica-tion of the book, eight new studies have been reported. Every one of these has verified the value of ascorbic acid. The APA report shows the same sort of negative attitude as that shown by the authorities toward ascorbic acid in relation to the common cold. There seems to be a sort of professional inertia that hinders progress.

CONCLUSIONS

Orthomolecular psychiatry is the achievement and preserva-tion of good mental health by the provision of the optimum molecular environment for the mind, especially the optimum con-centrations of substances normally present in the human body, such as the vitamins. There is evidence that an increased intake of some vitamins, including ascorbic acid, niacin, pyridoxine, and cyanocobalamin, is useful in treating schizophrenia, and this treatment has a sound theoretical basis. The APA task force report *Megavitamin and Orthomolecular Therapy in Psychiatry* discusses vitamins in a very limited way (niacin only) and deals with only one or two aspects of the theory. Its arguments are in part faulty and its conclusions are unjustified.

REFERENCES

1. Pauling, L.: Orthomolecular psychiatry. Science 160: 265-271, 1968
2. Hoffer, A.: Niacin Therapy in Schizophrenia. Springfield, Ill., Charles C. Thomas, 1962
3. Osmond, H., Hoffer A.: Massive niacin treatment in schizo-phrenia: review of a nine-year study. Lancet 1:316-319, 1962
4. Hoffer, A., Osmond H.: Treatment of schizophrenia with nicotinic acid: a ten-year follow-up. Acta Psychiatr Scand 40:171-189, 1964
5. Cleckley, H.M., Sydenstricker, V.P., Geeslin, L.E.: Nicotinic acid in treatment of atypical psychotic states associated with malnutrition. JAMA 112:2107-2110, 1939
6. Sydenstricker, V.P., Cleckley, H.M.: The effect of nicotinic acid in stupor, lethargy and various other psychiatric dis-orders. Am J Psychiatry 98:83-92, 1941
7. Kubala, A.L., Katz, M.M.: Nutritional factors in psycho-logical test behavior. J Genet Psychol 96:343-352, 1960
8. VanderKamp, H: A biochemical abnormality in schizo-phrenia involving ascorbic acid. Int J Neuropsychiatry 2:204-206, 1966
9. Herjanic, M., Moss-Herjanic, B.L.: Ascorbic acid test in psychiatric patients. J Schizophrenia 1:257-260, 1967

10. Pauling, L., Robinson, A.B., Oxley S.S., et al: Results of a loading test of ascorbic acid, niacinamide, and pyridoxine in schizophrenic subjects and controls, in Orthomolecular Psychiatry: Treatment of Schizophrenia. Edited by Hawkins, D., Pauling, L. San Francisco, W.H. Freeman and Co., 1973, pp 18-34

11. Orsenberg, L.E., Lilljeqvist, A-C., Hsia, Y.E.: Methylmalonic aciduria: metabolic block localization and vitamin B_{12} dependency. Science 162:805-807, 1968

12. Lindblad, B., Olin, P., Svanberg, B., et al: Methylmalonic acidemia. Acta Paediatr Scand 57:417-424, 1968

13. Walker, F.A., Agarwal, A.B., Singh, R.: Methylmalonic aciduria: response to oral B_{12} therapy. J Pediatr 75:344, 1969

14. Rosenberg, L.E., Lilljeqvist, A-C., Hsia, Y.E., et al: Vitamin B_{12} dependent methylmalonicaciduria: defective B_{12} metabolism in cultured fibroblasts. Biochem Biophys Res Commun 37:607-614, 1969

15. Williams, R.J.: Biochemical Individuality. New York, John Wiley & Sons, 1957

16. Pauling, L., Itano, H.A., Singer, S.J., et al: Sickle cell anemia, a molecular disease. Science 110:543-548, 1949

17. Hawkins, D., Pauling, L. (eds): Orthomolecular Psychiatry: Treatment of Schizophrenia. San Francisco, W.H. Freeman and Co., 1973

18. Hawkins, D.: Orthomolecular psychiatry: treatment of schizophrenia. Ibid, pp. 631-673

19. Osmond, H.: The background to the niacin treatment. Ibid, pp. 194-201

20. Horwitt, M.K.: Ascorbic acid requirements of individuals in a large institution. Proc Soc Exp Biol Med 49:248-250, 1942

21. Herjanic, M.: Ascorbic acid and schizophrenia, in Orthomolecular Psychiatry: Treatment of Schizophrenia. Edited by Hawkins, D., Pauling, L. San Francisco, W.H. Freeman and Co., 1973, pp. 303-315

22. Stone, I.: The Healing Factor: Vitamin C Against Disease. New York. Grosset and Dunlap, 1972

23. Pauling, L.: Evolution and the need for ascorbic acid. Proc Natl Acad Sci USA 67:1643-1648, 1970

24. Pauling, L.: Vitamin C and the Common Cold. San Francisco. W.H. Freeman and Co. 1970

25. Milner, G.: Ascorbic acid in chronic psychiatric patients: a controlled trial. Br J Psychiatry 109:294-299, 1963

26. Denson, R.: Nicotinamide in the treatment of schizophrenia. Dis Nerv Syst 23:167-172, 1962

27. Ananth, J.V., Ban, T.A., Lehmann, H.E.: Potentiation of therapeutic effects of nicotinic acid by pyridoxine in chronic schizophrenics. Can Psychiatr Assoc J 18:377-382, 1973

28. Edwin, E., Holten, K., Norum, K.R., et al: Vitamin B_{12} hypovitaminosis in mental diseases. Acta Med Scand 177:689-699, 1965

29. Pfeiffer, C.C., Iliev, V., Goldstein, L.: Blood histamine, basophil counts, and trace elements in the schizophrenias, in Orthomolecular Psychiatry: Treatment of Schizophrenia. Edited by Hawkins, D., Pauling, L. San Francisco. W.H. Freeman and Co. 1973. pp. 463-510

30. Task Force Report 7: Megavitamin and Orthomolecular Therapy in Psychiatry. Washington, DC, American Psychiatric Association, 1973

31. Ananth, J.V., Ban, T.A., Lehmann, H.E., et al: Nicotinic acid in the prevention and treatment of methionine-induced exacerbation of psychopathology in schizophrenics. Can Psychiatr Assoc J 15:15-20, 1970

32. Hoffer, A., Osmond, H., Callbeck, J.M., et al: Treatment of schizophrenia with nicotinic acid and nicotinamide. J Clin Exp Psychopathol 18:131-158. 1957

33. Greenbaum, G.H.C.: An evaluation of niacinamide in the treatment of childhood schizophrenia. Am J Psychiatry 127:89-93, 1970

34. Kelm, H.: The Hoffer-Osmond Diagnostic Test (HOD), in Orthomolecular Psychiatry: Treatment of Schizophrenia. Edited by Hawkins, D., Pauling, L. San Francisco. W.H. Freeman and Co. 1973, pp. 327-341

35. Pauling, L.: No More War! New York. Dodd, Mead and Co. 1958

16
Treatment of Schizophrenia*

A. HOFFER

SCHIZOPHRENIA SYNDROME

One of the major advances in the practice of medicine occurred when physicians realized that combinations of a few symptoms and signs pointed toward a single disease or condition. This constellation of complaints and observations is called a syndrome. The syndrome may result from a small number of causes. Its recognition leads to more accurate diagnosis and treatment. Individual symptoms on the other hand may be caused by a variety of conditions.

As long as symptomatic treatment only is available it is impossible to use treatment directed against the cause of the disease. For example, fatigue is almost an ubiquitous symptom of many diseases. It is therefore impossible to order specific treatment for fatigue.

Increased hunger and thirst as symptoms are not any more helpful in determining treatment. If, however, these are associated with weight loss and with increased excretion of urine, one will suspect diabetes. This combination leads to an investigation of carbohydrate metabolism, e.g., sugar-tolerance tests, urine tests for sugar and acetone. Thus diabetes is diagnosed or excluded and specific treatment is provided.

Syndromes are also useful in psychiatric diagnosis. In the same way they do not pinpoint the cause of the syndrome but will narrow the search for causes. Generally syndromes refer to organ dysfunctions or to metabolic diseases. Psychiatric syndromes point to different forms of cerebral disturbances. I consider every psychiatric disease a manifestation of a cerebral disorder. Psychiatry, then, is that branch of medicine which deals with cerebral disorders which cause changes in perceiving, thinking, feeling, and behaving. In the same way a liver disorder may produce jaundice, fever, loss of appetite, and colored pigments in the urine, while a lung disorder may produce shortness of breath, coughing, sputum.

Schizophrenia is a syndrome of a brain disorder of a particular kind. This was recognized several hundred years ago, especially and most clearly by Conolly (1830) who defined insanity as a disorder of perception combined with an inability to judge whether the misperceptions are real or not. This leads to

bizarre or strange behavior. Conolly recognized the three main aspects of brain function, perception, thinking, and behavior.

The brain is an organ which perceives, thinks (including memory), feels, and orders behavior. When its metabolism is disordered, this is expressed by changes in perception of one or more of the senses (illusions and hallucinations) in thinking, in mood, and in behavior. The basic changes which produce the schizophrenic syndrome are changes in perception and in thought. Arising from these primary changes (in a sequential sense) are the secondary changes in mood and behavior.

There are other syndromes which are not schizophrenic. If the main changes are in mood with no changes in perception and thinking, the diagnosis is depression for which there may be several reasons. If the schizophrenic syndrome is accompanied by signs of mental confusion such as disorientation and severe memory loss, the syndrome is said to be an organic confusional state.

As medical diagnosis is clinically never as sharp and precise as one would like, it may be difficult to distinguish between these syndromes if the symptoms and signs are vague as they sometimes are.

Diagnosing this syndrome is usually fairly easy provided the clinician is aware of the importance of perceptual changes and is not afraid to diagnose schizophrenia. Why should any psychiatrist fear schizophrenia? Because for most psychiatrists it carries a very pessimistic prognosis since with standard treatment (tranquilizers) very few patients recover. Very often a recovery immediately throws into doubt the diagnosis of schizophrenia for these clinicians. The diagnosis depends upon a very careful mental examination for the presence of illusions, hallucinations, and thought disorder (content or process or both). This may be done by the usual discussion interview between patient and doctor, or by the use of rapid perceptual tests such as the HOD test (Kelm, Hoffer, and Osmond, 1967), EWI (El-Meligi and Osmond, 1970), and the Green test (1970) for subclinical pellagra. These tests are the best available for detecting the cerebral functions disordered by metabolic faults. A physician with these tests is a better diagnostician than a psychiatrist who does not use them. However, all they do is confirm the diagnosis of the schizophrenic syndrome. They do not tell us the nature of the disorder. For this a different type of test, usually biochemical, is required.

Over the past 80 years various kinds of cerebral disturbances

*Reprinted with permission: *Orthomolecular Psychiatry*, Vol. 3, No. 4, 1974, 280-290.

have been described. About 1910 the main diagnostic problem in mental hospitals was to distinguish between general paresis of the insane (GPI), pellagra, scurvy, and dementia praecox (schizophrenia). When the causes of GPI, scurvy, and pellagra were discovered and treatment developed, these three schizophrenic syndromes disappeared from psychiatry. They fell into the domain of neurologists and nutritionists (M.D.'s). Unfortunately for psychiatry, each schizophrenic syndrome for which a cause is discovered is taken away as rational treatment develops. It seems as if only syndromes of unknown origin and useless treatment remain within the grasp of psychiatrists. Perhaps this is why there has been a general attitude of doom and gloom in psychiatry for the past 100 years, interrupted briefly by flashes of optimism when newer treatments developed. The tranquilizer era was characterized by a hypomanic euphoria, as was the advent of psychoanalysis into North America over 20 years ago. The tranquilizer euphoria is slowly settling down into the usual pessimism of psychiatrists when they are forced to recognize the schizophrenic syndrome.

Another schizophrenic syndrome taken from us is phenylpyruvic oligophrenia (PKU). This was first identified among a group of chronic schizophrenic patients by a characteristic urinary change. It is today treated by pediatricians, and only their failures eventually come under the care of psychiatrists, especially those specializing in retardation. Down's syndrome was excluded from the syndrome because of its appearance in infancy and because of the characteristic facial changes, not because of clear-cut differences in the mental state. They may have the characteristic schizophrenic syndrome.

Schizophrenic syndromes may also be produced by a variety of chemicals such as atropine (belladona), the amphetamines, other stimulant drugs, and the hallucinogens. These syndromes still are treated by psychiatrists, but there is a trend away from psychiatry as general practitioners become more knowledgeable about these syndromes. Thus at City Hospital, Emergency Department, Saskatoon, patients whose schizophrenic syndrome results from LSD intoxication are often treated by the interns on duty by the intravenous injection of 100 mg or more of nicotinic acid, and there is no need to request a psychiatric consultation.

However, the majority of schizophrenic patients are considered to be ill because of a functional disturbance with no known cause. The term functional originally applied to the psychosocial environment, but more recently there is a growing awareness of the fact that psychosocial factors shape and are caused by the illness and are not its cause.

I have divided these syndromes of "unknown" cause into three major groups: 1. the vitamin dependencies, 2. the cerebral allergies, and 3. those of unknown origin. I suspect that group three is a rather small group. I will therefore discuss the treatment of the dependencies and the allergies. This discussion will be rather general and brief since the details of megavitamin, mineral, nutritional, and allergy therapy will be discussed in other presentations.

TREATMENT

The Vitamin Dependencies

Vitamins are organic molecules which form components of enzymes. These catalyze the reactions in the body by which food is broken down into its basic units and which are used to construct those molecules required for structural purposes and for the production of energy. Nearly every chemical reaction requires a catalyst. They are required in rather small quantities since the same molecule can be used over and over. The majority of people probably have requirements for every vitamin which can be expressed by the usual bell-shaped curve so common for all biological phenomena, i.e., 95 percent of the population will have optimum vitamin requirements which fall within two standard deviations of the mean. About $2\frac{1}{2}$ percent will require more. But each vitamin will have its own distribution frequency. An individual may require more of one vitamin and have normal requirements of the others.

The reasons why individuals require much more than the average is not known, but it is likely there are a number of factors lying between the vitamins in the food and their delivery to the cells of the body. If a person with average requirements for any vitamin lives on a diet which contains less than his requirement, he will in time develop a deficiency state which may produce a characteristic syndrome such as scurvy, beri beri, or pellagra, or a generalized state of ill health with no characteristic syndrome, such as a vitamin E deficiency. The error is in the diet and not in the person. The deficiency states are the ones recognized by nutritionists.

If a person has an above-average requirement for a vitamin and consumes a diet which provides only average amounts, he will also develop a deficiency state which is just as real as the other deficiency. There is a relative deficiency. It has been called a dependency. The problem is in the person and not in the diet. Over a dozen dependencies have been described for pyridoxine and for vitamin B_{12}. It is likely that for each vitamin some patients will be found who have a dependency for that vitamin. There is an enormous range of variation ranging from 10 mg of vitamin B_3 for many people to 3,000 mg per day for a few. Anyone who has followed the work of Roger Williams (1971), L. Pauling (1968), F. Klenner (1973), and others cannot doubt that there is a very wide range of need for vitamins.

The reasons for the range in need are unknown, but there is some evidence that at least for vitamin B_3 a prolonged deficiency can lead to permanent dependency. In the mid-thirties it became known that for dogs maintained on pellagra-producing diet, for a long time thereafter megadoses of vitamin B_3 were required to keep them free of pellagra. The early pellagrologists were amazed to find that some adult pellagrins required maintenance doses of 600 mg of vitamin B_3 to keep them free of pellagra, a dose 60 times as high as that considered necessary by many nutritionists to prevent pellagra. A third line of evidence comes from prisoners-of-war. Maintained on starvation diets for 44 months, Canadian soldiers kept in Japanese prison camps in Hong Kong suffered from a variety of avitaminoses. These soldiers have remained physically and mentally ill since then (Richardson, 1964). The exceptions are a group of a dozen veterans, all as ill as the rest, who have been taking nicotinic acid, 3 grams per day, and have been well since. One patient, G.P., has been on this dose since 1960 and has been well the whole time with the exception of a two-week period in 1962 when he went on a holiday and forgot to take his nicotinic acid with him.

Patients who are vitamin dependent may have difficulty absorbing vitamins. Several schizophrenics who did not respond well to large oral doses of nicotinic acid have shown much better responses to the parenteral administrations of much lower quantities. I have suggested that schizophrenia is a vitamin B_3 dependency (Hoffer and Osmond, 1966). A more accurate statement is that a proportion of schizophrenics are vitamin B_3 dependent, that is vitamin B_3 dependency is a cause of the schizophrenic syndrome. I believe that the majority of schizophrenics fall into this category, but an accurate estimate is not possible. However, it is clear that a substantial number of schizophrenics are vitamin B_6 dependent, i.e., vitamin B_6 dependency is a cause of some schizophrenic syndromes. Vitamin B_3 and B_6 dependency ought to be very similar clinically since both are involved in the production of nicotinamide adenine dinucleotide (NAD), the active enzyme made from vitamin B_3. Vitamin B_3 is a precursor, and vitamin B_6 is required for the transformation of tryptophan into NAD. The absence of pyridoxine produces pellagra, as does the deficiency of vitamin B_3. A few patients may be both vitamin B_3 and vitamin B_6 dependent.

Treatment of course will be different. This illustrates once more that identity in the clinical syndrome does not accurately determine treatment.

Vitamin B_{12}-dependent states have been described where 1,000 times the usual daily requirement is needed. Newbold (1972) found several schizophrenics who were low in vitamin $B_{12}b$ and responded well to injections of vitamin $B_{12}b$. Kotkas (1972) has been using large quantities of both folic acid and vitamin B_{12} for his patients.

(1) *The vitamin B_3 dependencies.* These produce the schizophrenic syndrome and allied conditions. Treatment therefore must depend upon megadoses of either nicotinic acid or nicotinamide, but other vitamin supplements may be required.

Because of the variability of the syndrome it is impossible to prescribe the same treatment for every patient. To the normal variability between individuals one must add the effect of the disease, its duration, previous treatment, and so on. Therefore it seems more efficient to start with a general program of treatment shown by past experience to be most helpful to the largest number of patients. Patients who respond will require minor changes in therapy as they improve, while more complicated programs will be required for the treatment failures.

I therefore divide my patients into phases for which there is a particular treatment. Phase One treatment is given Phase One patients. Phase Two patients are Phase One treatment failures or failures from other programs. They require more vigorous treatment, usually in hospital. Phase One treatment given Phase Two patients is generally futile. Unfortunately all the so-called "controlled" studies by nonorthomolecular physicians have made no attempt to match treatment and patients. They should not have been surprised they did not find the same therapeutic response as do orthomolecular physicians. They have ignored this serious criticism of their work and have erroneously claimed vitamin B_3 was ineffective for the treatment of schizophrenia. The worst offenders have been Dr. Ban and his colleagues who were asked by the Canadian Mental Health Association to disprove the claims that vitamin B_3 therapy was efficacious for some schizophrenic syndromes.

Phase One

Phase One patients are acute schizophrenics ill one year or less or are subacute, i.e., have suffered one or more relapses from which they have recovered or have greatly improved. They are able to cooperate or have families who can insure their cooperation. They seldom need to be in hospital. Sometimes chronic mild schizophrenics highly motivated to get well will respond to Phase One treatment. The acute patients are generally the ones most likely to recover spontaneously. The natural remission rate is believed to be about 35 percent. I am increasingly doubtful this is correct, because I have seen a number of such patients said to have recovered from a schizophrenic illness. They consulted me up to 20 years later. During this period, when considered by hospital records to be normal, they suffered from periodic episodes of depression, tension, paranoid ideas and illusions, and so on. But they did not re-experience hallucinations, and their behavior remained within socially acceptable limits. They had not been well, they did not consider they were well nor did their families. Yet in the follow-up statistics they were recorded as recovered.

1. Supernutrition — This is basic. The no-junk diet will generally provide this. Junk food is any food adulterated with sucrose, starch, or white flour. The standard diet for relative hypoglycemia is good, but patients who are allergic to dairy products or meat should be cautioned either to avoid these foods or not to increase their consumption. One of my patients became much worse on this diet, because he greatly increased his consumption of beef to which he was found to be allergic. Any food which the patient likes excessively or loathes should be suspect.

2. Vitamin B_3 — Nicotinic acid and nicotinamide, both forms of vitamin B_3, are precursors of NAD. The dose range of nicotinamide is 3-6 gm per day. Higher doses may cause nausea and vomiting. The dose range for nicotinic acid is usually 3 gm per day and up. Generally patients can go much higher before developing nausea. The correct dose is that dose which will yield improvement and will not produce unpleasant or dangerous side effects. Dr. Ross (this meeting) describes the details of the use of vitamin B_3.

3. Other vitamins — Patients may require ascorbic acid to decrease the frequency of colds and infections, or any of the other vitamins such as pyridoxine, thiamine, pantothenic acid, folic acid, vitamin B_{12}, vitamin E, and vitamins A and D. For each nutrient the optimum dose must be used. There are as yet few firm indications for these vitamins. The few indications which suggest the specific vitamin are:

thiamine: depression.

riboflavin: visual problems, lesions at the corner of the mouth.

Pyridoxine: pyroluria (malvaria), allergy, hyperactive behavior, convulsions, malabsorption (a flat curve on five-hour glucose-tolerance curve, Silverman, 1974).

vitamin E: cardiovascular and peripheral vascular problems, aging.

pantothenic acid: general fatigue, allergies.

vitamins A and D: allergies.

4. Tranquilizers, antidepressants, and other standard drugs are used as indicated in optimum doses. The dose is decreased as the patients begin to recover. Generally lower dosages are required so that fewer troublesome side effects and toxicities are encountered.

5. Duration of treatment. Phase One treatment is continued as long as patients continue to improve. Patients should be started on Phase Two therapy if they have reached an unsatisfactory

Table 1. Summary of Treatment Phases

	Patients	Treatment	Duration	Results
Phase One	Sick less than one year, cooperative	Supernutrition Megavitamins Minerals Drugs	Up to 2 years	About 75% recovery
Phase Two	Sick longer than one year, unable to cooperate	As above plus ECT	Up to 3 years	About 50% out of Phase Two
Phase Three	Chronic	As described	Up to 5	About 50% out of Phase Three

plateau of improvement or if they have not improved. How long one will wait depends upon clinical judgment but it may range from one to 12 months.

Phase Two

Phase Two patients have not responded to Phase One treatment, or have been continually ill for more than one year. They are also patients too sick to cooperate with treatment at home because they are suicidal, homicidal, or engage in behavior impossible to cope with by their family or community. They usually must be treated in hospital. The main difference between Phases Two and One is that they are now given a series of electroconvulsive treatment (ECT) which may be unilateral for less severely ill or bilateral for chronic patients or a mixture of both. The series varies from about five to 15. The number is determined by the clinical response. The chemotherapy started in Phase One is continued, but generally larger doses of vitamins are given and parenteral administrations are used more frequently.

After the series of ECT is completed, the patient is kept in hospital until memory has been restored to a level compatible with living in the community; usually about five to nine days are required. On megadoses of vitamins there is much less confusion and memory loss. Patients may now continue to improve until they are well.

Phase Three

These are patients who have failed to respond to Phase Two treatment. It also includes patients who have been sick for many years. The prognosis of this group varies. It is best for chronic patients who have not been kept in mental hospitals for many years and is poorest for those who have.

These patients will require a good deal of support whether or not they recover for it is not easy to regain one's way in life after many years of illness. The prolonged illness and treatment creates problems, attitudes, and habits that are difficult to eradicate even if the schizophrenic syndrome should be immediately removed.

Phase Three patients may be given the following treatments:

(a) penicillamine usually combined with another series of ECT. The dose is ½ to 1 gm per day for up to 30 days.

(b) several series of ECT at intervals of one-half to two years. Each series raises the patient to a higher plateau of recovery.

(c) any new treatment which has been helpful for some patients provided that it will not harm the patient.

It has become clear over the past two years that a major proportion of the Phase Three patients are schizophrenic syn-

dromes caused by cerebral allergies. This is why they have not responded to any chemotherapy. Megadoses of some vitamins have anti-allergy properties, but it is obvious that patients who are continually exposed to an offending food or other allergen cannot become well until the allergenic food or chemical is removed from them. A quick summary of the three phases is shown in Table 1.

(2) *The vitamin B_6 dependencies.* Irvine (1961) and Hoffer and Mahon (1961) reported that a substance which stained mauve in color in paper chromatogram occurred more frequently in psychiatric patients, especially schizophrenics, than in any control population. Hoffer and Osmond (1961) compared subjects who excreted this mauve factor against controls using clinical description, the HOD test, response to treatment, and concluded that the mauve-factor excretors resembled schizophrenics more than any other diagnostic syndrome. Malvaria was suggested as the name for this new schizophrenic syndrome.

Recently Irvine, Bayne, and Miyashita (1969) identified mauve factor as kryptopyrrole (KP). It is a very toxic pyrrole. Pfeiffer (1972) and his colleagues have shown that KP binds pyridoxine and when present in excess must produce an increased need for pyridoxine, i.e., a pyridoxine dependency. Patients with too much KP or over 20 ug per 100 ml must therefore be given megadoses of pyridoxine or up to several grams per day. Pfeiffer recommends that extra quantities of zinc and manganese ions should be given along with pyridoxine. For these vitamin B_6-dependent schizophrenic syndromes vitamin B_6 must be considered the primary vitamin.

As I have stated earlier, both vitamin B_6 and vitamin B_3 are related to NAD. It is therefore not surprising that vitamin B_3 will also be therapeutic for the pyridoxine-dependent syndromes. However, there will be patients who recover on vitamin B_6 alone. Pfeiffer has suggested that KP-positive patients be called pyrolurias. This is a sensible recommendation and should replace malvaria as a diagnostic term. Fortunately his description of the treatment of this condition is presented in this volume.

SCHIZOPHRENIC SYNDROMES RESULTING FROM CEREBRAL ALLERGIES

Randolph (1961, 1966, 1970) used the technique developed by Rinkel (1944) for diagnosing cerebral allergies on the basis of personal experience with 500 patients. Randolph concluded: (1) any food can produce a cerebral reaction, (2) multiple-food

Relation Between Effect of Allergogenic Food and Depth of Hangover

Pick Up Intensity	Hangover
1. Active, buoyant, alert, stimulated.	A. Sniffly, itchy, queasy, absentminded, tired.
2. Hyperactive, keyed up, energetic, irritable.	B. Wheezy, rash, cramps, brain fogged, aches, puffy.
3. Jittery, argumentative, aggressive, drunk-like.	C. Confused, indecisive, morose, lethargic.
4. Uncontrollably excited, agitated, maniacal.	D. Depressed, stuporous, disoriented, amnesic.

susceptibility is the rule, (3) usually foods consumed every three days are involved, (4) other chemicals in the environment, such as insecticides, hydrocarbons, sprays, perfumes, and so on, can produce similar reactions, (5) these cerebral reactions are often labeled neurotic or emotional. Randolph called these psychiatric reactions ecologic mental diseases. This work has been propelled into psychiatry by Rees (1973), Newbold et al. (1973).

Fortunately Dr. Philpott, Dr. Green and Dr. Glaisher will describe in detail the vast importance of the cerebral allergies in the production of psychiatric diseases.

Randolph has outlined a clear relationship between the effect of foods to which a subject is allergic (allergogenic) and the intensity of the response. Randolph suggests that we have not only an allergic reaction, but an addiction. The reaction which comes on when the offending food is not available is the withdrawal or hangover effect. His scheme is shown above.

Intensity levels 2 and 3 describe the hyperactive syndrome in children, and level 4 well describes mania whether it is a manic-depressive or schizophrenic mania. Levels C and D are rarely recognized as cerebral allergies. Patients' clinical condition will vary from intensity level 1 to 4 and from A to D in the hangover level. Randolph concluded, "any mental or behavioral aberration in which causation has not been demonstrated deserves to be investigated from the ecologic standpoint." Crook (1970) listed the following symptoms which were present in patients with allergies, unreality, depression, bizarre and irrational behavior, nervous tics, and inability to concentrate. Crook concluded "The net result of this hyper group of symptoms is to make the unfortunate youngsters who manifest them definitely unpleasant little people to have around. They are apt to be reprimanded and punished by parents and teachers and rejected or ignored by their siblings and contemporaries."

The schizophrenic syndrome caused by cerebral allergy is not unique clinically. There is no way of distinguishing cerebral allergy by an examination of the mental state. From the 40 or so cases I have diagnosed there seems to be two clinical differences:

1. The cerebral allergies have a fluctuating course, their history is characterized by a series of recoveries or improvement followed by severe relapses in a few weeks or months. The chronic schizophrenics who did not respond to a four-day fast or to elimination diets were unremitting schizophrenics who had never experienced any significant recovery. On Phase Three therapy they improve slowly and may require many years of treatment.

2. The cerebral allergic patients generally have more insight, are more cooperative to treatment while the other schizophrenics more often show the typical lack of insight or schizophrenic thought disorder which can be so puzzling to everyone.

The cerebral allergies are diagnosed by several tests:

1. The usual epidermal challenge tests which may be surface penetration, or intradermal, are generally unreliable for foods but are very accurate for nonfood allergins such as pollens, dusts, fumes, etc.

2. Serological tests have been used by Ulett and Itil (1973).

3. A period of fasting from four to seven days. This may or may not be accompanied by treatment with laxatives and enemas to increase the elimination of food from the intestines. This is followed by introduction of single foods. If the patient is allergic he will respond by quickly developing his basic symptomatology, by an elevation of pulse rate, or by severe physical symptoms. Thus several patients who had become free from nearly continuous hallucinations by a fast suffered a resurgence of hallucinations within an hour of eating the allergogenic food, usually milk. One patient also developed violent abdominal cramps and severe diarrhea, another developed a skin rash.

A few patients were very much improved following a four-day fast even though they did not develop any reaction to any food thereafter. It seems as if the four-day fast may have some therapeutic value independent of allergies.

4. Elimination diets.

5. Rotation diets.

6. Provocative test. These are described by Philpott, Green, and Glaisher at this meeting.

Treatment of cerebral allergies must include the elimination of the allergogenic foods and chemicals for many months or years. They may then be introduced in small quantities on a rotation basis but may never be compatible with the person. (I am now investigating the desensitization procedure developed by Dr. I. Glaisher which may allow the use of small quantities of foods to which the patient is allergic.)

Rees (1974) suggested that rigid rotation diets may be harmful for some people if the offending food is used since each consumption of that food reinforces the allergic reaction. She suggested instead that the offending food not be used at all and that the rest of the diet should depend upon as wide a variety of foods as possible consumed in small quantities and in a random fashion.

Some of the vitamins in megadoses appear to have anti-allergy properties. So many are involved it appears as if any nutritional imbalance can sensitize people toward allergies. Two commonly used chemicals, alcohol and sucrose (table sugar), seem to have remarkable properties for inducing or aggravating allergies.

Many patients who go onto a sugar-free diet promptly lose their allergies to a variety of foods. Ulett and Itil (1973) have suggested that alcohol acts as a carrier for cereal grain-derived proteins and so increases the likelihood of producing allergies. The common alcoholic beverages are therefore very efficient in producing allergies (addictions).

The vitamins which appear to have anti-allergic properties include: (1) Nicotinic acid which releases histamine and heparin from most cells and decreases the concentration of these substances in the body. Since allergic-shock reactions depend upon massive release of histamine, a subject on nicotinic acid will suffer much less. There is less histamine stored and able to be released. (2) Ascorbic acid will combine with histamine and detoxify it. Large doses must be used. (3) Vitamins A and D as used by Reich (1971). (4) Calcium pantothenate appears to reduce intensity of allergic reactions. (5) Pangamic acid has anti-asthma properties according to Cott (1974). Pyridoxine also has anti-allergy properties, perhaps because it improves malabsorption.

However, it is illogical to expect these substances to cure allergies. They are very helpful in controlling minor allergic reactions provided that the major offenders are removed from our internal environment.

RESULTS OF TREATMENT

Over the years I have accumulated a number of megavitamin failures — patients who have not responded permanently to any treatment ever given them. Over the past four months I have treated about 60 of these failures with the four-day fast. Over 40 were normal by the fifth morning. When the offending food was given them they promptly relapsed. They are now well as long as they keep away from the offending food. Most of them no longer require any medication, including vitamins. Out of the responsive group, 75 percent were allergic to dairy products. Two were allergic to both beef and milk products. These two were chronic relapsing schizophrenics, both ill over 20 years and with at least 20 admissions to mental hospitals or psychiatric wards. One was allergic to smoking. I found very few cereal grain allergies, in contrast to Philpott whose population of patients included many cereal grain allergies. Perhaps this is due to different feeding habits of these different areas.

In addition I have placed a large number of patients on dairy-free diets, and many of them have been promptly freed of depression, tension, fatigue, and so on.

A couple of case histories will illustrate these recoveries. Mrs. G.C., age 21, was admitted to hospital June, 1971, as an emergency. She complained that her body seemed strange. As a child she was shy and passive and described herself as neurotic. After puberty she forced herself to be more outgoing, but was irritable and easily upset. In 1969 she began to use hallucinogenic drugs each week, but after one year took no more. She then began to feel strange and became very depressed. Her first child was born 3½ months before I saw her. During her pregnancy she felt normal. Mental state showed visual illusions, voices, and she heard her own and her husband's thoughts. She was very paranoid and believed her husband was poisoning her food. She complained of ideas of killing her baby and husband. She was very depressed, nervous, and tired. I diagnosed her as an acute schizophrenic and gave her Phase Two treatment.

After six ECT and megavitamin therapy she improved. She improved substantially. From then on she was on the whole megavitamin approach with vitamin B₃, ascorbic acid, thiamine, and pyridoxine. She also took antidepressants, tranquilizers, and lithium as required. But at no time did she recover and stay well more than a few weeks. She required nine ECT in June, 1972. She began to improve and by June, 1973, was nearly normal. The summer of 1973 she remained well, but in the fall her depression began to return. By February, 1974, she was withdrawing more

and more. She had developed unpleasant nausea from her nicotinic acid and November, 1973, was started on 1 gram per day of a slow-release preparation.

On March 1, 1974, I found her extremely depressed, suicidal, and ideas she would have to kill her baby. I promptly admitted her to hospital. The next day she started a four-day fast. On the evening of the fourth day she was normal. The fifth morning she had a severe relapse half an hour after one glass of milk. Later she was found allergic to peanuts. Since then she has been well and requires no medication. I have advised her her schizophrenic syndrome was caused by a cerebral allergy.

A second patient, age 19, under treatment four years, was on the entire orthomolecular program including several series of ECT. Her perceptual symptoms and thought disorder cleared, but she remained tense and depressed. May 13 she started a four-day fast and four days later was normal. Milk produced a rapid relapse. She is now normal on a dairy-free program.

My last example illustrates an aspirin allergy. The patient, age 54, had recently been discharged from a hospital in Eastern Canada. This was her third admission in three years. She fled from her husband because of her paranoid ideas about him to live with her sister in Saskatoon. A few days later I saw her. She complained of voices which told her her husband was unfaithful, which made fun of her. She was convinced her husband was plotting to get rid of her and had hired someone to follow her and was depressed.

At the end of a four-day fast she was normal. On returning to food there was no relapse, but on the second evening she had a mild headache and took two aspirins. Within the hour she had relapsed. Her hallucinations returned within 15 minutes. Then it turned out she had been using aspirins for four years to control pain in her hip. One week after I saw her she returned to her husband well. She required no medication and has remained normal.

DISCUSSION

The discovery of the schizophrenic syndrome due to cerebral allergy clarifies an important issue not only in treatment but for research. A substantial proportion of my megavitamin failures were cerebral allergic. They were also the kind of patient who used to comprise a large proportion of chronic patients in mental hospitals and still do make up a large proportion of the chronic nonresponders. These patients had also failed to respond to standard tranquilizer and antidepressant chemotherapy. These are the patients most accessible for research, and they have been used heavily for nearly all biochemical studies. Since this is a mixed population composed of schizophrenic syndromes due to a variety of causes, it is no wonder it has been so difficult to find significant differences between them and control groups. Our malvaria studies showed clearly that the highest proportion of malvarians occurred in the acute and subacute populations, while chronic patients seldom had kryptopyrrole in their urine.

One can therefore no longer reason from these studies of the past unless the groups have been clearly described and separated. The same applies to clinical studies. Treatments which work well for acute and subacute cases, which are mainly the vitamin-dependency group, will not do as well for chronic groups with a heavy loading of cerebral allergics. They will require different treatment.

CONCLUSION

Orthomolecular psychiatry uses a broad-spectrum approach to treatment which gives proper consideration to supernutrition, to vitamins up to megadoses, to optimum mineral metabolism, and to the cerebral allergies. This rational approach is aided when necessary by temporary use of tranquilizers, antidepressants, anti-anxiety, and other chemotherapeutic substances used by standard psychiatric practitioners.

REFERENCES

Conolly, J.: Indications of Insanity. Reprinted 1964 by Dawsons of Pall Mall, London, 1830.

Cott, A.: Preliminary Report on Vit. B_{15}. Academy of Orthomolecular Psychiatry, Detroit, 1974.

Crook, W.G.: The Allergic Tension Fatigue Syndrome, Allergy of the Nervous System. Ed. Speer, F., C.C. Thomas, Springfield, Ill., 1970.

El-Meligi, M., and Osmond, H.: E.W.I., Manual for the Clinical use of the Experiential World Inventory. Mens Sana Publishing Co., New York, 1970.

Green, R.G.: Subclinical Pellagra (its diagnosis and treatment). Schizophrenia 2, 70, 1970.

Hoffer, A., and Mahon, M.: The presence of unidentified substances in the urine of psychiatric patients. J. Neuropsychiatry 2, 331, 1961.

Hoffer, A., and Osmond, H.: Malvaria: A new psychiatric disease. Acta Psychiat. Scand., 39, 335, 1963.

Hoffer, A., and Osmond, H.: Nicotinadmide adenine dinucleotide (NAD) as a treatment for schizophrenia. J. Psychopharmacology 1, 79, 1966.

Irvine, D., Apparently non-indolic Ehrlich positive substances related to mental illnesses. J. Neuropsychiat. 2, 292, 1961.

Irvine, D.G., Bayne, W., and Miyashita, H.: Identification of kryptopyrrole in human urine and its relation to psychosis. Nature 224, 811, 1969.

Kelm, H., Hoffer, A., and Osmond, H.: Hoffer-Osmond Diagnostic Test Manual. Modern Press, Saskatoon, 1967, available from Northland Stationers, 62 - 33rd Street East, Saskatoon, Saskatchewan.

Klenner, F.R.: Response of peripheral and central nerve pathology to megadoses of the vitamin B complex and other metabolites. J. Applied Nutrition 25, 16, 1973.

Kotkas, L.: Personal Communications, 1972.

Newbold, H.L.: The use of vitamin $B_{12}b$ in Psychiatric Practice. Orthomolecular Psychiatry 1, 27, 1972.

Newbold, H.L.: Philpott, W.H., and Mandell, M.: Psychiatric Syndromes Produced by Allergies: Ecologic Mental Illness. Orthomolecular Psychiatry 2, 84, 1973.

Pauling, L.: (a) Orthomolecular Psychiatry. Science 160, 265, 1968, (b) Orthomolecular Somatic and Psychiatric Medicine, Sonderdruck aus der Zeitschrift Vitalstoffe - Zivhisationskrank - heiten 1, 1968. (c) Vitamin Therapy: Treatment for the mentally ill, Science 160, 1181, 1968.

Pfeiffer, C.: Neurobiology of the Trace Metals Zinc and Copper. Int. Review of Neurobiology. Supp. 1 Academic Press, New York, 1972.

Randolph, T.G.: Ecologic Mental Illness Levels of Central Nervous System Reactions. The Third World Congress of Psychiatry, 1, 379, 1961.

Randolph, T.G.: Clinical ecology as it affects the psychiatric patient. Int. J. Soc. Psychiatry 12, 245, 1966.

Randolph, T.G.: Domiciliary chemical air pollution in the etiology of ecologic mental illness. The Int. J. Soc. Psychiatry 16, 243, 1970.

Rees, E.: Discussion. Third Annual Meeting, Academy Orthomolecular Psychiatry, Detroit, 1974.

Reich, C.: The Vitamin Therapy of Chronic Asthma. J. Asthma Research 9, 99, 1971.

Richardson, H.J.: A study and survey of the disabilities and problems of Hong Kong veterans. Department of Health and Welfare, Ottawa, Canada, 1964.

Rinkel, H.J.: The technique and clinical application of individual food tests. Ann. Allergy 2, 504, 1944.

Silverman, L.: Personal Communication, 1974.

Ulett, G.A., and Itil, E.: Alcoholism and Allergy. 126th Ann. Meeting Amer. Psychiatric Assn., Hawaii, 1973.

Williams, Roger: Nutrition Against Disease. Pitman Publ. Corp., New York, 1971.

17
Treatment of Learning Disabilities*

ALLAN COTT

Orthomolecular treatment has been described in a previous chapter, but its definition at this point bears repetition. Dr. Linus Pauling, in his classical paper on Orthomolecular Psychiatry (1968), defined this approach as the treatment of illness by the provision of the optimum molecular composition of the brain, especially the optimum concentration of substances normally present in the human body. The implications for much needed research in the more universal application of orthomolecular treatment are clear. There is rapidly accumulating evidence that a child's ability to learn can be improved by the use of large doses of certain vitamins, of mineral supplements, and by improvement of his general nutritional status through removal of "junk foods" from his daily diet.

With orthomolecular treatment, results are frequently quick in starting and the reduction in hyperactivity often dramatic, but in most instances several months elapse before significant changes are seen. The child exhibits a willingness to cooperate with his parents and teachers. These changes are seen in the majority of children who failed to improve with the use of the stimulant drugs or tranquilizer medications. The majority of the children I see have been exposed to every form of treatment and every known tranquilizer and sedative with little or no success even in controlling the hyperactivity. Concentration and attention span increases, and the child is able to work productively for increasingly larger periods of time. He ceases to be an irritant to his teacher and classmates. Early intervention is of the utmost importance, not only for the child, but for the entire family since the child suffering from minimal brain dysfunction is such a devastating influence on the family constellation. He is the matrix of emotional storms which envelop every member of the household and disrupt both their relationship to him and to each other.

Based on empirical data, the application of orthomolecular principles can be successful in helping many learning disabled children. Positive results have been obtained when the treatment regimen consisted of the following vitamins - niacinamide or niacin, 1-2 grams daily depending upon body weight; ascorbic acid, 1-2 grams daily; pyridoxine, 200-400 mg daily; calcium pantothenate, 200-600 mgs daily. The vitamins are generally administered twice daily. Magnesium oxide powder is frequently used for its calming effect on the hyperactivity. Half teaspoon of

the powder is added to the vitamin intake twice daily along with 1 tablet of calcium gluconate or calcium lactate twice daily.

These are starting doses of the vitamins for children weighing 35 pounds or more. If a child weighs less than 35 pounds, 1 gram daily of niacinamide and ascorbic acid are used in ½ gram doses administered twice daily. If the child shows no signs of intolerance after two weeks, the dose is increased to 1 gram twice daily. In the smaller child the pyridoxine and calcium pantothenate are started at 100 mgs twice daily and gradually increased to twice the amount. In a child weighing 45 pounds or more, an optimum daily maintenance level of approximately 3 grams of niacinamide and 3 grams of ascorbic acid is reached. Frequently, vitamin B_{12}, vitamin E, riboflavin (B_2), thiamine (B_1), folic acid and L-glutamine can be valuable additions to the treatment. No serious side effects have resulted in any of the hundreds of children treated with these substances. The side effects which occur infrequently (nausea, vomiting, increased frequency of urination or bowel movements) are dose related and subside with reduction of the dose.

It has been shown that proper brain function requires adequate tissue respiration, and Dr. O. Warburg (1966), Nobel laureate in biochemistry, described the importance of vitamins B_3 and C in the respiration of all body tissues in the maintenance of health and proper function.

It has been the author's belief that those children and adults in all diagnostic categories who benefit from the massive doses of vitamins are not always suffering from vitamin deficiencies but rather from a genetic vitamin dependency. In August, 1970, Dr. L.E. Rosenberg of the Department of Genetic Research of Yale University reported that of the dozen known disorders involving genetic vitamin dependency, pyridoxine (vitamin B_6) is involved in five. Genetic dependency is described as a condition in which normal levels of vitamins are insufficient for the body and can be treated successfully only by massive doses of vitamins. Rosenberg found that in many instances up to 1,000 times the usual vitamin requirements are needed to prevent the disease from expressing itself. Laboratory findings with animals have shown a direct relationship between vitamin intake and learning enhancement. It has been found by some researchers that injections of vitamin B_{12} markedly enhanced learning in rats.

Control of the child's diet is an integral part of the total treatment, and failure to improve the child's nutritional status

*Reprinted with permission: *Orthomolecular Psychiatry*, Vol. 3, No. 4, 1974, 343-355.

can be responsible for achieving minimal results. Greater concern must be shown for the quality of the child's internal environment in which his cells and tissues function if we are to help him attain optimal performance. The removal of offending foods from the diet of disturbed or learning disabled children can result in dramatic improvement in behavior, attention span, and concentration. Since many disturbed and learning disabled children are found to have either hypoglycemia, hyperinsulinism, or dysinsulinism, cane sugar and rapidly absorbed carbohydrate foods should be eliminated from their diets. It has been the universal observation of those investigators who assess the child's nutritional status that they eat a diet which is richest in sugar, candy, sweets, and in foods made with sugar. The removal of these foods results in a dramatic decrease in hyperactivity. Most children do not drink milk unless it is sweetened with chocolate syrup or some other syrupy additive. All the beverages which they consume every day are spiked with sugar – soda, caffeinated cola drinks, highly sweetened "fruit juices," and other concoctions which are sold to them on TV commercials. The child who drinks any water at all is indeed rare.

The appalling fact about the constant consumption of these "junk foods" is the parents' belief that these foods are good for their children. Parents must realize that they litter their children's bodies by making these unnatural junk foods available to them and incorporating them in their daily diet. The children will not voluntarily exclude these foods from their diet, they must be helped to accomplish this. These foods should not be brought into the house. The child must learn the principles of proper nutrition and proper eating from his parents. The dissemination of this knowledge is far too important to entrust it to the writers of TV commercials whose aim is to sell rather than educate.

Dr. Jean Mayer (1970), Professor of Nutrition at Harvard University, speaking at a symposium on hunger and malnutrition, stated that "studies at Harvard among resident physicians suggest that the average physician knows little more about nutrition than the average secretary, unless the secretary has a weight problem and then she probably knows more than the average physician." "We did find that there is a difference between older physicians and younger in relation to this problem. The older doctors do not know more about nutrition than their younger colleagues, but they are conscious of this lack. All in all, it seems that most physicians tend to be happy about this state of affairs." Dr. Mayer complained that "only a half dozen or so medical schools in the U.S. include a nutrition course in the curriculum. Nutrition education should be centered on foods — their size, shape, color, caloric value, etc. . . . we must relate such vital information to the everyday uses of all people."

The author has taken many dietary histories which revealed that the usual "nutritious" breakfast for some children consists of a glass of soda or "coke" and a portion of chocolate layer cake! For the child with hypoglycemia, such food assures a drop in blood glucose level for several hours, during which time that child's brain function is impaired so that he cannot learn well even if he does not suffer from learning disabilities. At best, the breakfast menu of the majority of learning disabled children is poorly balanced and varies from the above extreme by the substitution of sugar-frosted cereals. The glucose in the bloodstream is one of the most important nutrients for the proper functioning of the brain, and the maintenance of a proper glucose level is essential in the creation of an optimum molecular environment for the mind.

Orthomolecular treatment has many advantages which make it especially suitable for large numbers of children. Treatment can be directed by parents and paraprofessionals, reducing to a minimum the occasions upon which the child must be brought to a specialist for therapy. It is inexpensive, as it does not depend upon complex machinery or psychotropic drugs. Of great importance is the role it could serve as a preventive as well as a therapeutic measure, because it could easily be included in prenatal and infant care programs everywhere. These are important considerations in view of the evidence that neurologically-based and biochemically-based learning disabilities are especially frequent among children from low-income areas. U. Bronfenbrenner (1969) points out that a low-income mother's "exposure to nutritional deficiency, illness, fatigue or emotional stress can be far more damaging to her child than was previously thought. The neurological disturbances thus produced persist through early childhood into the school years, where they are reflected in impaired learning capacity."

The relationship of severe malnutrition to infant mortality, disease, and retardation in physical development are all well documented. In recent years evidence has accumulated that malnutrition has adverse effects on mental development and learning as well. Mild malnutrition can result in the child who is a "picky eater," who chronically gags when he swallows some foods, or swallows it readily and then vomits. Recent studies utilized such reported differences within young twin pairs to show that subtle variations in eating habits in the first year can be related to differences in mental abilities later in life.

While the chronic ingestion of lead has yet to be clearly associated with hyperactivity in children, two recently reported studies of mice and rats show that lead poisoning causes definite changes in brain biochemistry, that such changes may lead to behavioral disorders including hyperactivity (Michaelson, 1973).

At the University of Cincinnati Medical Center, Drs. I. Arthur Michaelson and Mitchell U. Sauerhoff administered varying concentrations of lead solution to nursing mother rats and then measured the neurochemical changes in 90 babies. They found 15 percent - 20 percent decreases in brain dopamine. At Johns Hopkins University, Drs. Ellen K. Silbergeld and Alan M. Goldberg (1973) tested the effects of lead ingestion on mouse behavior. After administering lead solutions to nursing mothers the investigators found that the offspring were retarded in development and suffered behavior disorders — hyperactivity and aggression.

The environmental pollutants are often heavy metals such as lead, mercury, or cadmium. The pollution of our environment, and particularly the cities, with lead has already reached a disturbingly high level. In 1967 in Manchester, England, a group of children were found to have lead levels of 30+ micrograms per 100 ml of blood. Professor D. Bryce Smith of the University of Reading wrote recently in the journal, *Chemistry in Britain*, that no other toxic chemical pollutant has accumulated in man to average levels so close to the threshold for overt clinical poisoning. Whenever lead poisoning has been diagnosed, it has always been possible to trace it to some definite source. In children, it may be chewing on old paint work or toys containing lead. There has been no known case of lead poisoning from the widespread general pollution to which everyone is exposed. This is why the apparently alarming situation to which Professor D. Bryce Smith draws attention has caused little concern. Lead pollution does not seem to be doing any serious damage, the complacent argument runs, so why worry about it? However, this position begins to look more and more vulnerable in the face of mounting evidence that lead could have harmful effects at levels well below those which cause overt poisoning.

In 1964, Sir Alan Moncrieff and others at the Institute of Child Health in London found that a group of mentally retarded children had distinctly more lead in their blood than a group of normal children. In fact, nearly half the retarded children had higher blood levels than the maximum level in the other group. It does not, of course, follow that lead was responsible for the children's mental retardation. It could well have been their retardation which made them more prone to chew on substances with a lead content. Nevertheless, the possibility that lead at levels too low to cause obvious poisoning could result in mental retardation could not be ignored and acted as a spur to the search for some measurable effect of low levels of lead in the human body.

In 1970, Dr. Sven Hernberg and his associates found that lead affected the functioning of an enzyme, ALA Dehydratase, which is involved in haem synthesis. Furthermore, he showed that in the test tube any level of lead affected the activity of ALA Dehydratase to some degree. In October, 1970, a research group led by J.A. Millar fed lead to baby rats and found that the activity of ALA Dehydratase was affected not only in their blood, but in their brains as well. They wrote in their report in *The Lancet*, "The finding of decreased ALA Dehydratase activity in the blood of children with lead levels falling within the normal range and the possibility that similar biochemical changes are present in the brain also, emphasizes the danger of exposure to even very small amounts of lead during childhood and suggests that a downward revision of acceptable levels of blood lead in children is desirable." In addition to the lead discharged into the atmosphere in vehicle exhaust, one absorbs lead from foods and water.

It is now a well-known clinical fact that susceptibility to the harmful effects of lead is highly variable. Lead in heavy concentrations in the tissues (and some of the hundreds of children I have examined have concentrations as high as 85 ppm) can interfere with metabolic reactions which activate other metals such as copper, iron, manganese, and potassium.

In the author's studies of the trace metals in children's hair, it was found that they show a higher concentration of lead than do adults. In the adult groups it has been reported that pregnant women show a greater susceptibility than other adult members of the population. Now that attention has been focused on the level of lead in the tissues of many middle-class Americans who may be exposed to lead by-products in gasoline exhaust fumes, many new cases of borderline lead toxicity are appearing without the usual explanation of lead ingestion. While there is a close correlation between the level of atmospheric lead and the levels of lead accumulated and stored in the body, there is a wide diversity in the susceptibility, not only to symptoms, but also to the accumulation of this toxic trace metal. Recent experiments again give evidence that nutritional factors, particularly dietary calcium, may be important determinants in the capacity of the body to absorb and retain lead. Animals receiving lead in their drinking water showed a greater absorption of lead when their diet was deficient in calcium. This group of animals absorbed four times as much lead as compared to the group which received a normal dietary calcium intake.

PRENATAL INFLUENCES

Ashley Montagu, in his book *Life Before Birth*, states that life begins at conception and that the happenings in the interval between conception and birth are far more important for our subsequent growth and development than has until recently been realized. The thinking about this period of the child's life had for so many years for the majority of people been rather simplistic. It was stated with confidence that the child was safe, warm, and snug in the mother's uterus, shielded and protected from all external influences while he floated in his fluid-filled sac which by its hydraulic effect made him safe even from physical pressures. It was believed that the placenta acted as a "barrier" against the transmission of toxic substances from the mother's blood stream.

Not until the past decade of research has it been learned that during the prenatal period — the nine months between conception and birth — a human being is more susceptible to his environment than he will ever be again in his life. What happens to him in the prenatal period can help sustain normal development or hinder him from ever achieving his full genetic potential. The events which take place before his birth can exert a lifelong influence, for part of the child's environment consists of his mother's immediate state of health, her general physical condition, her age at the time of conception, and how fatigued she becomes each day. A pregnant woman's nutrition must be more than merely adequate, it must be the best that her circumstances allow.

Montagu emphasizes that "a mother's nutrition is the most important single environmental influence in the life of her unborn child and it is by means of the food she eats that a mother can have the most profound and lasting effect on her child's development — by the simple act of improving her diet where improvement is necessary she can greatly influence the development of her child toward normal healthy growth." A study of malnutrition and pregnancy is cited from which a surprising finding emerged — that none of the mothers in either group, the well fed or the poorly fed, showed any signs themselves of malnutrition or deficiency diseases, yet the diet of the pregnant woman can be so seriously inadequate that her child is endangered and yet not produce any recognizable symptoms that might give warning to her or her doctors.

This finding corroborates Roger J. Williams' (1971) report that greater concern must be shown for the quality of the internal environments in which our cells and tissues function, because these environments can vary through the full spectrum from those which barely keep cells alive up through hundreds of gradations to levels supporting something like optimal performance. It is an obvious undeniable conclusion that an unborn child should be given the advantage of growing to term in an optimum molecular environment. Proper diet based on wholesome foods, vitamin and mineral supplements, and the elimination of "junk foods" helps to create such an environment for prenatal development and growth — cigarette smoking, stimulant drugs, diuretic drugs, tranquilizers, dieting with or without the use of amphetamine-containing appetite suppressors do not.

In the author's clinical practice, detailed prenatal histories and the histories of labor and delivery reveal that some complications of pregnancy and delivery occurred in a majority of the children who show evidence of brain injury, behavior disorder, or learning disabilities. Clinical impressions are always open to all the possibilities of error found in such retrospective evaluations (Pasamanick et al., 1956).

Dr. Benjamin Pasamanick (1956) and his coworkers, in a series of papers describing their research in these areas, postulated "a continuum of reproductive casualties extending from fetal deaths through a descending gradient of brain damage manifested in cerebral palsy, epilepsy, mental deficiency and behavior disorders in childhood." In a 1958 report, Dr. Pasamanick extended the continuum of reproductive casualties to include reading disorders in childhood. In this study, reported in the *Journal of the American Medical Association* (March 22, 1958), they compared the prenatal and birth records of 372 white male children with reading disorders born in Baltimore between 1935 and 1945 with the records of a similar number of matched controls. The results of the study "appear to indicate that there exists a relationship between certain abnormal conditions associated with birth and the subsequent development of reading disorders in the child."

Those children with reading disorders had a significantly larger proportion of premature births and abnormalities of the prenatal and delivery periods than their control subjects. They found that the toxemias of pregnancy and bleeding during pregnancy constituted those complications largely responsible for the differences between the two groups. The investigation suggested that some of the learning disabilities in children constitute a component in the continuum of reproductive casualties, which Pasamanick had previously hypothesized to be composed of a lethal component consisting of stillbirths and neonatal deaths and a sublethal component consisting of cerebral palsy, epilepsy, mental deficiency, and behavior disorders in children.

Impressions leading to similar conclusions formed from the author's clinical experiences based on detailed histories of hundreds of learning disabled children. The interview with the parents generally begins with the request that they describe the pregnancy. With very few exceptions in the hundreds of pairs of parents interviewed, the opening response is "The pregnancy was perfectly normal." It is appalling to contemplate the disasters which can await the child in what women have been led to believe are quite the usual and therefore normal experiences of pregnancy. Many mothers report with a feeling of pride their accomplishment of having carried a pregnancy to full term and delivered a baby of normal weight without having gained a single pound in the nine months of the pregnancy! Nausea and vomiting occurs in the great majority of mothers and is accepted as a normal occurrence. Many mothers attempt to minimize the importance of "morning sickness" by adding (usually accompanied by a smile or a chuckle), "but I was sick every day with all my pregnancies."

Many mothers reported dieting severely throughout the pregnancy at the demand of their doctor, because he preferred that his patients have small babies. Amphetamines were frequently prescribed to suppress the appetite or to combat fatigue. Tranquilizer and sedative medications were used freely throughout the pregnancies, but the most frequently prescribed medication seemed to be the diuretic drugs which mothers took throughout the pregnancies and which were in very few cases taken along with an increase in potassium — rich foods. Anemia during pregnancy is frequently reported.

The frequency of the occurrence of complications during the perinatal period (delivery) is higher in children with learning disabilities. The most commonly encountered history is that of a prolonged period of labor and a difficult delivery. In a study reported by Dr. Mary Hoffman in *Academic Therapy* (Vol. VII, No. 1-Fall 1971), 25 percent of a group of children who were failing students were products of difficult deliveries, while this occurred in only 1.5 percent of the histories of the able students. Cyanosis occurred in 11 percent of the learning disabled and in only 0.5 percent of the able students. Prolonged labor, blood incompatibility, premature births, postmature births, breech deliveries, and induced labor were also found to be highly significant factors in the historical background of children with learning disabilities, since these casualties occurred far more frequently than in able children.

The examination of a child who suffers from a disorder of speech, communication, or learning cannot be considered complete without a visual examination, for the investigation of sight and vision is as important as any other part of the total examination and more important and revealing than many other routines. A major number of the children treated by the author have all had examinations which included electroencephalograms, but very few have been examined for vision by a vision specialist. If an examination has been done, it was performed for sight, and if the child demonstrated 20/20 vision on the Snellen Chart, the parents were informed that there was nothing wrong with the child's eyes. This may be true for distance eyesight, but overlooks all the near-point visual activity so important to the dynamic visual process of reading (Wunderlich, 1970). The child who has a school or learning problem must have an examination performed by a specialist who investigates the function of the eyes as well as their structure. Such a specialist could be an ophthalmologist (an M.D. specializing in diseases of the eye) or an optometrist specializing in developmental vision. At the present time few ophthalmologists perform these examinations, so one is more apt to find a developmental vision specialist among optometrists. Sight is the ability of the eye to see clearly. It refers only to the ability to resolve detail. Vision is the ability to gain meaning from what is seen (Wunderlich, 1970).

Too often parents are lulled into a false sense of security when they are told that their child's eyes are "fine" for here, also, early detection and treatment will produce a more rewarding response and the more successful will be the results of the remedial efforts. There can be significant deviations from normal vision even if a child has 20/20 on the Snellen Chart. Farsightedness can be overlooked in a distance vision screening examination and can cause difficulties when a child does near work. Trouble can be caused if one eye is different from the other in refractive power. Convergence of the eyes noseward for looking at things up close is of vital importance in centering with two eyes on a near-point task. Convergence bears an important relationship to focusing, and the two processes are combined. If this link is not proper, a child can be out of focus and be completely unaware that he is, just as a child who sees a separate image with each eye has no way of telling us about this since he believes that everyone sees in this way. The out-of-focus child cannot tell us about his blurred vision until he can be helped to see in sharp focus with the aid of lenses. The author has seen many children who had not seen near things in sharp focus or looked at the world through binocular vision until the eyes had been treated successfully by a developmental optometrist or by an ophthalmologist interested in developmental vision. Yet these children are daily trying to learn to read when the printed page presents nothing but a blur. Hyperactivity is frequently reduced when the visual systems work efficiently.

Lack of smooth eye muscle control makes a difficult task of trying to follow successive words in a line of print as the eyes sweep across a page. Often the eyes will not make the repeated necessary convergences if the focusing is not proper, and the child will skip words in the line, lose his place, or not be able to find the first word on the next line and as a result will not comprehend what he reads.

Developmental visual training is another vital link in the creation of an optimum molecular environment for the mind. Neither improved nutrition, vitamin and mineral supplements, enriched educational opportunities, or visual and perceptual motor training alone can be successful in fully helping the child with learning disabilities. All must be used in a coordinated program to develop each child's potential. Because research cannot at this time give an unequivocal or full answer to the question of what effect malnutrition or malnourishment has on intellectual development is not a valid reason to delay programs for improving the nutritional status and eating practices of mothers and infants. Information demonstrating the benefits of good nutrition in improved health, physical growth, and improved learning already justifies such efforts.

We cannot afford the luxury of waiting until causes can be unquestionably established by techniques yet to be developed. We cannot postpone managing as effectively and honestly as possible the 5 million or more children who desperately need help now.

REFERENCES

Bronfenbrenner, U.: "Dampening the Unemployability Explosion." Saturday Review, Jan. 4, 1969.

Cott, Allan: "Orthomolecular Approach to the Treatment of Learning Disabilities." Schizophrenia, Vol. 3, No. 2, 95-105, Second Quarter, 1971.

Cott, Allan: "Megavitamins: The Orthomolecular Approach to Behavioral Disorders and Learning Disabilities." Academic Therapy, Vol. VII, No. 3 (Spring 1972).

Hoffman, Mary S.: "Early Indications of Learning Problems." Academic Therapy, Vol. VII, No. 1 (Fall 1971).

Mayer, Jean: Medical Tribune-World Wide Report, Monday, Jan. 19, 1970.

Michaelson, I. Arthur, and Sauderhoff, Mitchell, W.: "Lead Poisoning." Medical World News, Sept. 7, 1973.

Montagu, Ashley: Life Before Birth. New American Library. 1964.

Office of Child Development and the Office of the Assistant Secretary for Health and Scientific Affairs, Dept. of H.E.W.: "Report of the Conference on the Use of Stimulant Drugs in the Treatment of Behaviorally Disturbed Young School Children." 1971.

Pasamanick, Benjamin, Rogers, Martha, E., and Lillienfeld, Abraham M.: "Pregnancy Experience and the Development of Behavior Disorder in Children." Journal of the American Psychiatric Association, 613-618, Feb. 1956.

Silbergeld, Ellen K., and Goldberg, Alan M.: Medical World News, p. 7, September 7, 1973.

Warburg, O.: "The Prime Cause and Prevention of Cancer." Lindau Lecture 1966. (Nobel Laureate 1931 and 1944 for work with respiratory enzymes.)

Wendle, William F., Faro, Maria D., Barker, June N., Barsky, David, and Gutierrez, Sergio: "Developmental Behaviors Delayed Appearance in Monkeys Asphyziated at Birth." Science, Vol. 171. No. 3976, 1173-1175, 19, March 1971.

Williams, Roger, J., Heffley, James D., and Bode, Charles W.: "The Nutritive Value of Single Foods." Paper presented to the National Academy of Sciences, April 28, 1971.

Wunderlich, Ray C.: Kids, Brains and Learning. Johnny Reads Inc., St. Petersburg, Florida, 1970.

18

The use of Vitamin B₁₂b in Psychiatric Practice*

H.L. NEWBOLD

INTRODUCTION

The recorded history of the use of vitamins in the treatment of mental illness goes back more than 2000 years, to a period long before lime juice was made required fare in the British Navy in 1795 [1]. The British rediscovered the forgotten Roman fact that fruits containing ascorbic acid would prevent, as well as cure, scurvy.

Prior to this discovery, British sea captains, in their instruction manuals, were advised to provide recreation and music of a stimulating nature, as well as uplifting conversations, to treat the depressions which occurred with scurvy. Perhaps there are lessons to be learned from this ancient attempt at curing mental illnesses through environmental manipulations, when in reality a chemical defect existed.

Well known is the work of Goldberger during the 1930's which resulted in the virtual disappearance of the widespread psychosis associated with pellagra. Cleckley, Sydenstricker and Geeslin (1939) [2] reported alleviation of severe psychiatric symptoms with the use of moderately large doses of Nicotinic Acid (0.3 to 1.5 grams per day). None of these patients had the physical stigma associated with pellagra.

In 1952 Hoffer and Osmond began using massive doses of Nicotinic Acid (3 to 30 gm. per day) and ascorbic acid (3 to 9 gm. per day) for the treatment of schizophrenia. Since then they have published their findings [3, 4, 5] and have done much to popularize what they termed megavitamin therapy, now expanded into orthomolecular therapy by Linus Pauling (1968) [6].

The latest impetus for the use of vitamins in the treatment of mental disorders comes from a paper published by Linus Pauling (1968) [6] in which he points out the wide variations of vitamin requirements for individual organisms.

Since most chemical reactions in living organisms require catalyzation by enzymes, vitamin levels are of critical importance. If there is a genetically defective enzyme system, the vitamin level for ideal function may be much higher than the accepted norm. Some defective enzyme systems can apparently be forced to function at a normal level with an increase in the vitamin required for that particular chemical reaction.

The Michaelis-Menten [7] equation illustrates this principle:

$$R = \frac{d\,[S]}{dt} = \frac{k\,E\,[S]}{[S] \div (1/K)}$$

Only several parts of this equation are of particular interest to illustrate my point.

(S) is the concentration of the substrate. E is the total concentration of the enzyme. K is the equilibrium constant for the production of the enzyme complex ES. k is the reaction rate constant for the breakdown of the complex into the enzyme and the reaction products.

If K = 2 is the normal constant for the formation of an enzyme complex, then only normal amounts of, say, vitamins will be required for the chemical reaction to proceed in the normal fashion.

If there be a genetic defect, however, and K = 0.01, then it will be necessary to increase the vital substance, say a vitamin, by a factor of 200x for the rate of the chemical reaction to proceed at a normal rate. Thus, a very large increase in the vitamin level of the organism can "force" the chemical reaction.

Causes of Vitamin B₁₂ Deficiency

It is well known that a deficiency of vitamin B_{12} can cause demonstrable lesions both in the spinal cord and in the brain proper. A vitamin B_{12} deficiency with change in the central nervous system may precede the actual appearance of anemia by several years.

Vitamin B_{12} deficiency may be produced by a low intake of the extrinsic factor, when patients follow a vegetarian diet, for example. Autoimmune reactions may block or bind the intrinsic factor so that vitamin B_{12} cannot be absorbed [8]. Also autoimmune reactions may be directed against the pareital cell, destroying its ability to produce the intrinsic factor [9].

A defect in the protein molecule which transports the vitamin B_{12} from the blood into the tissue may result in an effective tissue deficiency of vitamin B_{12} even when the serum B_{12} level is normal [10].

Of course, it has long been known that a vitamin B_{12} deficiency may result from infestation by the fish tapeworm *diphyllobothrium* or from excessive bacteria in the gut, such as may occur in the blind loop syndrome.

*Reprinted with permission: *Orthomolecular Psychiatry*, Volume I, #1.

Various drugs may bring about a deficiency of vitamin B_{12}; Dilantin is probably the most important offender.

Serum B_{12} Studies

A number of studies have been done in which the B_{12} serum concentrations of psychiatric patients have been performed. No attempt will be made here to review all these papers, but in general the percentages have run from 0.02 percent to a high of 16 percent (including borderline values). Of interest are the recent findings of Edwin (1965) [11], Hansen (1969) [12], Hutner (1967) [13], Shulman (1967) [14], Buxton (1969) [15], Murphy (1969) [16], Carney (1969) [17] and Philpott (1971) [18].

It has been estimated by Edwin [8] that approximately 0.5 percent of the general population in his area of Norway suffer from pernicious anemia.

This author is about to present the serum B_{12} levels on a total of 221 psychiatric patients.

Population Selection

Each of the 221 patients with low serum B_{12} reported here consulted me for a psychiatric problem. It should be pointed out that only one of the patients represented here is less than 16 years old. Previous to developing an interest in serum B_{12} levels, I saw a high percentage of young psychiatric patients. However, immediately preceding the present study, I began limiting my practice to the adult psychiatric population.

There is a further selection in patients presented here in that the author deals primarily with patients suffering from severe emotional illnesses. This means that the most frequent diagnosis represented is the syndrome of schizophrenia. As a rule, the author sees only patients who have failed to improve with previous psychiatric help. Most of the patients consulted three or four other psychiatrists before seeing me. It is apparent from these remarks that the patients represented here are not a cross-section of the categories usually treated by the general practice psychiatrist.

Of further interest is the fact that 93 of these patients are from the New York/Boston area and 128 of the patients come from North Carolina and the states adjacent to it. An interesting contrast in the serum B_{12} levels was discovered in these two geographic representations in the present study.

Results of Serum B_{12} Studies

The reader is referred to Table I.

Of the total of 93 patients seen from the New York/Boston area, 16.1 percent had what is generally considered a borderline low serum B_{12} level (150 picograms per millilitre to 200 picograms per millilitre). 17.2 percent of these patients had a serum B_{12} level of less than 150 picograms per millilitre. When we total low B_{12} level patients, including all with serum B_{12} levels less than the normal 200 picograms per millilitre, we find that 33.3 percent of this New York/Boston population had abnormally low serum B_{12} levels.

Table 1

New York Total 93		
159-200 pcg/ml	= 15	16.1%
less than 150 pcg/ml	= 16	17.2%
Total Low	= 31	33.3%
N.C. Total 128		
150-200 pcg/ml	= 8	6.3%
less than 150 pcg/ml	= 12	9.4%
Total Low	= 20	15.7%
Total 221		
150-200 pcg/ml	= 23	10.9%
less than 150 pcg/ml	= 28	12.7%
Total Low	= 51	23.6%

Of the patients from the general area of North Carolina, 6.3 percent had serum B_{12} levels of between 150 and 200 picograms per millilitre, 9.4 percent of the patients had serum B_{12} values of less than 150 picograms per millilitre, giving an overall total figure of 15.7 percent of these patients with serum B_{12} levels below the norm of 200 picograms per millilitre.

When the two different populations are averaged together, we find that 10.9 percent of the patients had a serum B_{12} level between 150 and 200 pcg/ml and 12.7 percent of the patients had a serum B_{12} level less than 150 pcg/ml, giving a total for the entire group of 23.6 percent of patients with serum B_{12} levels less than 200 pcg/ml.

Comments on Contrasting Geographic Serum B_{12} Levels

One can only speculate on the causes for the difference in the serum B_{12} levels of the patients from the New York/Boston area and those from North Carolina and the adjacent states. The figures from the North Carolina area come from at least three different laboratories but the great majority of the tests were performed at the Washington Reference Laboratory in Washington, D.C.

Most of the serum B_{12} levels from the New York area were performed at the Reference Laboratory, North Hollywood, California. A scattering of the tests from the New York area was performed at a number of different laboratories.

One might speculate what differences in diet in the two geographic areas might cause a difference in the serum B_{12} levels; however, this seems unlikely. Apparently, diet has very little effect on the serum B_{12} level unless a vegetarian diet is being followed. A few of the author's patients in the North Carolina area were from the Seventh Day Adventist religion and did not eat meat. None of these patients happened to have low serum B_{12} levels, however.

There were a few alcoholics in each geographical group, but if anything, the alcoholics seen in the New York area were better nourished and less desperately ill than those of the North Carolina area. Certainly there are genetic differences in the groups of patients seen in the two geographic areas. The N.C. area was heavily weighted with patients of English, Scottish-Irish and German ancestry, whereas in the New York area there was a high percentage of persons of Jewish and pure Irish ancestry. As a group, it is the author's opinion that the people of New York are generally sicker than those from the N.C. area and had been ill for a longer period of time. In the author's opinion, the group from New York in general represented a more aggressive population and one with an overall higher intelligence.

Although these patients were not tested for fish tapeworm, there is no reason to think that fish tapeworm would be any more common in the New York area than in the N.C. area and blind loops of intestine should not be more common in the New York group.

Since the absorption of vitamin B_{12} from the gut is largely dependent upon certain intact enzyme systems, which are inherited, one might speculate that the New York group is genitcally different from the N.C. group.

Clinical Experience with B_{12}

If one scans the literature concerning vitamin B_{12}, it is relatively easy to pick up studies in which psychiatric populations have been tested for serum B_{12} levels; however, less information is available giving the results of therapy with vitamin B_{12}. In general, reports by Smith (1960)[19], Strachan (1965) [20] and Shulman (1967) [21], were enthusiastic about the use of vitamin B_{12} in senile and confusional states; however, Hughes (1970) [22] gives a negative report.

I would like to present some clinical cases illustrating my experience with vitamin B_{12}, with the hope that more physicians will become alert to the possibilities of the therapy of mental illness of certain patients with the use of injected vitamin B_{12}.

Case 1. The first patient illustrating the use of vitamin B_{12} shows a most dramatic improvement with the medication.

He is a 33-year old white male who is a Ph.D. candidate at one of the country's major universities. Because he was not making progress in therapy, the patient was referred to me by his analyst for a chemical work-up.

Two years prior to seeing me, the patient had experienced a psychotic break. At that time he sat in his room and talked to himself for several days. He was completely out of touch with reality. For about two weeks he had experienced what he described as a snapping sensation in his head. He explained that space had been greatly foreshortened, that he felt like a midget. The streets seemed extremely short.

At the start of his psychosis he was so frightened that he left his apartment and began running up and down the street. He was convinced that a blood vessel had broken in his head. His attention span was quite short.

After three or four days of totally psychotic behavior, he was admitted to one of New York's most respected hospitals, where he was placed on Chlorpromazine (Thorazine). After a few days the more florid aspects of his psychosis were under control. After discharge from the hospital, he was maintained on Chlorpromazine, which was gradually reduced. He was taking only 50 mgs. at bedtime when he consulted me.

During the two years following his hospitalization, the patient had felt very lethargic. Work on his Ph.D. thesis had been impossible. He felt lonely and insecure and it was very difficult for him to interact with other people.

The patient's wife left him after his psychotic break. This only added to his feelings of inadequacy and insecurity. His head still felt as if it were not clear. His emotions seemed locked within him. He secretly harbored anger toward most people. It was difficult for him to drag himself to class. In class, he was unable to participate in an active way. His memory was poor and he felt depressed. It was quite difficult for him to comprehend and remember what he read.

At the time he consulted me, the patient's affect was flat and he spoke in monotones. He was oriented in significant spheres. No definite perceptual defects were present. He had vague paranoid feelings. A clinical examination of his memory and recall were normal.

A chemical work-up revealed an ATP level of 5.10 mgs/%, an NAD level of 1.04 mgs/%. A salt dumping test was negative, as was a six-hour glucose tolerance test. A routine blood count and urine was normal. BUN was 18.7, PBI 8.0 mgs/%, T3 was 24%, T4 was 4.8%. Serum B_{12} level was 103 picograms per millilitre. An HOD test was negative. A hair test for minerals revealed a lead level of 4.1 mgs/%, a normal iron level of 4.6 mgs/%, a normal manganese level of 0.26 mgs/%, a normal calcium level of 40 mgs/%, a normal magnesium level of 6.67 mgs/%, a slightly depressed potassium level of 3.5 mgs/%, a normal copper level of 2.6 mgs/%, a slightly depressed sodium level of 9.5 mgs/% and a somewhat elevated zinc level of 18.8 mgs/%.

The patient was requested to take a computerized Minnesota Multiphasic Personality Inventory but he was unable to concentrate on the test and refused to take it because the attempt at concentration made him angry and upset.

Following his laboratory tests, the patient was given $B_{12}b$ (Hydroxocobalamin) 1000 mgs. intramuscularly on June 4, 1971. When he returned to the office on June 9, 1971, he reported no change in his condition. A second intramuscular injection of hydroxocobalamin 1000 mgs. was administered at that time. When the patient reported to the office again on June 17, 1971, he spoke of a remarkable improvement of his condition. At that time his memory was much improved and he found that he was learning well. He was participating in class activities and for the first time in two years, was hard at work writing his Ph.D. thesis. He still felt angry occasionally with people but this did not bother him as before. The sense of depression had lifted. Clinically, the patient had developed a normal affect and he was able to relate well with me.

During the five months I have been seeing this patient, he has, with two exceptions, maintained an excellent level of improvement. The nurse at the office of his local medical doctor administered hydroxocobalamin 1000 mcg. intramuscularly twice weekly.

When this interval between injections was gradually increased to once weekly, the patient maintained his feeling of well-being. However, on the two occasions when we have tried to increase the injection interval to ten days, the patient quickly became tired, depressed and had difficulty concentrating. Each time the symptoms lifted promptly upon decreasing the interval between injections to seven days.

It would have been most interesting to have observed the effect of vitamin $B_{12}b$ on this patient at the time of his original psychotic break.

Case 2. The second patient chosen to illustrate a point in the therapy with vitamin B_{12} is a 38-year old white woman with a many-year history of recurrent periods of severe depression and of disabling physical complaints, for which a clear anatomical diagnosis could not be made. She had been helped temporarily by psychotherapy. Of particular significance was the fact that her serum B_{12} level was 231 picograms per millilitre.

In spite of this normal serum B_{12} level, I decided to give the patient a trial on hydroxocobalamin. The decision was based on Linus Pauling's article (1968), in which he pointed out that some gentically defective enzyme systems might function more effectively on vitamin levels much higher than the accepted norms.

At the time the hydroxocobalamin injections were started the patient was being carried on diazepam (Valium) 5 mgs. four times daily and chlorprothixene (Taractan) 10 mgs. five times daily. This combination of medications had been arrived at through trial and error. The medication enabled her to avoid some of her acute distress but she was not able to function even close to adequately in her role as a housewife.

Approximately a year ago, she was administered her first injection of hydroxocobalamin 1000 mcg. She experienced an immediate increase in her energy and feeling of wellbeing. She reported, however, at the time of her visit a week later, that the improvement lasted only about two and a half days. Interestingly enough, this is about the length of time one can expect high tissue levels of B_{12} after an injection of hydroxocobalamin.

Instructions were given to her family physician to repeat the hydroxocobalamin injection every two and a half days. At the time of the patient's next visit to me, she was markedly improved. She was less depressed. Her energy level was greatly improved, and she was rapidly losing her physical complaints.

Approximately two weeks later the patient was still improving in all spheres. On her own, she soon began experimenting by letting herself go three or four days on occasion between injections of hydroxocobalamin. Each time, she noticed a definite reduction in her energy level and her feeling of wellbeing.

This patient was maintained on hydroxocobalamin injections 100 mcg. every two and a half days for approximately ten weeks, at the end of which time her interval between injections was gradually increased, so that now her injections come only about every two weeks. She has continued her improvement. In addition to the large family which she cares for, she has been employed full time in a very stressful position.

This patient was tried on many combinations of medications, including various injections, prior to her receiving hydroxocobalamin. No previous treatment had given her even temporarily satisfactory remissions. It is felt that this patient has an enzyme defect which requires larger than normal amounts of hydroxocobalamin.

Case 3. This patient is a 28-year old white male who has spent most of the last ten years of his life in a State hospital. He had two courses of electroconvulsive treatment. After the first course, he was considerably improved but soon relapsed. He was somewhat improved after the second course but quickly relapsed. Prior to my seeing the patient, he was on heavy doses of chlorpromazine (Therazine), niacin and ascorbic acid.

He was fed the usually inadequate state hospital diet. The patient was extremely negativistic, was completely out of touch with reality. He could not carry on a conversation, he had numerous delusions, a very short attention span and his behavior was characterized by frequent outbursts of anger, so that it was almost impossible for him to have even brief visits at home.

The patient was found to have a serum B_{12} level of 155 picograms per millilitre and was started on injections of hydroxocobalamin 1000 milligrams twice weekly. His other medication was continued. The patient showed no appreciable response for the first six to eight weeks after beginning the hydroxocobalamin. At that time, he began gradually becoming calmer and less negativistic. For example, it was no longer necessary to have him forcibly restrained for his injections of hydroxocobalamin. Soon, he was able to go out on passes with his family with less difficulty. For the first time in many years, he expressed an interest in his clothes. His weight increased and he began to lose the wild, dishevelled look of madness which had been so characteristic of him previously. His attention span increased so that he was able to work for long periods in occupational therapy and complete complex drawings. His grasp of reality remained spotty.

In my judgment, there has been a modest improvement in his condition, though he still remains schizophrenic.

Since this patient was also receiving niacin and ascorbic acid, it is possible he was one of those patients slow to respond to this therapy and that his improvement simply happened to correspond to the time when hydroxocobalamin was begun.

This patient may have had a marked vitamin B_{12} deficiency in spite of his modestly low serum B_{12} level of 155 pcg/ml. If he happens to be one of those patients, like case 2, who requires high levels of B_{12} for his optimum function, then the level of 155 pcg/ml may be extremely low for this particular individual.

Case 4. The next patient was the only juvenile included in the present series. This 6-year old white child came from a family with a strong history of schizophrenia. At the time I saw him, he was quite hyperactive and immature for his age. He was pale and thin and had a very short attention span. The patient was shy and withdrawn.

A serum B_{12} level revealed 140 mcg/ml. At the time hydroxocobalamin was started, the patient was taking ascorbic acid 500 mgs. three times daily, a multivitamin capsule once daily and calcium gluconate 1 gram daily as well as methylphenidate HCl (Ritalin) 5 mgs. twice daily. He was given diphenhydramine HCl (Benadryl) 25 mgs at bedtime for sleep. The patient had improved somewhat on this regime, which had been followed for a number of months. He was unable to tolerate larger doses of methylphenidate HCl (Ritalin).

It can easily be understood that both the patient's mother and I were reluctant to give a child of 6 years old intramuscular injections. However, his level of improvement was not adequate and in view of the low serum B_{12} level, it seemed mandatory that he receive the vitamin. He was accordingly given hydroxocobalamin 1000 mcg. intramuscularly one time a week. He reacted violently to having the injection, so that it was necessary to hold him and forcibly administer the medication. Since this seemed likely to interfere with the rapport between us, the patient was sent to his pediatrician for future injections.

The next week, when the patient returned, the mother reported that he had been a great deal calmer for approximately three days following the injection. In that period, he was more tractable, he slept better, he was less hyperactive, less clinging to her, more outgoing and generally much more pleasant to live with. It is interesting to note that the mother reported that the pale, sickly color of his skin improved a great deal for several days after the injection.

Because the mother gave a history of the patient having relapsed approximately three days following his injection, it was decided to start him on hydroxocobalamin 1000 mcg/ml intramuscularly twice weekly. With this increase in frequency of administration, the patient maintained his new level of improvement throughout the week. For a little more than a year, the patient has continued receiving his injections of hydroxocobalamin.

On several occasions, I have attempted to space the injections over a longer period of time; however, the former symptoms always return when the interval between injections is increased. I might add that this mother is generally reluctant to have the child on medication and has attempted, several times, with this and other medications, to gradually discontinue them on her own. However, she has always returned to the schedule of injections twice weekly because of the return of symptoms.

Later, this patient was taken off Ritalin and placed on daenol acetamidobenzoate (Deaner) 300 mgs. in the morning. He showed a rather definite improvement with the substitution of Deaner for Ritalin. Since being given the Deaner, again attempts have been made to reduce the frequency of hydroxocobalamin. However, the symptoms always become worse when the hydroxocobalamin interval is increased. It is therefore continued and will be continued apparently indefinitely at this level.

The patient is now progressing quite well. He is attending school and for the first time able to keep up with his peer group.

Other Patients. It is understandably difficult to evaluate the role of hydroxocobalamin in treating patients with mental illnesses. The author has had other patients who, he suspects, have improved with the addition of hydroxocobalamin to their psychochemotherapeutic regime; however, other modalities were used in treating the patients and the percentage of improvement attributable to vitamin B$_{12}$ injections was difficult to assess. Some patients with low serum B$_{12}$ did not significantly improve with the addition of injections of hydroxocobalamin to their therapeutic regime.

Certainly it is theoretically possible that brain damage can proceed to the point of being irreversible in vitamin B$_{12}$ deficiency. The administration of vitamin B$_{12}$ in certain patients would simply prevent further insults to the central nervous system.

It is believed that vitamin B$_{12}$ is needed in at least ten different enzyme systems throughout the body. It is important in the formation of RNA.

Of interest is the fact that B$_{12}$, along with folic acid, is needed in the biosynthesis of methyl groups [23].

The author had one adverse reaction to the administration of hydroxocobalamin 1000 mcg. intramuscularly. This patient was a highly abnormal 18-year old boy who was mentally defective. He was a behavior problem. It was very difficult to maintain him outside of the hospital even with the use of tranquillizers. His serum B$_{12}$ level was normal but I decided to give him a trial with an injection of hydroxocobalamin. About forty minutes after the injection, the patient became highly restless, irritable and negativistic. This disturbed state lasted for approximately two days.

The author is not aware of any other instances of any such reactions to vitamin B$_{12}$ injections. It is of interest to note, however, that some patients when placed on massive doses of niacin become hyperactive and irritable and it is necessary to place them on some tranquillizer such as Valium for a few weeks to control the over-stimulated central nervous system.

CONCLUSIONS

1. This first conclusion is not, properly speaking, a conclusion which arises from the information presented in this paper. However, the information is placed here because, with the ever mounting volume of medical literature, many physicians have time only to read the conclusions at the end of a paper.

In England, Foulds and others (1970) [24] have started a movement to remove the conventional form of vitamin B$_{12}$ (cyanocobalamin) from the market. These authors feel that the cyanide radical is toxic for some patients and has produced optic nerve atrophy.

They propose that vitamin B$_{12b}$ (hydroxocobalamin) be substituted for cyanocobalamin. This seems wise for several other reasons. The body must transform cyanocobalamin into hydroxocobalamin before it is available for metabolic processes. Also hydroxocobalamin maintains high serum B$_{12}$ levels longer than does cyanocobalamin.

2. From a psychiatric office practice, a consecutive group of 221 patients has been tested for serum B$_{12}$ levels. Of this group, 10.9 percent showed vitamin B$_{12}$ serum levels of between 150 and 200 pcg/ml. The level between the 150 and 200 pcg/ml is considered by some authorities to be borderline and by others to be low.

3. From the group of 221 patients tested, 12.7 percent had serum B$_{12}$ levels less than 150 pcg/ml.

4. Of the psychiatric patients tested, 23.6 percent were found to have borderline or low serum B$_{12}$ levels.

5. An interesting contrast was found between the serum B$_{12}$ levels in the psychiatric patients of the New York area as opposed to those in the Western Northern Carolina area. Of 93 patients tested in the New York area, 16.1 percent were found to have serum B$_{12}$ levels between 150 and 200 pcg/ml, whereas in the North Carolina sample of 128 psychiatric patients, only 6.3 percent fell in this category. In the New York area, 17.2 percent of the patients had serum B$_{12}$ levels less than 150 pcg/ml, whereas the North Carolina group showed 9.4 percent in this group.

Of the total low B$_{12}$ determinations, the New York group showed 33.3 percent and the North Carolina group showed 15.7 percent.

6. Several case histories illustrating the value of hydroxocobalamin (vitamin B$_{12b}$) for the use in the treatment of psychiatric patients were presented.

It is my impression that hydroxocobalamin is of definite benefit to a small but significant percentage of psychiatric patients. Quite clearly, at least two (of the 221 patients) had dramatic improvements in their psychiatric illnesses following the use of B$_{12b}$.

7. I would suggest that all people and especially patients with psychiatric complaints, should be tested for serum B$_{12}$ levels. When the serum B$_{12}$ level below 200 picograms per cc. is discovered, the patients should be given at least monthly injections of hydroxocobalamin 1000 pcg/ml during the remainder of their

lives. Surely this is worthwhile in view of the possible consequences of demylinazation of the spinal cord and the brain proper in states where the serum B_{12} level is low.

8. I feel that every psychiatric patient should be given a clinical trial of injections of hydroxocobalamin, regardless of his serum B_{12} level. If the patient feels improved after the injections, the proper interval between injections should be determined by trial and error. This is in accordance with the author's clinical experience, and agrees with the theoretical postulations put forth by Linus Pauling (1968) [6].

N.B. Although cyanocobalamin (B_{12}) may be given even intraveinously or intramuscularly, hydroxocobalamin (B_{12b}) should only be injected intramuscularly.

REFERENCES

1. Encyclopaedia Britannica, 1958, Vol. 20, p. 232. Williams, R.J. and Deason, G.: Proc. Nat. Acad. Sci. U.S., 57, 1638, 1967.
2. Cleckley, H.M., Sydenstricker, V.P. and Geeslin, L.E.: J. Amer. Med. Assn. 112, 2107, 1939.
3. Hoffer, A.: Niacin Therapy in Psychiatry, Charles C. Thomas Co., Springfield, Ill. 1962.
4. Hoffer, A. and Osmond, H.: Lancet 1, 316, 1962.
5. Hoffer, A. and Osmond, H.: Acta Psychiat. Scand. 40, 171, 1964.
6. Pauling, Linus: Int. J. Neuropsychiat. 2, 234, 1966.
7. Michaelis, L. and Menten, M.: Biochem. z. 49, 333, 1913.
8. Samter, Max (Ed.): Immunological Diseases: pg. 1230, Little Brown & Co., Boston, 1971.
9. Turk, J.L.: Immunologin in Clinical Medicine: pg. 161, Appleton-Century-Crofts, New York, 1969.
10. Hakami, N., Neiman, P.E., Canellos, G.P. and Lazerson, J.: Neonatal Megaloblastic Anemia Due to Inherited Transcobalmin II Deficiency in Two Sibling: Vol. 285, No. 21, pg. 1163, New England Journal of Med., 1971.
11. Edwin, E., Holten, K., Norum, K.R., Schrumpf, A. and Skaug, O.E.: Acta Med. Scand. 177, 689, 1965.
12. Hansen, T., Rafaelsen, O.J. and Rodbro, P.: Lancet 2, 965, 1966.
13. Hunter, R., Jones, M., Jones, T.G. and Matthews, D.M.: Brit. J. Psychiat. 113, 1291, 1967.
14. Shulman, R.: Brit. J. Psychiat. 113, 241, 1967.
15. Buxton, P.K. Davison, W., Hyams, D.E. and Ervine, W.J.: Gerontologia Clinica 11, 22, 1969.
16. Murphy, F., Srivastava, P.C., Varadi, S., and Elwis, A.: Brit. Med. J. 3,559, 1969.
17. Carney, M.W.P.: Behavioral Neuropsychiatry, Vol. 1, No. 7, p. 19, October 1969.
18. Philpott, W.H.: Personal communication, 1971.
19. Smith, A.D.M.: Brit. Med. J. 2:1840, 1960.
20. Strachan, R.W. and Henderson, J.G.: Quart. J. Med. 34, 303, 1965.
21. Shulman, R.: Brit. J. Psychiat. 113, 252, 1967.
22. Hughes, D., Elwood, P.C., Shinton, N.K. and Wrighton, R.J.: Brit. Med. J. 2, 458. 1970.
23. Best, C.H. and Taylor, N.B.: The Physiological Basis of Medical Practice: Williams & Wilkins Co., Baltimore, 1966.
24. Foulds, W.S., Foleman, A.G., Phillips, C.I. and Wilson, J.: Lancet p. 35, Jan 3, 1970.

19
Pangamic Acid: B₁₅*

ALLAN COTT

Vitamin B_{15} (pangamic acid) was discovered, isolated, identified, and synthesized in the laboratory of E.T. Krebs, Sr., and E.T. Krebs, Jr., in San Francisco, California, in 1951.

Pangamic acid was first isolated from aqueous extracts of kernels from apricot stones, and later it was crystallized from rice shoots, rice bran, brewers yeast, bull blood, and horse liver. Subsequently it was identified with vitamin B_{15}. It is still not known whether pangamic acid is synthesized in the body, or is taken in with food and then enters the circulation and tissues (Garkina, 1962). It has been demonstrated to be a remarkably safe substance for which no undesirable side effects have been recorded. Its toxic dose for man is 100,000 times the therapeutic dose (Krebs, 1971).

Experiments were conducted on 350 rats weighing 140-250 g. Vitamins C and B_6 were injected one at a time in a 5 percent solution; B_{15} was used in a 40 percent solution. The lethal dose of B_6 consisted of 1,200-2,500 mg/kg. Calcium pangamate in a dose of 2,000 mg/kg did not have any toxic effect. This corresponds to data in the literature that vitamin B_{15} is practically nontoxic. The lethal dose of vitamin C was 3,000 mg/kg (Alpatov et al., 1971).

It has been well established experimentally that vitamin B_{15} increases the rate of phosphorylation of creatinine to phosphocreatinine. The latter is a high-energy compound that upon hydrolysis back to creatine and phosphoric acid yields a high level of energy for the mediation of muscle contraction, nerve conductivity, and membrane permeability.

It has been listed in the Merck Index (7th Edition), Dorland's Illustrated Medical Dictionary (23rd and 24th Editions), and Tabors Cyclopedic Medical Dictionary (10th Edition, 1965). While its discovery has received little notice, as has been the fate of other vitamin discoveries made in this country, it has been accorded much attention abroad. In recent years many countries have contributed a substantial literature on B_{15} in French, German, Italian, Japanese, Portuguese, Russian, and Spanish. Many of these studies were done in prominent universities and in the medical institutions and hospitals associated with the USSR Academy of Sciences. The Russian papers published by the McNaughton Foundation (Garkina, 1967) report clinical trials conducted on more than 1,000 patients suffering from cardio-

vascular diseases. A positive effect of B_{15} was observed in 80-90 percent of all patients treated. The calcium salt of Pangamic acid was administered by intramuscular injections in daily doses of 15-20 mg for 20-30 days, or in daily intra-abdominal injections of 40-50 mg, or in daily doses of 50-100 mgm taken orally.

Experimental and clinical studies by a number of workers have revealed that the physiological role of pangamic acid in the organism is based on its lipotropic activity, on its stimulation of oxidative metabolism in cell tissues, and on its detoxifying activity (Udalov, 1965). Udalov (1965) found an increased excretion of 17-ketosteroids in the urine of patients and a concomitant decrease in the content of ascorbic acid and cholesterol in the blood. Bertelli et al. (1957) injected vitamin B_{15} into mice and noted a decrease in serum ascorbic acid content.

These workers assumed that the decrease in the content of ascorbic acid and cholesterol was due to their utilization for the synthesis of corticosteroids. They also point out the significance of pangamic acid as a new methyl donor in the biosynthesis of many biologically important compounds. Udalov and Sokolova (1962, 1965) performed experiments with rats kept on a protein-deficient diet in which pangamic acid served as the sole source of methyl groups. In these experiments it was shown that the administration of pangamic acid almost completely prevented fatty infiltration of the liver. Udalov (1965) has shown that pangamic acid can serve as a methyl donor in the methylation of amide groups of nicotinic acid with the formation of N-methyl-nicotinamide in men kept on a protein-deficient diet. The conclusion is drawn that the apparent universality of action of pangamic acid is due to its methylating activity and its activity in the respiratory processes taking place in the cells and tissues of living organisms (Udalov and Sokolova, 1962, 1965).

In recent years numerous works had appeared on drug treatment for children suffering from severe disorders of behavior and communication. The search for new drugs affecting the activity of the central nervous system is mainly directed toward finding drugs with a general stimulatory activity. During the first year of life almost one half of the O_2 taken up by the child in the resting state is utilized by the brain. Numerous clinical and experimental data have shown that lowered respiration in the brain or in some of its segments may lead to various disturbances in mental activity (Himwich, 1951). The reports of Garkina (1962) and Dokukin (1967) draw attention to the antihypoxic properties of

*Reprinted with permission: *Orthomolecular Psychiatry*, Vol. 4, No. 2, 1975, 116-122.

calcium pangamate (B_{15}) in oxygen starvation in the brain.

Two Russian investigators, M.G. Blumena and T.K. Belyakova of the Moscow City Psychoneurological Clinic for Children and Adolescents, found improvement in speech in 12 of a group of 15 children diagnosed retarded after the oral administration of 20 mg of vitamin B_{15} three times daily. All children in this group displayed little interest in their environment, "lacked initiative and were rather passive." Four children in the group hardly verbalized, and none used language as a means of communication. Included in the experiment was a second group of six children whose mental state was characterized by "increased excitability, motor de-inhibition and tendency to affective outburst." Both groups were treated for one month during a period free of schooling. The use of drugs was suspended four to five days prior to the treatment with vitamin B_{15}. The efficacy of the treatment was controlled by constant clinical observation, and psychological tests were performed every 10 days.

After one month 12 of the first group of 15 children showed considerable improvement in speech development. The vocabulary of the four children who were virtually nonverbal prior to treatment was "considerably enriched." Some of them began to form disyllabic sentences. The general mental state and intellectual activity of the majority of the children in the group improved. Concentration improved and interest in toys and games developed.

The effect of vitamin B_{15} on the children in the second group was considerably less pronounced. Little improvement in their mental state was noted (Blumena and Belyakova, 1965).

The following case histories are presented in the form of reports from parents. The first group of reports described the reaction of children who have been diagnosed as autistic types, or rather children who suffer from severe disorders of learning, behavior, and communication.

Case #1, Jimmy, Age 7

His mother writes: "You know that Jimmy is emotionally disturbed and has a vocabulary of five or six words. I started giving Jimmy 200 mg of vitamin B_{15} for the past three weeks. I have noted a change in two areas. He has increased his vocabulary using words like candy, banana, chicken, dinner, couplets like 'get that,' 'get this.' He is constantly making sounds like he is trying to communicate. He has begun playing games with his brothers and sisters. He seems to want to be in their company now. Previously he never acknowledged his siblings' presence and never cared to be in their company. Jimmy is on no other medication at the present time."

Another letter three months later describes the following progress.

"Jimmy tries to dress himself and with my guidance can dress himself completely. He communicates a feeling of hunger to me by saying 'dinner.' Recently when one of his toys broke he handed it to me and said the word 'broke'. Today he said 'mom' for the first time. Jimmy's teacher visited him at home and was telling me that Jimmy had a different look in his face and that he seemed to be looking almost like a 'normal kid,' because some of his strange expressions and behavior are disappearing."

Case #2, Jimmy, Age 4

"Jimmy had a reaction almost immediately to the introduction of B_{15}. He became downright noisy. He still constantly is making sounds even in his sleep, at times you could hear a humming sound. He seems very pleased at his new noisiness also. He likes to hear himself, and he enjoys hearing himself played back on the tape recorder. He is saying a few more words, but now each word he tries is a different one. He says daddy quite clearly now and has said mommy once or twice."

One month later, Jimmy's mother wrote that her supply of vitamin B_{15} was exhausted, and eight days later the change in Jimmy was drastic. She described that:

"Jimmy can no longer sit still, his arms are going constantly, he can't even sit long enough to eat. He seems terribly distressed, almost as though he were in pain. He has lost eye contact and has become impatient and at times destructive. He punched the baby quite hard at least four times today. All this is completely unlike the Jimmy of a few weeks ago. It is a terrifying thing to see him go through this. He had come to be a peaceful, happy, easy child and generally a cooperative pleasant one. He had excellent eye to eye contact, but now he looks frightened and runs to us for assurance frequently. I know the B_{15} was administered originally to stimulate speech and in that area he has improved, but obviously it has been doing a lot for him which we did not realize fully until this recent relapse. His old symptoms of head-banging have recently returned also."

A letter dated 30 days later described how in 24 hours his crying had stopped and in 48 hours most of the bizarre behavior which had returned began to vanish.

"Within three days after he was back on the B_{15} he was again happy, his mood was pleasant and he slept well at night. This was absolutely the best Christmas we ever had with Jimmy. He enjoyed every minute of it. He enjoyed Santa instead of crying. None of his gifts caused him to become totally obsessed as in past years. He just seemed to enjoy everything as a normal child would. It feels good for me to use those words to describe our Jimmy."

The next letter from Jimmy's parents came seven months later. His mother wrote that:

"Jimmy is really starting to use words. Every day he has been saying words without the apparent effort it used to take. All the words are appropriate and relevant to what he is trying to express. He is just enjoying life so much now. He has a pleasant disposition and loves going out places. He is very patient and when he does get upset he is easily calmed down."

Two months later Jimmy's mother wrote again to say that he is doing better every day.

> "It's the most exciting thing I have ever experienced. He was repeating words and he answers questions now. He asks what's this and he names many things. There is no strange look when he tries to talk anymore, instead he has a big proud smile. He said something very special for me, 'I love mommy.' Frequently when I walk into his room I hear him talking to himself."

Case #3, Janet, Age 4

Janet's mother wrote that she had been vomiting daily after starting the vitamins, so she withheld everything but the vitamin B_{15} of which Janet would take 1½ tablets daily without nausea or vomiting. Within several days she said two sentences. When she reported this to me by telephone, I told her to increase the B_{15} to 3 tablets daily.

> "The following three days were the most exciting I have ever known. She spoke only in sentences, was eager to try everything and was quick to respond. Neighbors and other children commented on the remarkable difference. However, her teacher reported no change whatever in Janet's behavior or verbalizing at school and was slightly incredulous when I described Janet's improvement at home. Last Sunday when Janet was unaware of my presence I saw her cover her naked doll with her coat as she said 'that's all right baby, I know you are cold. I will cover you with my coat and make you warm.' "

The Russian literature on vitamin B_{15} reported its value in the treatment of a variety of forms of asthma. In taking case histories of my patients, I frequently came across the history of siblings who suffered from asthma and suggested that the child might benefit from the use of the vitamin B_{15} for treatment of the asthma. The following series of cases indicate that vitamin B_{15} is indeed a valuable treatment of asthma and other allergic conditions.

Case #4, Ellen, Age 12

Ellen's mother wrote:

> "In 1959, when Ellen was two and a half, she began to wheeze. Asthma was diagnosed, and she was started on antihistamines. Soon her attacks became more severe and occurred about once every two weeks lasting two to three days. The attacks continued on and off over the next year and a half during which time her pediatrician prescribed steam tents, antihistamines, ipecac to make her vomit, and adrenalin when necessary. She improved steadily, but in the spring of 1965 she was wheezing again and she began to have attacks of asthma severe enough to sometimes require adrenalin. She was also taking Tedral and antihistamines. Her pediatrician advised us to take Ellen to an allergist which we did. He treated her for a year at which time she did not improve. She had a series of desensitization injections, Tedral, antihistamines, and prednisone.

> "During the summer of 1966 while riding her bike she had such a severe attack that she was taken to the emergency room of the local hospital. There she was given oxygen and an injection of adrenalin, and again prednisone was prescribed. In 1966 skin testing found her to be allergic to trees, grasses, molds, ragweed, and dust. A series of desensitization injections were begun. She continued taking antihistamines for a runny nose and eyes, Tedral for wheezing, and was put on prednisone whenever she had a severe attack. During the year of 1966 she was out of school for at least half of the school year due to her recurring attacks of asthma. She was unable to take gymnasium classes and had to be driven back and forth to school since any physical exertion would make her breathing even more labored. In January, 1971, vitamin B_{15} was begun. We were very willing to try. We waited for spring and early summer for any results and this was always one of the times of the year when Ellen became very asthmatic. However, that spring and early summer we had seen a great improvement. She had taken Tedral for a slight wheeze only about six times, has not needed prednisone or adrenalin, has been very active riding on her bike, swimming, and going on long hikes. We consider this a miracle medication for Ellen."

The follow-up report written six months later states that:

> "Ellen has been taking the vitamin and continues to be virtually free of asthmatic attacks. During the summer when there was a great amount of mold, she did have watery eyes and a runny nose on occasion. This has been a great improvement for her. She continues to be able to walk long distances, ride her bike, and the past year has been taking modern dancing courses. As you know, these were activities which at one time Ellen was never able to do without getting short of breath or wheezing. As long as she takes her vitamin she has been free of asthmatic attacks."

Case #5, Johnny, Age 9

At age nine, Johnny was an accomplished performer on the stage and in the movies. His mother wrote to confess that when she started him on the vitamin B_{15} she had very little hope "since she and her husband had given up all hope of ever curing Johnny's croaking," as they called it. Her letter stated:

> "I was always afraid to send him out on cold or damp days. Now he is out in every weather and without a hat or all muffled up as he always was. Best of all, when he runs up the stairs now or plays basketball, etc., he breathes quite normally. Up to the time he started on the vitamins he had great trouble sometimes recording, as they always seemed to pick up his wheezing on tape. Now he tapes without the slightest difficulty. Singing was always impaired by the wheezing. Now he has a fine voice. If possible I would like

you to take another look at Johnny sometime next week to see for yourself the amazing recovery."

Case #6, Paula, Age 18

Paula, age 18, wrote the following report about her improvement.

"I first took the B_{15} in the winter of 1970. I took one pill when I had an asthma attack and it usually cleared the congestion, but the frequency of the attacks has not changed. In May, 1971, I went to California and discontinued the B_{15} because I had only two asthma attacks. When I returned to New York, I started wheezing again because I was allergic to the dog and the cat after being out of the house for three months. In December I started taking the B_{15} four times daily. Within three or four days the wheezing stopped.

"Before the B_{15} I used to have coughing and/or wheezing attacks which lasted from one to two and a half hours. I usually use my Medi-Haler, cough medicine, and hot tea to relieve it. These attacks used to occur two or three times a week. Since resuming the B_{15}, I have had only one such attack and it has lasted for half an hour.

"To get to my house I have to walk up a steep hill. I always become short of breath, but in winter and fall I wheeze heavily. I use the inhalor and it clears up within the hour.

"With the B_{15} I still have shortness of breath, but I rarely wheeze heavily. If I do wheeze it clears within 15 minutes. I have been attending an exercise group for two years. Last year I started wheezing after half an hour and could not always finish the 80-minute class. Since taking the B_{15} I have not wheezed once this year while exercising. For me the B_{15} seems to have a preventative effect. The inhalor and cough medicine can only be taken when the coughing and wheezing actually start, but the B_{15} when taken regularly controls the asthma. Another advantage of the B_{15} for me is that is does not cause an allergic reaction which occurred when I took other pills for asthma such as Tedral. This has been the first fall season since I had asthma that it has been under control. I attribute this control to the use of B_{15}."

Case #7, Scott, Age 10

Scott's mother writes that:

"Scott has shown little problems with allergies since being started on vitamin B_{15}. Previously he had problems breathing, especially when exposed to grasses, molds, ragweed, and other inhalants. Sometimes his eyes would water and itch."

She continued that: "Scott has been having injections for desensitization once every three weeks for the past year. In May the supply of B_{15} was exhausted and Scott did have several attacks and had to take Allerest. He also had a reaction to his injections and the doctor decided that he needed to come every two weeks instead of every three."

She concluded the letter by adding Scott had started taking the B_{15} again and has not had any problems since.

Case #8, Lisa, Age 11

Lisa's mother writes:

"Lisa has been on vitamin B_{15} since last February. This was the first summer in three years that she did not have any hay fever. If she is without B_{15} for more than a few days her behavior changes and she is constantly angry. Whenever she does have the B_{15} she is much more cooperative and appears to be alert."

Case #9, Tony, Age 9

Tony's mother wrote:

"Tony has become a very cooperative, agreeable, pleasant, and willing child. He has also become inventive and shows a great deal of initiative. I have no inkling as to the concentration span, and small muscle control appears no better. I don't know if this picture is because of lack of school pressures or participation in sports, the addition of vitamin B_{15}, or an accumulation of all of these things, but I am very thankful. At last he is a happy child. M.J. (Tony's brother) came home from a camping trip that very weekend with a cold and a slight trace of asthma. I did not take him to the doctor which I would normally have done. In one week he was completely without symptoms and has been so ever since. He took vitamin B_{15} twice a day."

The following patient has been diagnosed Cerebral Palsy. She is 16 years of age. The mother writes:

"It is difficult to measure a day-by-day improvement, but as I look back over the last year and a half I can truly say that I have noted great improvement. She seems to have much more assurance, better organization of thought, and expression in her excessive movements are better controlled. More concrete evidence is the fact that she is earning more money at the workshop because her production is better. Comparing hand samples, one sees a dramatic change. Since the addition of B_{15} to the megavitamins, the whole picture seems to be even more improved."

Pangamic acid is a classical example of a vitamin because it is almost impossible to escape the self-limiting mechanisms that prevent any toxic manifestations. A true drug is, by contrast, the exact opposite of a vitamin. It is toxic or at least irritative, stimulative, or depressive in any dose. Thus, it is really impossible to have a vitamin that is toxic or a drug that is nontoxic when each is used within the parameters of its optimal therapeutic response (Krebs, 1971).

The scientific and clinical progress of vitamin B_{15} has been characteristic of that of most important vitamins whose value becomes increasingly apparent as research and clinical application widen. This is in contrast to the history of all but a few drugs. Their lack of value becomes increasingly apparent as they are studied over the years. No vitamin has ever come into clinical application without the scope of its utility becoming more and more apparent with continuing studies (Krebs, 1971). While it appears that the potential therapeutic spectrum of pangamic acid is impressive, it becomes more so when one keeps in mind that it is a vitamin and not a drug. For this reason, it is most rationally handled as a physiological tool to be utilized for achieving specific physiological ends directed toward the prevention or amelioration of deficiencies grounded in the failure of the relevant metabolic pathways.

REFERENCES

Garkina, I.N.: "Pangamic Acid and its Derivatives." Vitamin B_{15} (Pangamic Acid), Properties, Functions and Use. Science Publishing House, Moscow, USSR. Translated by McNaughton Foundation, Montreal, P.Q., Canada, 1962.

Shpirt, Y.A. Y.U.: "Indications for Use and Efficacy of Calcium Pangamate in Internal Disease Clinic." Russian Publication by V/O Medexport, Moscow, USSR, 1968.

Alpatov, Dagaev, Sanotskin, Udalov, Luzhnikov, Pankov. Biological Abstracts. 50-81312, 1971.

Garkina, I.N.: "Pangamic Acid and its Derivatives." Vitamin B_{15} (Pangamic Acid), Properties, Functions and Use. Science Publishing House, Moscow, USSR. Translated by McNaughton Foundation, Montreal, P.Q., Canada, 1967.

Udalov, Y.U.F.: 1965.

Bertelli et al.: Soc. Ital. Biol. Sperirn. 63,885, 1957.

Udalov, Y.U.F., and Sokolova, M.N.: 1962, 1965.

Dokukin: The Effect of Pangamic Acid on Heart and Brain Hypoxia. Vitamin B_{15}. Properties, Functions and Use, Science Publishing House, Moscow, USSR, 1967.

Himwich, H.E.: "Brain Metabolism and Cerebral Disorders." Baltimore, Williams and Wilkins, 1951.

Blumena, M.G., and Belyakova, T.K.: "The Use of Vitamin B_{15} for Oligophrenic Children." Science Publishing House Moscow, USSR. Translated by McNaughton Foundation, Montreal, P.W., Canada. 1965.

Krebs, E.T., Jr.: Communication from John Beard Memorial Foundation to McNaughton, A.R.L., The McNaughton Foundation, Montreal, P.Q., Canada. Dated August 10, 1971.

20

Copper, Zinc, Manganese, Niacin and Pyridoxine in the Schizophrenias*

CARL C. PFEIFFER AND DONNA BACCHI

INTRODUCTION

Considering that "schizophrenia" is at present a biochemical wastebasket diagnosis, the enrichment of white flour with four nutrients, including niacinamide, has probably arrested more "schizophrenia" (i.e. pellagra) than all of psychoanalytic therapy. One would further predict that the proposed enrichment of all cereals with ten nutrients, including zinc, B_6, and folic acid will stop more "schizophrenia" (i.e. pyroluria and histapenia) than all of the various types of talking and drug therapy combined. In light of the biochemical advances that have been made within the past few decades to ameliorate many schizophrenic symptoms, the time has come to extol the biochemical approach as a major breakthrough in the treatment of the schizophrenias and to credit the biochemists and nutritionists with long overdue praise for their contributions to the reduction of mental disorders.

Derek Richter (1970) has pointed out that "cure" can seldom be applied to the schizophrenias, but still, since 1900 the schizophrenias have been diminished remarkably by the "subdivide and conquer" approach provided by the advance of the nutritional and biochemical sciences. The clinical systematists may reclassify and rename the multifarious clinical symptoms, but this does not enhance our knowledge of the etiology. Although additional names may be added to the list, the patients and their symptoms remain unchanged. Through the biochemical "subdivide and conquer" approach we now know that a niacin deficiency or dependency may enhance mental illness, that a combined B_6 and zinc deficiency or a severe copper excess may produce clinical symptoms of "schizophrenia", that mental disturbances associated with EEG abnormalities may indicate a B_{12} deficiency, and that other inborn errors of metabolism may predispose an individual to the development of a psychosis. With increasing evidence supporting the biochemical approach it is egregious that most psychotherapists still insist that too much or too little social attention in the formative years has made the schizophrenic what he is today. A better understanding of the evidence supporting the biochemical and nutritional approach to the schizophrenias will elucidate the problems afflicting many individuals currently labeled "schizophrenic" so that proper

diagnosis and better treatment can ensue.

In 1967, when we found that some schizophrenics had very low, while others had very high, blood histamine levels, we turned to trace metal studies to see if abnormalities might be present to account for these differences. The possibility was encouraged by the reports that histamine occurs in the mast cells with zinc, and, (other than the pineal gland and retina) the highest brain level of zinc occurs in the hippocampus (possibly in connection with the terminal vesicles of the mossy fibers where, again, histamine may be stored). In addition, diaminoxidase (histaminase) is a well-known copper-containing enzyme that is also stored in the mast cells with the trace metal zinc. Copper and zinc are biologically antagonistic and in animal studies using either or both these metals, it has been shown that any dietary excess of one will lead to a depletion of the other. A few reports indicate that zinc and manganese are biological synergists that work together to rid the body of excess copper, and that manganese poisoning results in Parkinson's disease — the symptoms of which may be mimicked as a side effect of any of the presently used antischizophrenic drugs. Manganese has many functions in the body. It is specifically needed for the action of choline acetylase, for normal thyroid function, for cartilage and bone growth and for the production of mucopolysaccharides.

Excess copper blood levels have been recorded frequently in groups of schizophrenics; these reports would be easier to categorize if the workers had studied the biochemical types of schizophrenics rather than "schizophrenia" as a homogeneous entity. Good precedence for this concept exists since approximately ten clinical, biochemical, and genetic syndromes have been separated from "schizophrenia" since 1900. The separations were effected by finding the cause of other disorders which mimic schizophrenia perfectly. The ten separations are now called dementia paralytica (brain syphilis), pellagra, porphyria, homocysteinuria, myxoedema (thyroid deficiency), amphetamine psychosis, vitamin B_{12} folic acid avitaminosis, food sensitivity (wheat gluten), temporal lobe epilepsy, and Klinefelter syndrome [Pfeiffer et al. (1970).]

The concept that some metals, now called trace elements or micronutrients, may be deficient in some types of schizophrenia is not entirely new, but biochemical analysis to direct treatment is a novel approach. Diagnosis and treatment of schizophrenic

*Reprinted with permission: *Journal of Applied Nutrition*, Volume 27, #2.

outpatient populations has led us to a subdivision in three different categories: 50 percent are histapenic (low blood histamine, high serum copper), 20 percent are histadelic (high blood histamine, low or normal serum copper), and a third group, constituting 30 percent of the schizophrenic population, which are normal in copper and histamine but excrete a substance in their urine called kryptopyrrole, depleting them of B_6 and zinc and manifesting itself in a myriad of clinical symptoms. Nutrient therapy consisting of controlled administration of needed trace elements and vitamins has proven effective in restoring the body's optimal dietary intake and in arresting the clinical and biochemical symptoms indicative of "schizophrenia".

HISTORICAL

A. Critical Review

Schizophrenics may have low levels of zinc and manganese; high levels of copper, iron, mercury, and lead may be found. The last two are, of course, poisons, but the poisoning may produce symptoms which mimic those of schizophrenia. This has been documented for mercury and lead. For the porphyric schizophrenic, the suggestion of a need for extra dietary zinc goes back to 1929, when Derrien and Benoit found a high level of zinc in the urine of the porphyric patient. They suggested that zinc deficiency might be the cause of the abnormal psychiatric symptoms. The excess loss of zinc via the chelating action of uroporphyrin has been confirmed by Watson and Schwartz (1941), Nesbitt (1944) and Peters (1961). In 1965, Kimura and Kumura found that brain autopsy specimens from schizophrenics contained approximately half the zinc found in brains of patients dying of other causes.

Other than indirect copper studies, very few studies of trace metals appear in the literature on schizophrenia. In fact, the use of trace metals as a possible treatment method in schizophrenia began in 1929. At that time, Dr. W.M. English of Brockville, Ontario, reported on the use of intravenous manganese chloride in 181 schizophrenic patients and found that half of them improved. As with both chlorpromazine and reserpine therapy, English reported a gain in weight in those patients who responded to manganese therapy. (Intravenous manganese produced a cutaneous flush like that of niacin!) This study was in part repeated by R.G. Hoskins of the Worchester Foundation, who published in 1934, but instead of using manganese chloride intravenously he used, for the most part, suspended manganese dioxide given intramuscularly. In the first instance, the intravenous route was unnecessary with water soluble and orally absorbed manganese chloride. In the second instance manganese dioxide is a nonabsorbable form, deposited intramuscularly, where it probably stayed for a very long time. Hoskins found no improvement in the small group of schizophrenics injected with manganese dioxide.

B. Copper Studies in Schizophrenia

One of the earliest studies of the implications of serum copper in schizophrenia is to be found in 1941. At that time, Heilmeyer et al. reported findings of elevated serum copper levels in 32 of 37 schizophrenics. In subsequent studies the same authors found similar serum copper elevation in groups of manic depressives, and epileptics, and also in cases of alcoholic intoxication, infectious disease, and cancer.

These original findings did stimulate some interest in copper research in schizophrenia, and the details were essentially verified by several workers in the subsequent years (Brenner, 1949; Jantz, 1950; and Bischoff, 1952). Brenner made an extensive study of the serum copper levels in childhood schizophrenia under different physiological and pathological conditions. In children with definite schizophrenic symptoms, he found highly elevated serum copper levels, in contrast to the findings for children with cerebral-organic disorders, postencephalitic processes, or mental retardation. Considerable serum copper elevation was also found by Brenner in 38 percent of an adult schizophrenic group. Brenner's conclusion was that such a copper elevation could be found only in a condition of endogenous aggravation but not at the time of a spontaneous remission. Such differences were not found by Munch-Petersen (1950) in a group of chronic schizophrenics.

A very careful and well controlled study on copper metabolism in schizophrenics was performed by Ozek (1957). Serum copper levels of 122 schizophrenics were determined. In 38 of these the ceruloplasmin levels were also measured, and, in addition, the erythrocyte copper levels in 56 patients were also determined. The experimental group was divided in four categories: acute, subacute, chronic and organic defects. Of the total, 66 percent exhibited copper levels above the normal (especially in the acute group) but this was considered by the author as a reflection of body response to some physiological disturbance. No difference in the erythrocyte or ceruloplasmin levels was detected.

Ackerfeldt (1957) was the first to report elevated serum oxidase levels in adult schizophrenics. Abood et al. (1957) also found abnormally high ceruloplasmin levels in two-thirds or more of 250 schizophrenics. However, these workers considered dietary factors, hepatic damage, and chronic infections as possible contributory factors. Some preliminary experiments performed by Ostfeld et al. (1958) indicated that excitement tends to elevate ceruloplasmin. Normal subjects receiving a synthetic hallucinatory agent demonstrated the same elevated ceruloplasmin level as psychotic schizophrenics. Other workers (Horwitt et al, 1957; Frank and Wurtmand, 1958; Scheinberg et al., 1957) were unable to find significant differences in ceruloplasmin oxidase activity in schizophrenic children and adults as compared to controls.

More recently Bakwin et al. (1961) compared the serum copper concentration of 91 schizophrenic children against a control group of 73 children, and were unable to detect any significant difference between the two groups. On the opposite side of this controversial study of the significance of elevated copper serum levels in schizophrenia. Swedish workers (Martens et al., 1959) reported favorable improvement in 28 schizophrenics after intravenous injection of purified ceruloplasmin. Barress et al. (1970) examined the effect of schizophrenics' urine extracts, as compared to extracts from postoperative controls, on the oxidative activity of ceruloplasmin, using as a substrate norepinephrine and 5-hydroxytryptamine. They found that the urine of schizophrenics contained a factor or factors which accelerates the ceruloplasmin catalyzed oxidation of norepinephrine, but inhibited the oxidation of 5-hydroxytryptamine.

A well-established fact is that ceruloplasmin synthesis is accelerated by estrogens, and women taking contraceptive pills uniformly exhibit elevated serum copper and lower zinc levels. It is also interesting to note that any biological state which elevates the serum copper is apt to increase the need of vitamin C. The schizophrenic state, late pregnancy, and particularly the use of the contraceptive pill produces states of elevated copper levels, which in turn may aggravate depression and disperception in schizophrenic patients on the pill. Natarajan Saroja (1971) administered mestranol to guinea pigs, the result was a marked reduction in the ascorbic acid concentration in their blood plasma (decreased 23 percent) and an even greater reduction in their blood capillaries (decreased 38 percent). Rivers and Devine (1972) found that in controls the total ascorbic acid concentrations were highest at ovulation and lowest during menses. Subjects on the pill had higher C concentrations during menses than when they were ingesting the drug. The results of the study indicated that oral contraceptives effectively prevent changes in plasma and total ascorbic acid concentration, probably due to the increased level of copper in the blood. Oral contraceptives depress plasma ascorbic acid levels and prevent the sharp increase in plasma ascorbic acid levels at times of ovulation. Thus, situations which cause a rise in serum copper demand extra vitamin C. It is then necessary to examine in man trace metals, such as iron and copper, which are known to oxidize vitamin C.

Porphyria appears in many cases to have a more than casual relationship to schizophrenia, and low ceruloplasmin levels have been reported (Yamada, 1965). Porphyrins act as chelating agents to increase urinary excretion of both copper and zinc. In summary, it seems that serum copper and ceruloplasmin levels deserve more attention than they have received in the past.

One might hastily and erroneously conclude that any involvement of excess copper in the schizophrenias is excluded by the above studies. This is not true since most of the previous workers have assumed that the schizophrenias are biochemically homogeneous. Most of the studies deal with single serum copper determinations on individuals. Longitudinal studies (to correlate possible changes in tissue and serum copper with psychiatric state as the patient improves) have not been done, even when improvement was obtained with D-penicillamine, the copper chelating agent. Metabolic studies are needed in depth as patients improve with various therapies. Finally the relationship of excess copper to zinc deficiency and iron excess needs to be unravelled, since many zinc-deficient patients (low serum zinc) seem to be loaded with excess copper and iron, as shown by hair analyses and by the longitudinal studies on serum copper when patients are treated with zinc and manganese.

C. Use of D-Penicillamine in Schizophrenia

Walshe (1956) used penicillamine to increase the urinary excretion of copper in patients with Wilson's disease. Therefore Greiner and Berry (1964) had a convenient and proven copper chelating agent to use in the treatment of abnormal melanin formation in schizophrenic patients. Copper is the trace element involved in the synthesis of the B-hydroxy group of catechol amines. This B-hydroxy group is present in Z-dopa, which is synthesized into melanin, the normal skin pigment. The histapenic patient is the blondest of the family and usually sunburns excessively when exposed. The pyroluric patient also reports that he cannot tan in the sun. The studies of the Canadian group culminated in a report (Nicholson et al., 1966) of a double-blind study in which five patients received D-penicillamine and a trace metal dietary supplement (Fister et al., 1958) while the five controls received placebo therapy. All of the D-penicillamine and trace metal patients improved while none of the controls benefited. The study has been repeated by many other groups (Table I), but only Ozek used the trace metal dietary supplement (without copper) recommended by Fister. This may be most important, since D-penicillamine also chelates zinc and increases zinc excretion via the urinary pathway. (The national diet would be the deciding factor in response to D-penicillamine therapy if an adequate trace metal supplement was not used.) One of the side effects of D-penicillamine therapy is loss of taste which is now ascribed to zinc deficiency.

Those diets supplying adequate zinc would, in all probability, cause less incidence of "schizophrenia" than diets lacking zinc. One can predict that the European diet would provide more zinc and manganese than the American, since in Europe many more soups, fresh vegetables, and wines are used rather than ice cream, frozen foods, soft drinks, and artificial fruit juices. In future studies of D-penicillamine, patients with high serum copper should be chosen for the study. Serum copper, zinc, and iron should be assayed weekly. The study should run 4 to 6 months, and a dietary supplement of at least zinc should be used.

Of interest is the convergence of three lines of study toward the study of copper balance in some schizophrenic patients. First, the observation that copper and zinc are chelated by urinary porphorins to such an extent as to produce a zinc deficiency; second, the occurrence of excess copper in some schizophrenics as shown by high serum levels; and finally, the beneficial effect of D-penicillamine therapy in a few hard to treat patients.

D. Methods

In general the methods used in this report have all been detailed in previous publications. A Perkin-Elmer 305 atomic absorption spectrophotometer was used to determine serum and urinary iron, zinc, and copper. Serum manganese was determined by the same method, using 4 ml of concentrated serum.

Urinary excretion of trace metals was determined for a 6-hour period, from 9:00 a.m. to 3:00 p.m. In this way accurate collections could be obtained in a 7½-hour work day. These patients and normals usually had a quantitative electroencephalogram taken every 10 minutes out of each hour for a 6-hour period after the control run.

The "normal subjects" were laboratory personnel, reformatory inmates, and others who passed a psychiatric interview and who also had a normal score on the Experiential World Inventory (EWI) [Osmond and El Meligi (1971)]. Outpatients with schizophrenia were referred by physicians mainly to determine their type with regard to high or low blood histamine level. Most patients had been hospitalized one or more times for their schizophrenia. Patients who had not been hospitalized were given the EWI and Minnesota Multiphasic Personality Inventory to ascertain their degree of psychopathology. The accurate method for precise assay of the degree of brain arousal and the EWI to determine the degree of disperception and thought disorder made possible the correlation of biochemical findings with the neurophysiological status and psychiatric state of the schizophrenic patient.

The outpatients consisted of the problem patients who had not responded to antipsychotic drug therapy. Various treatments were used to improve the psychiatric status of the patients. These were the conventional antischizophrenic drugs, vitamin supplements, lithium therapy up to the level of 1.0 meq/liter, and a trace element dietary supplement consisting of 10 percent zinc sulfate and 0.5 percent manganous chloride in distilled water. When used at the level of five drops a.m. and p.m., the last solution provides half of the zinc and manganese which should be present in an ideal normal diet. Similar dietary supplements are now available commercially (Ziman Fortified, Vicon Plus, and Plus 85).

Patients were studied at five week intervals over a period of 1 to 6 years. A 30-ml blood sample was taken at each visit. A 2-ml whole blood aliquot was used for histamine and polyamine determinations. The remaining serum was used for lithium, trace metal, and other determinations.

E. Results

The results are tabulated in the form of tables and figures wherein an attempt has been made to have the legends completely explanatory. Some tables represent several years of study on 300 schizophrenic out-patients, with a trace metal report on a longitudinal study of 240 patients.

Trace metal urinary excretion and plasma levels have been done on 6 hospitalized patients and 6 to 30 outpatient schizophrenic patients. In most instances, the trials have been repeated to determine the variability of a given patient and to increase the actual number of trials. Urinary excretion of the trace metals studied varies widely. Thus a series of 25 trials is sometimes necessary to produce a reasonably low standard deviation. The mean excretion of zinc, copper, and iron as given in Table II provides trends on which to base working hypotheses on the interactions of these trace metals in man. In the 6-year period covered by this study, many normal subjects have provided comparative data. These data are included in the appropriate tables.

Most of the trace metals have been cautiously tried for the effect on both zinc, copper and iron excretion and the quantitative EEG effect of stimulation or sedation. In general copper, chromium, cobalt and iron are stimulant to the brain while zinc, manganese, vanadium, and molybdenum are sedative. Fluorine and selenium are without effect on the quantitative EEG at the low doses tested. In addition, the amino acids which may chelate trace metals have been explored for their effect on the excretion of zinc, copper, and iron. D-penicillamine was the only standard chelating agent studied.

We tested for the effect of estrogens on serum levels of copper and zinc and found elevated serum copper with an accompanying depletion of serum zinc resulting from both normal estrogens and the use of the contraceptive pill. In a normal cycle, serum copper reaches a peak approximately one week before the menstrual period. This peak coincides with the peak of estrogen activity and may be responsible for the premenstrual tension, depression, and headaches indicative of high copper. A study of schizophrenic women before and after oral contraceptive use (Figures 1, 2) revealed a sharp rise in serum copper levels upon initiation of contraceptive therapy, with a resulting decrease in copper after discontinuation. It is also interesting to note that the mean normal serum copper levels for these women was considerably higher than that found in normal women (1.0-1.7 ppm).

The accumulated data for copper is as follows: Normals, one week before menstrual period, copper-1.2 mcg/ml (120 mcg percent ppm); one week after menstrual period 0.9; postmenstrual females on conjugated estrogens, 1.4; normals on birth control pills, 1.75; schizophrenics on conjugated estrogens, 1.82; normals in ninth month pregnancy, 2.20; schizophrenics on birth control pills, 2.88 (range 2.16-5.65!). Some young girls date their depression and disperception to the time when the birth control pill was prescribed to regulate their menstrual period or decrease dysmenorrhea. The increased intake of copper with contraceptive use, in addition to an inadequate amount of zinc, results in an imbalance of these trace metals in the body can possibly lead to clinical manifestations indicative of copper excess.

Our study of the amino acid methionine has shown it effective in ameliorating the symptoms characteristically found in the high histamine patients. Based on the over-methylation theory of schizophrenia, numerous studies have confirmed that methionine with or without an MAO inhibitor will worsen the degree of schizophrenia in most hospitalized schizophrenics. These patients have hallucinations and paranoia and might be expected to be low in blood histamine (Pfeiffer et al., 1969). Methylation of histamine is one pathway in the degradation of histamine, thus those patients low in histamine should worsen with methylating agents, such as methionine. However, the 20 percent of the schizophrenic patients that are high in histamine do benefit from the methionine-induced methylation of histamine.

Schizophrenic outpatients who were given single oral doses of 1.2 grams D-methionine, 1.2 grams L-methionine, 1.5 grams DL-methionine or placebo demonstrated a lowering of blood histamine by both isomers of methionine, with DL-methionine being the most active. The lowering of blood histamine by DL-methionine is constant and may be sufficient to ameliorate the symptoms of some high histamine schizophrenic patients. This lowering of histamine may correlate with CNS stimulant effect of methionine seen in rabbits and man.

DL-methionine has also been found to increase the excretion of copper, iron, and zinc in schizophrenic patients (Table IV). An oral dose of 1.5 grams DL-methionine (greater than the usual therapeutic dose) significantly increased urinary excretion of zinc, copper, and iron. Considering that most schizophrenics are burdened with copper, the use of DL-methionine, in addition to possibly reducing histamine in the histapenic patient, can be used to restore the bodily balance of copper, iron and zinc. Some of the vitamins also cause significant urinary excretion of trace metals over a 6-hour period (Table V). The similarity of trace metal excretion by "Hexanicotol" and "Linodyl" is of interest because they are presumably identical. Both are the nicotinic acid ester of inositol.

F. The major Schizophrenias '74: Histadelia, Histapenia, Pyroluria

The schizophrenias may have many biochemical facets, since, in the past, ten biochemical entities have been separated. We now suggest three major subdivisions to be used in diagnosis and treatment and to be considered for further research (Figure 3). The patients sensitive to wheat gluten are low in blood histamine and represent a special group of the histapenic patients. The histapenic patient is low in blood histamine, high in serum copper and has a low serum folate level. In addition, this group demonstrates low mean energy content (MEC) of their alpha waves and high ceruloplasmin. Ceruloplasmin has histaminase activity and all diaminoxidases contain copper. These patients are usually overstimulated, paranoid, and hallucinatory and respond well to niacin, B_{12}, and folic acid (2.0 mgm daily). Folic acid in conjunction with weekly B_{12} injections raises the blood histamine while lowering the degree of psychopathology, as evidenced by the decreased EWI score. Folic acid in doses larger than 2.0 mgm daily can produce myoclonic jerkings with accompanying seizures when combined with antipsychotic drug therapy. Occasionally in epileptics the drug at fault is diphenylhydantoin (Dilantin). This drug-induced folate deficiency is of the low histamine type which is characterized by paranoia and hallucinations. These patients also seem to be niacin-dependent and respond well to niacin therapy. D-penicillamine is also effective in the paranoid patient.

The histadelic group is characterized by suicidal depression and is a biochemical antithesis of the low histamine group. Their MEC and blood histamine are high, while their serum copper is normal or low. The blood histamine is contained in the basophils, so they frequently show basophil counts above 1 percent (Pfeiffer et al., 1971). It follows that those patients high in histamine should use diphenylhydantoin to produce an antifolate effect and thus lower their histamine level. Dilantin when given knowledgeably with calcium, methionine, and trace metal nutrients zinc and manganese, is effective therapy. Patients high in histamine have adequate niacin intake and do not benefit from niacin therapy. The low histamine patient receiving B_{12} and folic acid must be carefully watched for a histamine increase that may be so high as to induce a return of their depression. Regular blood histamine tests can insure against such a reaction.

The third and perhaps most interesting group contains those patients normal in histamine and in trace metals, except for those who are low or high in serum zinc. They have the mauve factor (kryptopyrrole) in their urine which depletes them of both zinc and B_6 (Pfeiffer et al., 1974). This may result in abnormal EEG's with single convulsions when first placed on neuroleptic medication. They respond best to large doses of pyridoxine a.m. and p.m. and dietary supplements of zinc because the pyrrole combines with pyridoxal (B_6) and then makes a complex with zinc to produce a combined deficiency. Some problem patients may have both the mauve factor and a histamine imbalance, making them more difficult to treat. Pyroluric patients may have any of the classical symptoms of schizophrenia, but their insight and affect are much better than other schizophrenic types.

Several workers have confirmed the original observations of Irvine (1961) and Hoffer/Osmond (1962) that abnormal mauve factor is excreted in greater frequency in the urine of schizophrenics. Other workers (Ellman et al., 1968) have labeled this finding a drug artifact noted only in patients on phenothiazines. Recently Irvine et al (1969) have succeeded in isolating and identifying the mauve factor as 2, 4 dimethyl-3-ethylpyrrole, an observation subsequently confirmed by Sohler et al. (1970). Neither Irvine nor Sohler could find any relationship of KP excretion to phenothiazine medication. Furthermore, 5 percent

of "so-called" normals, who are not on phenothiazines, excrete the mauve factor.

The dose of B_6 needed by the KP positive patient may be as high as 3,000 mg per day to prevent psychopathology and keep the urine free of KP. Our present quantitative test for KP measures the total assayable KP.

This clinical entity would undoubtedly have been discovered much earlier if the essential interrelationship between zinc and B_6 had been known. We have found that mauve positive patients excrete in their urine significantly more zinc and coproporphyrin (Table VII). A 50 mg oral dose of B_6 reduces urinary zinc excretion in both patients and normals while increasing copper. The decrease in zinc produced by the intake of B_6 is greater in schizophrenic patients than in normals; also, they characteristically excrete less copper than normals. Because of wide individual variation these changes are not statistically significant (Table II).

We now have over three years of experience diagnosing and treating over 300 of mauve positive pyroluric patients. The B_6 and zinc treatment is usually effective in producing a remission of their psychoses sometimes in 5 to 10 days. Manganese may be needed in addition to zinc and B_6. We have used a dietary supplement of zinc sulfate 10 percent and manganese chloride 0.5 percent at the rate of 6 drops a.m. and p.m. This supplies two-thirds of the zinc and manganese needed in a normal daily diet. Many schizophrenic patients are burdened with excess copper and this combination of trace metals mobilizes copper and iron to produce greater copper and iron excretion. Copper excretion is increased progressively by the combination of zinc, manganese, and B_6.

The etiology of the syndrome as a double deficiency syndrome has not been definitely established. Research is under way to provide more exact evidence. We do know that substitution of placebo capsules for the B_6 and zinc therapy may result in catatonia, muscle weakness and chills with fever. In such tests slow withdrawal is recommended.

Three possible nutritional and biochemical facets of the schizophrenias have been diagnosed and are currently being treated. Treatment may be supportive, but nutrition for prevention may decrease the future need for such treatment. The fortification of food and soft drinks with 10 to 15 nutrients removed from wheat might be earth shaking. Awareness of the dietary and environmental factors involved in excess copper and deficient zinc dietary consumption may preclude some latent schizophrenics syndromes. Simplistic referral to "schizophrenia" as an entity should be discouraged in the scientific literature.

RESEARCH NEEDS

Like a silent fifth column man is being burdened with excess copper which can, if unregulated, cause serious physiological and psychological complications (Table VIII). The prospective mother may find herself the unfortunate victim of repeated spontaneous abortion or of eclampsia. Successful conception in a woman burdened with copper may lead to passage of this excess copper across the placental barrier and can possibly affect her off-spring, who can become hyperactive. Accumulation of excess copper in childhood and adolescence may also be manifested in adulthood. Many individuals who get excess copper from their water and inadequate zinc from their diet may show paranoia or hallucinations. The water we drink may be loaded with excess copper.

It has been said that zinc deficiency in animals was not clearly evident until the galvanized animal cages were replaced by stainless steel cages. One can now suggest that zinc deficiency in man was not evident until galvanized water pipes were replaced by modern copper plumbing. The rats obtained their needed zinc by gnawing the cages, and we can obtain zinc by drinking water that has coursed through zinc-lined (galvanized) iron pipes. With our modern copper plumbing and slightly acid water we may get an excess of copper which antagonizes any zinc which may be supplied by our diet (see Table IX).

An overabundance of copper or iron can substitute for zinc, manganese and magnesium to produce a continuous level of overstimulation which can manifest itself clinically as insomnia, elevated blood pressure and restless, non-productive activity. Neurophysiologists have known for years that if the isolated nerve muscle preparation fires continuously, that some copper ions must have gotten into the nutrient saline solution. Many patients with psychiatric depression are also high in serum copper.

Acidic soft water, as from a well bored into shale or peat, can erode the plumbing to produce high levels of toxic heavy metals. River water (Potomac) in Washington, D.C. as it comes from the faucet has accumulated less copper (0.04 ppm) as compared to Princeton, N.J. well water, 1.25 ppm (Siegerman and O'Dom, 1972). Since zinc is not pure, galvanized piping can lead to excess cadmium in the drinking water, while copper piping with soldered joints can lead to an excess of copper and lead. In some areas of New Jersey soft well water will produce pin holes in copper piping in ten years time. The copper and lead goes into the drinking water!

Experimentation has confirmed that excessive amounts of copper in the blood can be toxic. Klein et al. (1972) studied patients undergoing repetitive hemodialysis and discovered significant hypercupremia following dialysis and contamination of tap water from the copper pipes. The directions for house dialysis now include a flushing of the water system for five minutes before dialysis is started. Large medical buildings present a problem because of their extensive copper piping. Pigs and sheep fed excess copper develop hemolytic anemia; this same anemia was found to afflict hemodialysis patients. When patients on dialysis accidently accumulated excess copper ions in their blood they displayed psychiatric symptoms of unreality, disperceptions and psychosis. (Halpern, 1971) (Table X).

Adequate blood ceruloplasmin inhibits intestinal absorption of copper. But, as in the case of Wilson's disease, where the serum ceruloplasmin is low, copper is absorbed in excess and diffuses into the tissues and may accumulate in high levels in the brain and liver producing severe mental illness and death. In our present environment we are saturated with excess copper so that only premature infants might be deficient. A comparison of schizophrenics and normals reveals that schizophrenics excrete less copper than do normals, this seems to correlate with knowledge that excess copper can produce mental illness. Also, this would validate the use of penicillamine in the treatment of schizophrenia. Penicillamine is a chelating agent of both zinc and copper, therefore, some source of zinc plus pyridoxine should be given all patients on penicillamine therapy.

In a case report from Australia by Walker-Smith and Bloomfield (1973) the death of a 14 month old male child has as its possible cause chronic copper poisoning. The child was brought to the hospital with ascites and jaundice and died of severe micronodular cirrhosis with some biochemical evidence of Wilson's Disease, highly unlikely at such a young age. The possibility of copper poisoning was investigated, and it was found that the farm on which he lived was supplied with new copper piping and that the drinking water contained 6.75 ppm copper, well above the USPH standard of 1.0 ppm — this water was clearly undrinkable. The family was tested, all excreted normal urine copper except the mother, who when given penicillamine excreted large amounts of copper. This suggests that copper transference could have begun in the neonatal period. The baby was bottle fed rather than breast fed, but the formula was made with high copper water. This tragic death was ascribed to the abnormally early occurrence of Wilson's Disease, to chronic copper poisoning, or to liver infection in utero with subsequent exposure to high copper levels. The extremely high level of copper in the drinking water would suggest chronic copper poisoning.

The present use of the copper chelating agent penicillamine in schizophrenia is an attempt to decrease the copper level in the treatment resistant schizophrenic patient. Fister et al. (1958) suggested that the patient on this therapy be given extra trace metals (except copper) once each week. This regimen was also followed by Nicholson et al. (1966). Others have ignored the finding that penicillamine chelates and may deplete zinc as well as copper (McCall et al., 1967). One of the side effects of penicillamine therapy is the loss of the sensation of taste, which is a sign of zinc deficiency (Henkin et al., 1971). We can confirm the fact that penicillamine chelates zinc out of the body as well as copper. Urinary iron excretion is, however, decreased (Table VI). This confirms the findings of Walshe and Patston (1965) who reported no effect on serum iron. Penicillamine also complexes with pyridoxine (B_6), so that many workers have recommended 50 mgm of B_6 per day as a supplement. If the penicillamine is given after meals to prevent nausea, then the B_6 (25 mgm) should be given before breakfast and 25 mgm before supper to minimize interaction with the penicillamine.

As mentioned previously, if one considers porphyric schizophrenia as one of the schizophrenias (frequently overlooked), records of zinc deficiency in schizophrenia can be traced back in 1929 when Derrien and Benoit, working at Montpelier in France, discovered that uroporphyrin chelated zinc and thus depleted zinc via the urinary pathway. They postulated that some of the psychic and neurological symptoms could be precipitated by the zinc deficiency, Peters (1961) found an increased urinary zinc and also copper in patients with acute attacks of porphyric schizophrenia. Perhaps the main cause of the acute attack is added copper ingestion or absorption, which then displaces zinc, followed by excessive excretion of both. Peters also suggests another trace metal deficiency (which might be that of manganese). Pyridoxine deficiency as suggested by Meltzer (1961), could also be a precipitating factor. In any event, the mauve factor is now known to be a pyrrole derivative (Irvine et al., 1969) which may come from the breakdown of myoglobin or hemoglobin. Thus mauve-positive patients may be mild porphyrics.

For copper and iron one can find many environmental factors which may overload the human system. Numerous studies show that 250 ppm additional copper sulfate in the feed of pigs and chickens will increase their growth rate, thus permitting faster production of edible meat products. While faster production is the grower's primary concern, excess copper in the human body can be toxic and can impair physical and mental health.

Copper sulfate is a widely used growth promoter in pig production in England and Europe, the customary amount being 250 mg Cu/kg. Canada and the United States have not allowed the use of copper. Manure from copper fed animals is unusable as fertilizer. In all animals, high dietary copper produces a marked increase in liver copper. Although copper sulfate may promote growth, the increased storage of copper in the liver will render the animal liver, liver products and intestines inedible because increased copper content of foods without adequate dietary zinc and manganese may cause various disorders. Animal liver is an important source of many nutrients and its inedibility will be a serious deficit to the human diet. Since the individual producer may add copper an upper limit of allowable copper in liver, liver sausage and liver capsules should be set.

From a biochemical point of view, surplus dietary copper is an added burden to the human body. Even those who refrain from eating meat may subject themselves to an extra copper burden. Soybeans and soybean products contain a significant amount of copper; if research can discover a way to grow soybeans in soil copiously supplied with zinc and manganese, those individuals relying on this product for their intake of protein will not be excessive in copper or nutritionally deficient in zinc and manganese.

Owing to vitamin publicity, many patients unwittingly take vitamins with iron and copper. Frequently the only clue to the presence of these elements is the letter M after the brand name. When vitamin C is present, as with a multi-vitamin, oral iron (and possibly copper) is better absorbed. Zinc and/or manganese deficiency may allow copper and iron to accumulate in the tissues, so that any depletion of zinc and manganese from our diet may allow copper and iron excess to occur. Food processing is designed to reduce trace metals, since removal prolongs shelf life. Fresh green vegetables turn slightly grey if the trace metals are present, but if they are removed the vegetables stay a bright green. The treatment of green vegetables with the chelating agent ethylene diamine tetraacetate (EDTA) prior to the freezing process reduces zinc and manganese in peas (Pfeiffer and Iliev, 1972). The processing of flour decreases zinc, manganese, and magnesium (Zook et al., 1970). Fortified or enriched flour in the United States has only the trace element iron added.

With some impoverished or deficient soils the level of trace elements may be definitely less in the food plants. Finally, a high grain diet with its high phytate content may sequester trace metals so that they are not available to the body tissues. Conversely, high doses of vitamin C keeps many trace metals in the reduced state so that excess absorption (as of iron) may occur.

One may ask why a double-blind study has not been planned and executed before this report. Double-blind studies are only valid to compare homogeneous populations. Historically, the schizophrenias have been biochemically very heterogeneous and apparently are still heterogeneous as shown by these exploratory biochemical studies. Trace metal serum levels show low-zinc patients, high-copper patients, and patients who get a rise in copper and iron when zinc and manganese are given. In addition, some patients are high or low in blood histamine while others may be low in spermine and very high in spermidine. The agitated, low-histamine patient is high in blood serum creatine phosphokinase, a muscle enzyme which leaks out with muscle exertion or excess stimulation. Faced with these biochemical abnormalities, some of which may be psychiatrically significant, one can only study numerous individual schizophrenics and put the similar biochemical categories together. The search for biochemically similar schizophrenic patients is exactly what we have attempted in this exploratory study and report.

For example, the anemias, hypertensions, and arthritic disorders are all now known to be biochemically heterogeneous. If we believed the anemias to be homogeneous, vitamin B_{12} would score very poorly when used in a double-blind experiment to determine its effectiveness in the relief of lassitude in pale people even if the best of our presently available mood questionnaires or expert interviewers were employed. However, when the simple objective criterion of erythrocyte counts is added as a yardstick, then only a few anemia patients respond to vitamin B_{12} while most do not. Finally, when the anemia is hypochromic macrocytic (a distinct category) then vitamin B_{12}-folate is highly specific for this small percentage of anemias. To our knowledge a double-blind study has yet to be done on pernicious anemia since with objective diagnostic criteria such studies are less pertinent. At present everybody understands the double-blind study but few are interested in longitudinal biochemical changes by which one can select biochemically similar patients for future double-blind studies on homogeneous populations.

CONCLUSION

The human body is a delicate organism, relying on the specific interaction of the ingested vitamins and trace elements to provide the energy needed to keep the organs functioning properly. Without adequate dietary intake, the delicate balance cannot be maintained and physical or mental illness may ensue. The schizophrenias are a series of biochemical disorders manifesting themselves clinically in sundry syndromes; we have suggested three, but there are undoubtedly more. The available evidence strongly indicates that individuals suffering from these mental disorders are deficient in or dependent upon the nutrients most of us assume are being supplied by our "well-balanced diet" and sufficient water consumption. A survey of the diet will reveal that food-refining, poor soil and needless carbohydrate intake are denying our bodies some essential nutrients. The biochemists and nutritionists have contributed much to the fight against these illnesses. We must realize that nutrition, body chemistry, and mental disease are intimately related.

Table 1. Trials of Penicillamine in Schizophrenic Patients

Date	No. Pats.	Study Type	Copper Serum	Urine	Trace Metal Supp.	Results	Investigators[a]
1962	5	Open	−	−		Pos.	Hoffer and Osmond (1962)
1964	6	Open				Good	Greiner and Berry (1964)
1966	5	Blind	+	+	Yes	Good	Nicholson et al. (1966)
1966	24	Open	+	−	No	Neg.	Hollister et al. (1966)
1967					No	Pos.	Helmchen et al. (1967)
1969	10	Blind	−	−	No	10%	Affleck et al. (1969)
1969	21	Blind	+	+	No	Neg.	Kanig and Breyer (1969)
1970	24	Open	−	−	Yes	Good	Ozek (1970, unpublished results)
1971	30	Blind	−	+	No	Neg.	Adler et al. (1971)
1971	30	Blind	−	−	No	60%	Mattke and Adler (1971)

[a]As many as ten publications have appeared since 1962. Only the Greiner and Ozek studies used the Fister trace metal supplement (without copper) which would provide for replacement of the other trace metals chelated by D-penicillamine. Future studies should concentrate on those schizophrenic patients who have high levels of serum or tissue copper.

Table II. Urinary Excretion of Copper, Zinc, and Iron[a]

Med. Oral Doses	Patients				Normals			
	No. Trials	Cu	Zn	Fe	No. Trials	Cu	Zn	Fe
Placebo	18	1.7	152	16	26	4.6	148	20
Calcium Lactate, 2.0 gm	9	1.5	163	33	−	−	−	−
Chromium Acetate, 5 mg	8	1.4	155	14	−	−	−	−
Ammonium Molybdenate, 5 mg	12	1.2	146	10	−	−	−	−
$ZnSO_4$, 50 mg	11	2.3	204	20	16	2.1	115	13
Zn Ac, 35 mg	13	3.7	108	22	10	3.6	138	15
$McCl_2$, 3 mg	11	5.5	137	47	10	1.2	325	12
$ZnMg$[b], 70 mg	18	6.6	140	10	10	15.7	133	20
$ZnMgMn$[c], 70 mg	21	7.8	108	13	−	−	−	−
B_6, 50 mg	21	3.9	89	15	14	7.4	105	10
ZnMn, 50/3 mg	12	11	147	15	12	9.1	154	15
ZnMn B_6, 50/3/50 mg	14	20	224	16	13	3.0	186	6
$CuSO_4$, 5 mg	16	2.5	126	36	15	1.4	151	42
$MgCl_2$, 200 mg	10	2.3	141	28	10	3.1	116	34
$FeSO_4$, 900 mg	9	0.4	262	116	13	6.5	123	21
Na_2SO_4, 200 mg	18	7.3	118	19	12	6.7	116	8
CPZ[d], 150 mg	27	9.3	122	19	−	−	−	−

[a]Urinary excretion (total mcg) over a 6-hour period, of copper, zinc, and iron after the oral administration of small amounts of various trace elements. Schizophrenics compared with normal male subjects. Schizophrenics excrete less copper and iron. Zinc increases copper excretion but zinc-manganese with B_6, 50 mg. results in the greatest increase in copper excretion. Sulfate ion and chlorpromazine also increase copper excretion. In both schizophrenics and normal pyridoxine (B_6) tends to conserve zinc insofar as urinary excretion is concerned. Both calcium and magnesium increase iron excretion, as does copper. Added iron causes increased iron excretion in schizophrenics but not in normals.

[b]1 Vicon-C.

[c]1 Vicon-C plus $MnCl_2$, 3 mg.

[d]Chlorpromazine

Table III. Summary Blood Serum Trace Metal Studies 240 Schizophrenic Outpatients

	No. Subjects	Percentage
Low Zinc[a] (>0.80 µg/ml)	27	(11%)
High Copper (<1.20 µg/ml)	47	(20%)
Low Iron (>0.60 µg/ml)	18	(8%)
High Iron (<1.50 µg/ml)	29	(12%)
Changes After Zinc Dietary Supplement		
Increased Copper and Iron	76	(32%)
Increased Copper	43	(18%)
No Change	48	(20%)

[a]Only 11% + 20% = 31% of the patients could be classified as low in zinc or high in copper, but with zinc supplementation the rise in copper (or both copper and iron) indicates many more may have excess copper and iron in their tissues.

Table IV. Effect of Dl-Methionine on Urinary Trace Metal Excretion

	No.	Zinc		Copper		Iron	
		0	6 Hr.	0	6 Hr.	0	6 Hr.
Males	16	98.6	154	3.9	9.4	6.2	17.0
S.D.		117	97	3.0	6.7	4.9	19.0
Females	16	63.9	107	3.3	6.6	4.0	17.9
S.D.		51	52	1.8	3.5	4.6	17.7

Legend Table IV: Patients were given 1.5 grams of DL-methionine. Mean urinary excretion is reported in mg% present before ingestion and six hours after taking the drug. In both females and males the methionine succeeded in increasing the urinary excretion of copper, zinc, and iron.

Table V. Urinary Exretion 6-Hour Period (Schizophrenic Patients)

		No. Trials	Zinc	Copper	Iron	Manganese in ngm
1)	Vitamin C, 2.0 gm	(12)	139.2 mcg	7.43 mcg	20.2 mcg	9.76
2)	Inositol, 2.0 gm	(12)	109 mcg	9.44 mcg	18.1 mcg	
3)	B_6, 200 mgm	(16)	120 mcg	6.00 mcg	29.6 mcg	13.10
4)	B_6, 300 mgm	(38)	123 mcg	8.80 mcg	17.0 mcg	
5)	Pangamic Acid, 700 mgm	(12)	137.2 mcg	4.50 mcg	20.5 mcg	
6)	L-cysteine, 900 mgm	(19)	208 mcg	7.20 mcg	21.0 mcg	
7)	Lecithin, 2.0 gm	(17)	160.6 mcg	5.20 mcg	27.8 mcg	
8)	"Hexanicotol", 3.0 gm	(17)	171.2 mcg	7.40 mcg	24.6 mcg	8.6
9)	"Linodyl", 3.0 gm	(12)	175.0 mcg	9.50 mcg	31.9 mcg	8.6
10)	Average of 8 & 9	(29)	172.7 mcg	8.27 mcg	27.6 mcg	8.6
11)	Placebo	(18)	152 mcg	1.70 mcg	16.0 mcg	

Legend Table V: The effect of several vitamins and other biochemicals on urinary trace metal excretion. Vitamin C, vitamin B_6 and inositol would appear to conserve zinc while l-cysteine would appear to increase zinc excretion. All preparations increased urinary copper excretion. "Linodyl" and "Hexanicotol" are identical, both being the nicotinic acid ester of inositol. "Linodyl" is marketed in Canada while "Hexanicotol" was formerly marketed in the U.S.A.

Table VI. Blood Histamine Nanogram/ml ±S.D.

		Number	
Normal	Male	(19)	46.3 ± 18
	Female	(10)	41.7 ± 14.5
Pyroluric	Male	(27)	52.8 ± 23.8
	Female	(27)	46.1 ± 11.7
Low Histamine	Male	(28)	20.2 ± 10.4 t* = 6.3 p = <0.001
	Female	(29)	27.6 ± 8.1 t* = 2.3 p = <0.05
High Histamine	Male	(29)	110.7 ± 16.5 t* = 12.8 p = <0.001
	Female	(26)	107.3 ± 24.4 t* = 7.9 p = <0.001
Hypoglycemic	Male	(35)	43.4 ± 25.1
	Female	(71)	49.3 ± 21.1

* Compared to normal group

Legend Table VI: Comparison of blood histamine levels in normals and hypoglycemic patients with 3 types of schizophrenic patients means ± standard deviation. The means of normals, pyroluric and hypoglycemic patients are similar and not significantly different.

Table VII. Urinary Content of Trace Metals and Coproporphyrin in Schizophrenic Outpatients

		All means are mcg % ± S.E.		
Schizophrenic Outpatients	An N = 45	Cu N = 45	Fe N = 45	Coproporphyrin N = 27
Mauve Positive	49.71 ± 6.95	3.18 ± 0.62	4.07 ± 0.56	121.11 ± 10.49
Mauve Negative	N = 35 29.66 ± 4.43	N = 35 3.31 ± 0.56	N = 35 5.20 ± 0.80	N = 12 38.50 ± 7.79

t for Zn – 6.34 (p <0.0001)

t for Coproporphyrin – 5.04 (p <0.001)

Legend Table VII: Urinary content of trace metals and coproporphyrin in mauve negative and mauve positive schizophrenic outpatients. All means are mcg% ± standard error of metal or coproporphyrin content in early morning urine sample. The mauve positivity was determined by the Irvine test before the development of the present quantitative test. Zinc excretion is greater in the mauve positive as is also the coproporphyrin excretion.

Table VIII. Possible Effects of a High Copper Burden in Man

1) Miscarriage

2) Eclampsia

3) Birth Defects

4) Cystic Fibrosis

5) Hemolytic Disease of the Newborn

6) Autism

7) Histapenic Schizophrenia

8) Essential Hypertension

9) Psychiatric Depression

10) Premature Aging

Table IX. Copper Content of Some Drinking Waters in Eastern United States[a]

City	Water Source	Dwelling	Copper Content PPM[b]
New York City	River	Apartment	0.07
Long Island	Well	Cottage	0.03
Cleveland	Lake	Motel	0.06
Boston	Well	House	0.12[c]
Greenwich	Well	House	0.35[c]
Greenwich	Well	House	0.37[c]
Wilton, Conn.	Well	House	1.60[c]
Wilton	Well	House	1.34[c]
Wilton	Well	House	0.68[c]
Wilton	Well	House	0.36[c]
Wilton	Well	House	0.40[c]
Wilton	Well	House	0.18[c]
New Caanan	Well	House	0.85[c]
Redding, Conn.	Well	House	4.20[c]
Belle Mead, N.J.	Well	Clinic	0.12
Bernardsville, N.J.	Well	House	0.54[c]
Princeton, N.J.	Well	House	0.05
Princeton, N.J.	Well	House	0.11
Princeton, N.J.	Well	House	0.04
Princeton, N.J.	Well	House	0.06[c]
Milwood, N.J.	Well	House	0.09
Trenton, N.J.	Well	House	5.60[c]
Stamford, Conn.	Well	House	5.20[c]
Boston	Well	House	0.64[c]
Atlantic City	River	House	0.01[c]
Dayton, Ohio	Well	House	0.56[c]
Washington, D.C.	River	Hotel	0.01

[a]All waters were collected in plastic containers and were acidified with copper free HCL prior to testing. The sample was the first collection of water in the morning.

[b]The United States Public Health Service rules that water containing more than 1.0 ppm of copper is unfit to drink. In earlier generations with lead plumbing, Grandfather, who drank the first cup out of the faucet in the morning, got lead poisoning. The possibility now exists in some urban homes for grandfather to get copper poisoning.

[c]Indicates a family in which at least one member has psychiatric problems.

Legend Table IX: The psychiatric, neurological and medical findings of hemodialysis patients when tap water is used. Copper in the tap water may turn the blood plasma green since copper accumulates preferentially in plasma. Symptoms have been described since 1964, but only 1969 was the syndrome correlated with excess copper or other heavy metals such as tin. In some instances, copper tubing and copperized plastic were involved (Barbour et al., 1971). Excess copper would be the most likely cause since some schizophrenics improve when their excess copper is removed. Cross references between the two columns are so rare as to suggest a dichotomay of diagnosis and thinking.

Table X. Dementia Dialytica: Clinical Mystery or Diagnostic Dichotomy?

Psychiatric Diagnosis Since 1964 (Peterson and Swanson) Termed "Dementia Dialytica"	Medical Diagnosis Since 1969 (Matter et al.) Tap Water Dialysis Increases Serum Copper

Neurological:

Speech disorder, slow articulation

Stuttering, aphasia, headaches

EEG: Slow waves with delta waves and spikes. (Alfrey et al., [1972])

Myoclonus, convulsions

Hypertension, restlessness

Increased heart rate and irregularities

Cardia standstill

Medical:

Hemolytic, anemia, Hematuria (Ivanovich et al., 1969)

Lowered hematocrit with right (Liver) or left spleen) upper quadrant pain (Manzler & Schreiner, 1970)

Green plasma!

Nausea, vomiting

Yellow watery diarrhea

Weakness, syncope

Psychiatric:

Inability to concentrate

Imparied memory

Personality changes

Psychotic behavior

"Disequilibrim syndrome" (unknown changes in vasoactive amines

JAMA 224: 1578 (1973)

Ibid 226: 190 (1973)

Psychiatric:

Unreality

Depression

Psychosis

Pathological:

Increased tin in brain autopsies

Psychiatric Theories:

1) Dependency increases aggressive feelings (Dependency on public finances)

2) Defences all brittle

3) Stress = Anxiety, Depression, Paranoia, Suicidal

4) Denial of aspects of reality

5) Decreased sex activity

Medical Theories:

1) Heavy metal intoxication

2) Copper intoxication (Mahler et al., 1971)

Table XI.

	Normals (8)	Schizophrenics (11)
	After Placebo	
Copper	4.46 ± 1.69	0.2
Zinc	128.00 ± 24.78	143.90 + 27.28
Iron	31.12 ± 7.03	16.18 ± 2.39
	After 500 MG. D-Penicillamine	
Copper	178.00 ± 37.96	174.00 ± 37.37
Zinc	299.71 ± 41.27	525.87 ± 132.66
Iron	9.28 ± 3.86	11.62 ± 3.08

Legend Table XI: Effect of Placebo or D-Penicillamine on six hour urinary excretion of copper, zinc, and iron in 8 normals and 11 schizophrenics — means ± standard error. The normal excretes more copper and less zinc. Penicillamine greatly increases copper excretion, but zinc excretion is more than doubled. Iron excretion is decreased.

Figure I

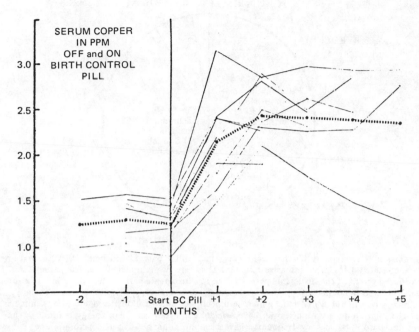

SERUM COPPER LEVELS OF SCHIZOPHRENIC WOMEN OFF AND ON THE BIRTH CONTROL PILL

The Y axis of the graph gives the level of serum copper as ppm/serum. The axis indicated months before and after the beginning of contraceptive therapy. Blood samples were taken at these monthly intervals. The dotted line represents the mean serum copper level of all the subjects tested.

Figure 2

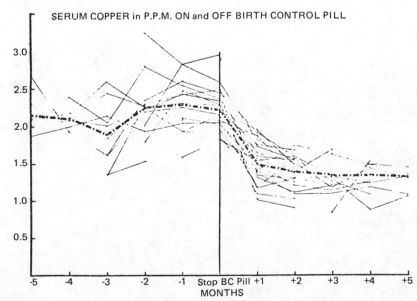

SERUM COPPER LEVELS OF SCHIZOPHRENIC WOMEN ON AND OFF THE BIRTH CONTROL PILL

The Y axis of the graph gives the level of serum copper as ppm/serum. The X axis indicates months before and after discontinuation of contraceptive therapy. Blood samples were taken at these monthly intervals. The dotted line represents the mean serum copper level of all the subjects tested.

Figure 3

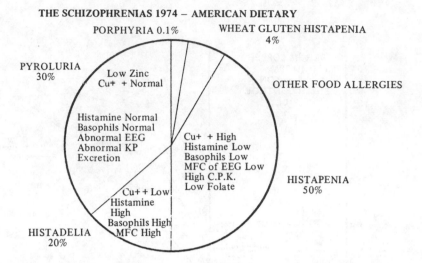

THE SCHIZOPHRENIAS 1974 – AMERICAN DIETARY

Legend Figure 3: The schizophrenias may have many biochemical facets, since, in the past, 10 biochemical entities have been separated. We now suggest that 3 major subdivisions may be considered for more intensive research. These are diagrammed above. The patients sensitive to wheat gluten are low in blood histamine and represent a special group of the histapenic patients. The few histapenic patients tested are low in serum folic acid but high in creatine phophokinase (CPK). These paranoid and hallucinatory patients do respond to vitamin B_{12}, folate and niacin therapy. The histapenic group is low in mean energy content of the alpha waves in the EEG and high in serum copper and ceruloplasmin. Ceruloplasmin has histaminase activity, and all diaminoxidases contain copper. The high blood histamine group have suicidal depression and high energy content in the alpha waves of their EEG. The blood histamine is contained in the basophils, so they frequently have basophil counts above 1%. Serum copper is low or normal circa 1 ppm. The pyrolurias are normal in histamine and normal in trace metals except for those who are low in serum zinc. The mauve factor (KP) (kryptopyrrole) in their urines depletes them of both zinc and pyridoxine. This may result in abnormal EEG's with occasional slow waves and isolated high voltage spikes. These patients may have single convulsions when first placed on neuroleptic medication. They respond best to large doses of pyridoxine A.M. & P.M. and added dietary source of zinc. Pyroluric patients may have any of the classical symptoms of schizophrenia, but their insight and affect are usually much better than other schizophrenic types.

REFERENCES

Abood, L.G., Gibbs, F.A. and Gibbs, E. (1957). Comparative Study of Blood Ceruloplasmin in Schizophrenia and Other Disorders. *AMA Arch. Neurol. Psychiat.* 77:643.

Ackerfeldt, S. (1957). Oxidation of N.N Dimethyl-p-phenylenediamine by Serum from Patients with Mental Disease. *Science* 125:117.

Adler, M., Mattke, D., and Nedelmann, K. (1971). Ueber die Wirkung des D-penicillamins bei Chronisch Schizophrenen. *Pharmakopsychiat. Neuro. Psychopharmakol.* 4:45.

Affleck, J.W., Copper, A.J., Forrest, A.D., Synthies, J.R., and Zealley, A.K. (1969). Penicillamine and Schizophrenia — A Clinical Trial. *Br. J. Psychiat.* 115:173.

Barbour, B.H., Bischel, M. and Abrahms, D.E. (1971). Copper Accumulation In Patients Undergoing Chronic Hemodialysis. The Role of Cuprophen. *Nephron* 8:455.

Barrass, R.C. and Coult, D.B. (1970). Interaction of Some Centrally Active Drugs with Ceruloplasmin. *Biochem. Pharmacol.* 19:1675.

Bawkin, R.M., Mosbach, E.H. and Bawkin, H. (1961). Concentration of Copper in Serum of Children Schizophrenia. *Pediatrics.* 27:642.

Bischoff, A. (1952). Ueber die Frage des Erhoten Kupfter — Spiegels im Serum Schizophrenen. *Montasschr. Psychiat. Neurol.* 124:211.

Brenner, W. (1949). Beitrage zur Kenntnis des Eisen — und Kupferstoffwechsels im Kindersalter. *Kinderheilk.* 66:14.

Derrien, E., and Benoit, C. (1929). Notes et Observations surs les Urines et sur Quelques Organes d'une Femme Encrise de Porphyric Aigue. *Arch. Soc. Sci. Med. Biol. Montpelier.* 8:456.

Ellman, G.L., Jones, R.T. and Rychert, R.C. (1968). Mauve Spot and Schizophrenia. *Amer. J. Psychiat.* 125:161.

English, W.M. (1929). Report on the Treatment with Manganese Chloride of 181 Cases of Schizophrenia. 33 of Manic Depression, and 16 of Other Defects or Psychoses at the Ontario Hospital. Brockville, Ontario. *Amer. J. Psychiat.* 9:569.

Fister, W.P., Boulding, J.E. and Baker, R.A. (1958). The Treatment of Hepatolenticular Degeneration with Penicillamine, with Report of Two Cases. *Can. Med. Assn. J.* 78:99.

Frank, M.N. and Wurtman, R.J. (1958). Some Sources of Error in the Ackerfeldt Test for Serum Oxidase Activity. *Proc. Soc. Exp. Biol. Med.* 97:478.

Greiner, A.C. and Berry, K. (1964). Treatment of Schizophrenia with D-Penicillamine. *Can. Med. Assn. J.* 90:663.

Heilmeyer, L., Keiderling, W. and Struve, C. (1941). Kupfer und Eisen Als Korpereigene Wirkstoffe und ihre Beduetung beim Krankheitsgeschenen. *Fisher. Jena.* Germany.

Helmchen, H., Hippius, H., Hoffmann, I. and Selbach, H. (1967). D-Penicillamine in der Schizophrenic-Behandlung. *Nervenartz* 38:218.

Henkin, R.I., Schecter, P.J., Hoye, R. and Mattern, C.F.T. (1971). Idiopathic Hypogeusia, with Dysgeusia, Hyposmia and Dysosmia: a new Syndrome. *J. Amer. Med. Assn.* 217:434.

Hollister, L.E., Moore, F.F. and Forrest, F. (1966). Antipyridoxine Effect of D-Penicillamine in Schizophrenic Man. *Amer. J. Clin. Nutr.* 19:307.

Horwitt, M.K., Meyer, B.J., Meyer, A.C., Harvey, C.C. and

Haffron, D. (1957). Serum Copper and Oxidase Acitivity in Schizophrenic Patients. *Arch. Neurol. Psychiat.* 78:317.

Hoskin, R.G. (1934). The Manganese Treatment of Schizophrenic Disorders. *J. Nerv. Ment. Dis.* 79:59.

Irvine, D.G., Bayne, W. Myashita, H. and Majer, J.R. (1969). Identification of Kryptopyrrole in Human Urine and Its Relation to Psychosis. *Nature* 224:811.

Jantz, H. (1950). Leberfunktionsprufungen bei Schizophrenie. *Zentralbl. Neuro.* 108:313.

Kanig, K. and Breyer, U. (1969). Zur Behandlung Schizophrenen Psychosen Mit D-Penicillamine. *Pharmakopsychiat. Neuro. Pharmakol.* 2:190.

Kimura, K. and Kumura, J. (1965). Polarigraphic Determination of Zinc Levels in the Brains of Schizophrenics and Control Patients. *Proc. Jap. Acad.* 41:943.

Klein, W.J., Metz, E. and Price, A. (1972). Acute Copper Intoxication *Arch. Int. Med.* 129:578.

Martens, S. (1966). *Effects of Exogenous Human Ceruloplasmin in the Schizophrenic Syndrome.* Tryckeri Balder AB. Stockholm.

Mattke, J.D. and Adler, M. (1971). Mode of Action of D-penicillamine in Chronic Schizophrenia. *Dis. Nerv. Syst.* 32:388.

Metzter, D.E. (1961). Metal Binding of Pyridoxal Derivatives and Possible Relationships to Tryptophan Metabolism. *Fed. Proc. Amer. Soc. Exp. Biol.* 20:234.

Munch-Peterson, S. (1950). On Serum Copper in Patients with Schizophrenia. *ACTA Psychiat. Scand.* Suppl. 25:423.

Nesbitt, S. (1944). Acute Porphyria. *J. Amer. Assoc.* 124:286.

Nicholson, G.A., Greiner, A.C., McFarlane, W.J. and Barker, A. (1966). Effect of Penicillamine on Schizophrenic Patients. *Lancet* 1:344.

Ostfeld. A.M., Abood. L.G. and Marcus, D.A. (1958). Studies in Cerulo-Plasmin and a New Hallucinogen. *Arch. Neurol. Psychiat.* 79:317.

Oezck, M. (1957). Untersuchengen uber den Kupferstoffwechsel im Schizophrenen Formenkreis. *Arch. Psychiat. & Ztschr. Ges. Neurol.* 195:408.

Oezek, M. (1970). Personal Communication to Mattke and Adler.

Peters, H.A. (1961) Trace Metals. Chelating Agents and the Porphyrias. *Fed. Proc. Fed. Amer. Soc. Exp. Biol.* 20:227.

Pfeiffer, C.C., Iliev, V., Goldstein, L. and Jennery, E.H. (1969). Serum Polyamine Levels in Schizophrenia and Other Objective Criteria of Clinical Status. *Schizophrenia Current Concepts and Research* PJD Publ. Hicksville, N.Y.

Pfeiffer, C.C., Iliev, V., Goldstein, L., Jenney, E.H. and Schultz, R. (1970a). Blood Histamine. Polyamines and the Schizophrenias. *Res. Commun. Chem. Pathol. Pharmacol.* 1:247.

Pfeiffer, C.C., Ward, J., El-Meligi, M., and Cott, A. (1970b). *The Schizophrenias: Yours and Mine.* Pyramid Moonachie, N.J.

Pfeiffer, C.C., Smyrl, E.G. and Iliev, V. (1972a). Extreme Basophil Counts and Blood Histamine Levels in Schizophrenic Outpatients as Compared to Normals. *Res. Commun. Chem. Pathol. Pharmacol.* 4:51.

Pfeiffer, C.C. (1972b). Blood Histamine. Basophil Counts and Trace Elements in the Schizophrenias. *Rev. Can. Biol.* 31:73

Pfeiffer, C.C. and Iliev, V. (1972c). A Study of Zinc Deficiency and Copper Excess in the Schizophrenias. *Int. Rev. Neurobiol.* suppl. 1. pp. 141-165.

Pfeiffer, C.C. and Jenney, E.H. (1974). Fingernail White Spots:

Possible Zinc Deficiency. *JAMA* 228:157.

Richter, D. (1970). The Biological Investigation of Schizophrenia. *Biol. Psychiat.* 2:153.

Rivers, J. and Devine, M. (1972). Plasma Ascorbic Acid Concentrations and Oral Contraceptives. *Amer. J. Clin. Nutr.* 25:684.

Saroja, N. (1971). Effect of Estrogens on Ascorbic Acid in the Plasma and Blood Vessels of Guinea Pigs. *Contraception* 3:269.

Scheinberg, I.H., Morell, A.G., Harris, R.S. and Bergen, A. (1957). Concentration of Ceruloplasmin in Plasma of Schizophrenics. *Science* 126:925.

Siegerman, H. and O'Dom, G. (1972). Differential Pulse Anodic Stripping of Trace Metals. *Am. Lab.* 59.

Sohler, A., Beck, R. and Noval, J.J. (1970). Mauve Factor Re-Identified as 2, 4, Dimethyl-3-ethylpyrrole and Its Sedative Effect on the CNS. *Nature* 224:138.

Walker-Smith, J. and Bloomfield, J. (1973). Wilson's Disease or Chronic Copper Poisoning? *Arch. Dis. Child* 48:476.

Walshe, J.M. (1956). Penicillamine. A New Oral Therapy for Wilson's Disease. *Amer. J. Med.* 21:487.

Walshe, J.M. and Clark, V. (1965). Effect of Penicillamine on Serum Iron. *Arch. Dis. Child* 40:651.

Watson, C.I. and Schwartz, S.J. (1941). A Simple Test for Urinary Prophobilinogen. *Proc. Soc. Exp. Biol. & Med.* 47:393.

Zook, E.G., Greene, F.E. and Morris, E.R. (1970). Nutrient Composition of Selected Wheats and Wheat Products VI. Distribution of Manganese, Copper, Nickel, Zinc, Magnesium, Lead, Tin, Cadmium, Chromium and Selenium as Determined by Atomic Absorption Spectroscopy and Colorimetry. *Cereal Chemistry* 47:720.

21
Ecologic Orientation in Medicine: Comprehensive Environmental Control in Diagnosis and Therapy*

THERON G. RANDOLPH

The chronically ill patient has long been a major medical problem. When the usual work-up fails, the dilemma is compounded. When the ordinary routines of therapy and/or psychiatrically orientated approaches also fail, especially when dealing with multiple alternating physical and mental complaints, a train of disasters often occurs. These include unnecessary overtreatment and the virtual abandonment of patients, on the one hand, and on the other, needless medical shopping and general dissatisfaction with the medical profession.

More is needed than the time-tested tools of the history, physical examination and laboratory work-up to reveal the interplay between environmental and bodily factors which characterize many chronic illnesses. It is apparent that the investigation of the patient's illness must be broadened to include measurements of these dynamic components as well as to demonstrate the inciting causes of symptoms syndromes. Although the regimen to be described draws from and supplements the clinicopathologic, the animal-experimental and the epidermiologic methods, it differs sufficiently to be considered as a fourth investigative technique. It is not basically new, except in the detailed nature of certain avoidances.

The program of comprehensive environmental control followed by single test re-exposures, heretofore presented only preliminarily [1, 2], supplements the traditional medical investigation. It applies to a wide range of physical and related mental syndromes [3, 4] in many of which pathologic changes are minimal or absent. It demonstrates their inciting causes and opens a sound therapeutic approach to many of them. Its techniques do not depend upon elaborate instrumentation but are applicable at the level of clinical practice. Its findings do not require confirmation by means of laboratory or animal experimentation. However, its use does necessitate abandonment of certain long-cherished medical attitudes and practices as well as acquisition of a point of view not currently taught.

SPECIFIC ADAPTATION IN THE PRESENCE OF INDIVIDUAL SUSCEPTIBILITY

Understanding of the program of comprehensive environmental control requires a brief review of the process of adapta-

Reprinted with permission ANNALS OF ALLERGY, Volume 23, Pages 7-22, January, 1965.

tion to specific environmental incitants. Similar to the general adaptation syndrome [5], adaptation to specific external agents also consists of non-adapted, adapted and non-adapted sequential stages [6, 7].

Non-adapted stage I reactions are not ordinarily diagnostic problems, since immediate post-exposure effects associated with widely-spaced environmental exposures are usually readily apparent as far as their etiology is concerned. In contrast, specifically adapted stage II reactions, characterized by delayed withdrawal-type symptoms associated with frequently repeated exposures, are diagnostic problems. In fact, ubiquitous environmental materials perpetuating such chronic reactions are much more common than currently diagnosed. Since these hidden cause and effect relationships are usually multiple, they are most clearly demonstrated when a wide range of possible incitants selected on the basis of probability are avoided simultaneously, then returned singly. This course changes specifically adapted responses of unsuspected origin and manifesting as chronic illness to non-adapted stages. Specific re-exposures then induce immediate acute (stage I) test reactions which demonstrate specific etiology.

For reasons not well understood, some persons become susceptible to certain environmental agents. The presence of such a susceptibility — individualized to the host and specific to the incitant — tends to increase the relative impact of a given substance and to accelerate the developmental stages of specific adaptation. The designation individual susceptibility is used in preference to the term, allergy, because certain chemical incitants of adaptive responses [8, 9] and perhaps foods [8, 10, 11] do not apparently involve antigen-antibody responses with which allergy has become closely associated. Specific susceptibility is measured clinically in terms of the immediacy and severity of test or non-adapted reactions. Both the terms, individual susceptibility and adaptation are used descriptively, no attempt being made in this presentation to interpret either in respect to their possible underlying mechanisms.

The demonstration of these ecologic relationships must be emphasized. Little is gained and much may be lost in assuming the presence of maladaptation to a given agent. Indeed, these excellent terms — ecology and adaptation — are not to be applied in medicine in a speculative or philosophical sense. If such relationships cannot be demonstrated, they cannot be assumed to exist.

121

BODILY CENTERED VERSUS ECOLOGIC MEDICINE

The development of ecologically orientated medicine could be accelerated by placing less emphasis on the bodily defenses of adaptation and more attention on the specific aspects of the process. Selye [5] failed to emphasize specific features of adaptation in focusing on the similarities of the body's response to a wide range of stressors in his general adaptation syndrome. Although this generalized concept has been useful in describing the sequential stages of the process and has aided in understanding its mechanisms, it has failed as a guide for physicians in their daily practices. This failure apparently stems from differences in points of view of physiologists and clinicians. It might be said that a physiologist views adaptation as an open book consisting of three successive stages. In contrast, a physician first sees his patient when the subject's adaptation to one or more incitants is already failing. The doctor's job is to identify the impinging materials — a task which might be likened to being plunged into a book, somewhere between its middle and latter parts. The physician is badly in need of a guide to aid him in identifying the materials to which his patient has been maladapting. A clinically orientated concept of adaptation in the presence of individual susceptibility [6, 7] supplies it.

To paraphrase Smut's holistic doctrine of nature and evolution [12], the determing factors in adaptation as applied to medicine are wholes, not their constituent parts. This means that a person is reacting as a biologic unit, not his constituent parts, as emphasized in today's anatomically demarcated specialties, nor in terms of his constituent physiologic and chemical bodily processes, as most commonly thought. Furthermore, the environment is to be considered as comprising various external incitants as wholes, such as specific foods rather than their constituent parts — protein, fat, carbohydrates, vitamins and minerals. Neither is interest focused on the chemical formulae of these materials, although there is great concern with the chemical environment in general [9].

Although analytical approaches to the body and its intake and surroundings have provided much useful information, such fragmented investigations have also obscured dynamic inter-relationships which have an important bearing in medicine. In contrast to the vogue for over-generalization of concept and over-analysis of medical investigation, it must not be forgotten that the whole living body is actually exposed to and reacts to specific foods, chemically derived products and other environmental agents as these are encountered in their intact forms. For instance, the ecologically-minded physician is primarily concerned with a patient's adaptational status to coffee, wheat, corn, milk, egg, potato and other common foods, including the tendency for cross-reactions to biologically related foodstuffs. He is also concerned with chemical fumes, drugs, food contaminants and other chemical contactants, including the tendency for cross-reactions to other materials of common genesis. Although he is interested in other aspects of the biologic and physical environment, such as pollens, spores, animal and insect emanations and fibers, as well as man's responses to cold, heat, sunlight, radiation and other physical exposures, these are not his chief concern. For, in general, members of the human race are adapting more satisfactorily to these materials to which their forebearers have long been exposed, than to relatively new foods such as coffee, cereal grains, potato, citrus, et cetera, and, expecially, new aspects of the chemical environment (fossil fuels and their combustion products and derivatives).

In short, dynamic ecologic relationships — individualized to the subject and specific to the incitant — have been obscured by bodily orientated overgeneralizations of concept and relatively static analytical views of both the body and its surroundings. More attention to individuality and specificity of the adaptation process, and more synthesis as contrasted with analysis, are needed to uncover inter-relationships between man and his environment that reflect in his health.

IN THE DIRECTION OF MORE SYNTHESIS IN MEDICINE

Maladaptation to specific materials to which one is regularly exposed and susceptible presents as both physical and mental illnesses. These manifestations may be mild or severe, acute or chronic, depending upon multiple variables.

Whether a susceptible person reacts to a given incitant appears to depend on quantitative variations in the degree of individual susceptibility on the one hand, and dosage of the incitant on the other. As judged clinically, the resulting symptoms response is a product of these two factors. Obviously, a susceptible person does not react if not specifically exposed. If one is only slightly susceptible to a given substance, a relatively large exposure is necessary to produce symptoms. This is illustrated in part a, Figure 1, in which it is assumed that a detectable reaction arises as a result of a product of 100 or over and that the factors involved are measurable. In this instance, a specific susceptibility of two and an exposure of 60 results in a reaction. But when one is highly susceptible (let us assume a relative value of 40) a very small exposure — a value of three — is sufficient to induce a reaction, as illustrated in part b of the chart. Although such amounts are usually considered "harmless" or "insignificant" or present only in "trace" amounts, the important point to emphasize is that such minimal exposures are illness-producing for the specifically susceptible. Indeed, it is with these small amounts that this presentation is largely concerned.

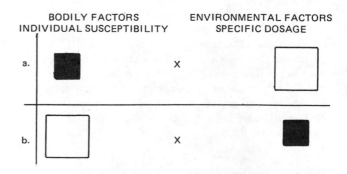

Fig. 1. This chart illustrates interrelationship between bodily and environmental factors assumed to be important in specific adaptation. Clinical observations suggest that an individual's response is a product of his degree of susceptibility and the specific dosage to which he is exposed. Based on the assumption that a product greater than 100 is associated with a clinically detectable reaction, this product might result from many different combinations. One extreme (a) represents the slighly susceptible person exposed to a massive dose; the other (b) a highly susceptible person reacting to a relatively small dose.

There are also highly significant variations in the same susceptible individual at different times, depending principally on the frequency of dosage and the stage of specific adaptation. These combinations largely determine whether a patient's illness is chronic or acute. Furthermore, this relationship may occur at any quantitative level of susceptibility or dosage, as previously described. For example, each frequently repeated exposure to an incitant to which a high degree of susceptibility exists tends to stimulate the chronically reacting, specifically adapted person. In fact, cumulative exposures often induce an addiction-type response in which the victim not only fails to suspect the inciting agent, but in which he literally goes after it or some mixture containing it as often as necessary to remain stimulated. But if such a susceptible person avoids these oft-repeated specific exposures sufficiently long to recover from the effects of the last dose, he becomes non-adapted to this material and reacts acutely upon re-exposure to it [6, 7, 10]. Thus, variation in the frequency of given exposures, whether by chance or design, largely determines the chronicity or acuity of this type of illness.

Planned variations in the frequency of given exposures are used to change chronic illness to acute illness. Deliberate re-exposures under conditions most conducive to the patient's safety and to observations of resulting clinical responses [13] demonstrate the inciting causes of many illnesses. Such planned variations are the keys to the ecologist's armamentarium. Their clinical significance demands that the technique to be described or other methods based on the principles of specific adaptation be incorporated as integral parts of the medical investigation. Indeed, the applications of these principles will hasten medicine's transition from artistry to science.

Once the inciting causes of illness have been demonstrated, one may choose between the desirability of an ecologically orientated therapeutic approach to illness, which avoids exposure to incriminated materials, and bodily orientated symptomatic therapy. These programs may be combined later if desired. However, the important point to stress is that the patient must be observed in respect to his intake and environment either before or after symptomatic therapy. These programs are not to be undertaken concurrently. Why? Because symptomatic therapy and the administration of drugs are becoming increasingly synonymous. And maintenance drug therapy is not only an important part of the causative environment, but, significantly, it also obscures observation of reactive symptoms.

COMPREHENSIVE ENVIRONMENTAL CONTROL

The most accurate method of demonstrating the inciting causes of illness is to observe the patient while potential, probable and suspected environmental incitants are avoided simultaneously. The program of comprehensive environmental control to be described, usually: (1) Clears or greatly reduces the previous level of chronic symptoms; (2) Reverts adapted and partially adapted responses to nonadapted ones; and, (3) Favors accurate observation of acute diagnostic responses following specific re-exposures. Incriminated incitants are then avoided as detected. This planned avoidance and retesting of the patient in respect to his intake and surroundings is neither purely diagnostic nor therapeutic, but bridges the two with features of both.

The presently recommended diagnostic-therapeutic program

developed as a result of trying and discarding various other limited approaches. One by one, skin testing with food extracts, basic elimination diets and ingestion tests [10] performed by avoiding and returning one food at a time were given up in favor of the present program. In the course of performing over 50,000 individual food ingestion tests (in which common foods were avoided for several days prior to observing the effects of the test ingestion of one of them), two types of reaction were finally differentiated. One, reactions to given foods *per se*; the other, reactions to chemical additives and contaminants of various foods. The two coexisted so frequently that testing with foods of known cultural and processing pedigrees became necessary [9]. Moreover, the frequency of reactions to chemical fumes encountered either in the home or in transit to the office [9] necessitated making observations under more controlled conditions [13].

Although the writer first employed fasting as a diagnostic-therapeutic procedure in 1950, initial patients were not fasted long enough or under sufficiently controlled circumstances to clear their specific "withdrawal effects." Re-instating the fast for a longer period in 1955 at the suggestion of Dr. Donald S. Mitchell [14] and incorporating hospital control of the chemical environment in a so-called "ecologic unit" [13] resulted in the present program which has been carried out on over 1000 chronically ill patients.

DIAGNOSTIC ASPECTS OF COMPREHENSIVE ENVIRONMENTAL CONTROL

The General Program

Untreated patients are observed while fasting on spring water in hospital quarters in which air pollution and contactant exposures are minimized [13].

Either prior to hospitalization or immediately thereafter, the gastrointestinal tract is emptied by means of a saline purge. All nail polish, lipstick, perfumes, hair oils and lacquers, and other cosmetic residues are removed. Subjects drink only spring water and use dextrose-free non-iodized salt in moderation. If desired, potassium chloride may be used as recommended by Mitchell [11]. Patients wear only cotton, linen, wool or silk — if known to be tolerated — and leather footwear. Synthetic clothing (textiles or plastic), slippers, handbags, suitcases and toilet articles are removed from the room.

All drugs, cosmetics, perfumes, scented soaps and shampoos, detergent-containing shampoos, personal deodorants, dentifrices, mouth washes, back-rub solutions, powders, creams, cleansing preparations and medicated douches and enemas are avoided. Previously used drugs are usually stopped abruptly, although barbiturates, steroids and certain other potential or actual addictants are either tapered-off prior to admission or during the first few days of hospitalization. Tobacco is best stopped abruptly; with the avoidance of foods, the desire to smoke is usually reduced. Each patient is provided with an individual thermometer, so as to avoid the use of disinfectants. Unscented tolerated soap may be used.

Observations are carried out in a special area of the hospital in which recently operated patients, the use of tobacco, flowers (cut or artificial), perfumes, institutional deodorants and odorous housekeeping techniques are not permitted. The air of such quarters is filtered mechanically and electrostatically for the removal of dust, pollens, spores and animal and insect debris, as well as through activated carbon window air-conditioning units* for the removal of chemical odors and fumes. The area is heated either electrically or by means of hot water central heating. Steam heating systems using chlorinated water are relatively less desirable because of the volatility of the chlorine. Room heating or ventilating units containing fans or motors which become heated are avoided because of their volatility. Oil-impregnated glass wool filters and certain oiled filtering equipment as well as some plastic duct systems may also be causes of reactive symptoms. However, the most troublesome air pollutants arise from gas stoves and gas or fuel-oil space heaters. These devices should be removed from the quarters used for this purpose, whether or not these devices are currently in use in rooms, kitchens and laboratories [9]. Care should also be taken that odors do not arise from other floors via stair-wells, elevator shafts, laundry chutes and ventilating systems.

Despite these restrictions, there are certain other inhaled and contacted substances associated with the bed and room that may perpetuate chronic symptoms. The most troublesome of these — rubber draw sheets, rubber-containing or plastic-covered mattresses and pillows and plastic-covered or sponge rubber upholstered furniture — are avoided routinely. In specific cases, reactions have also been traced to the plasticized surfaces of bed linens, bleach and detergent residues, gas drier residue, cornstarch, and mineral oil preparations employed for dust control. Since most of these latter avoidances are not in keeping with hospital routines, the most satisfactory control is accomplished in a common area in which the staff is familiar with the needs and cognizant of the aims and nature of this work [13]. Sometimes it is necessary to bring in non-plasticized bed linens, laundered only with soap and dried in the open air. These rooms are furnished with wood or metal furniture, upholstered with cotton padding and covered with natural fabrics. Recently laundered feather pillows (if not treated with insecticides) are often tolerated, but a recently laundered cotton blanket rolled up in a pillow case is preferred. Smoking or the wearing of perfumes by anyone entering this area is not permitted.

Patients are weighed at the same time each morning after urinating and before breakfast. Weight loss during the fast follows an "S" shaped curve, being slow at first, then rapid and associated with a diuresis, and then more slowly at the time of termination of the fast.

Withdrawal-type symptoms usually begin at the end of the first day or sometime during the second day of fasting. Although these are apt to be most troublesome during the second and third days, they may reach a peak on the fourth day, following which they tend to taper off. During this time, the sense of smell is apt to be hyperacute, sometimes manifesting as parosmia. Despite withdrawal effects consisting of the patient's former chronic manifestations, these may be relatively more severe and sometimes more advanced than those previously experienced [3]. Withdrawal effects from regularly eaten foods *per se* are usually absent by the end of the fifth day of fasting; those from avoided chemical additives and contaminants of food, air, water supplies, biological drugs and especially those from synthetic chemical drugs subside more slowly. The type of clinical response is also

*Furnished for this study through the courtesy of the Whirlpool Corporation, St. Joseph, Michigan.

related to the time required for clearing of withdrawal reactions, in that psychotic and musculo-skeletal reactions tend to subside relatively more slowly than lesser symptom levels [3].

Indications for breaking the fast are a relative absence of or a marked decrease of previous chronic symptoms, satisfactory sleep, and stabilization of the pulse rate at significantly lower levels for a period of 24 hours. Most commonly excessive hunger, insomnia, foul taste in the mouth, coated tongue, excessive perspiration, chilling sensations, weakness, aching and rapid weight loss have disappeared by this time. However, the pulse may remain elevated for longer periods, only reverting to lower levels after compatible feedings have been started.

SUSCEPTIBILITY TO FOODS PER SE

The fast is broken by a meal of chemically uncontaminated unsuspected fish or shell fish. Salmon canned in glass, crayfish (lobster tail) or fresh fish, fowl or meat known not to have been chemically contaminated [9] are usually employed. Other common foods, formerly consumed in some form once in three days or more frequently and known not to have been contaminated by chemical additives [9], are then returned one at a time. Approximately double- to triple-size portions are cooked with spring water in glass or stainless steel containers and served at regular mealtimes. The order of testing is unimportant, except that it is helpful to rotate the use of highly probable and less probable foods, so as to reduce the possibility of cumulative reactions from different foods. However, wheat and corn cereals are each used in two successive meals in order to accentuate cumulative effects for diagnostic purposes. Corn and beets are followed respectively, by corn sugar (dextrose or glucose) and beet sugar (sucrose of beet origin), since a person may react to the chemical contaminants of these foods present in their sugars but not in their native sources. Beef and milk as well as chicken and eggs are also tested in successive meals.

The pulse rate is recorded for a full minute prior to each feeding and at 30, 60 and 90 minutes after the completion of the test meal, as described by Coca [15] and confirmed by others [16, 17]. Skipped beats are recorded as if present. Although the majority of patients may be taught to record their own pulse accurately, this is not possible in all cases. The type and timing of objective and subjective symptoms are observed by the patient and another person.

Interpretation of Ingestion Tests

As previously emphasized [10], the interpretation of individual food ingestion tests depends principally on clinical observations. Clinically detectable evidence of a reaction to a food formerly eaten regularly and frequently but avoided completely for four to ten days prior to the test feeding is usually noted by the experienced observer within the first hour. There are two phases of the test reaction. The first phase may be so mild in character and so transient in duration as to be missed. This is commonly followed by a relative improvement for several hours prior to the more apparent delayed phase of reaction [3, 10].

Commonly but not invariably, these positive clinical findings are associated with an elevation of the pulse rate [15, 16, 17]. A critical level above which this acceleration is significant cannot be stated, as the range between the daily minimal and maximal pulse rate of a person decreases as the value of the minimum increases. This relationship, pointed out by Corwin and associates [16] provides a convenient means for estimating the normal daily range of the pulse if an individual's daily minimal rate is established. In the presence of unmistakable clinical symptoms, an interpretation of the pulse findings is not needed. In the absence of early demonstrable symptoms, a pulse acceleration above this normal range may presage either a delayed clinical response or the existence of a low grade specific susceptibility. The latter may manifest clinically only when a given food is used cumulatively. At times, however, there may be no significant changes in the pulse rate in the presence of a clinical response. Occasionally, especially in coffee tests, a bradycardia may be associated with clinically positive reactions.

The most commonly incriminated foods in the approximate order of probability are: coffee, corn, wheat, milk, egg, potato, yeast, orange, tomato, beef, pork, legumes, oat, chocolate, beet, carrot and cane. However, any food used once in three days or more frequently should be suspected and tested.

Food allergy may also be investigated satisfactorily by means of provocative food tests [18] which correlate closely with individual food ingestion tests and which also apparently depend on the precipitation of acute non-adapted test responses [19]. However, when susceptibility to given foods and the chemical environment coexists, as often occurs, comprehensive environmental control followed by observing the effects of single test re-exposures is preferable.

SUSCEPTIBILITY TO CHEMICAL ADDITIVES AND CONTAMINANTS OF DIET

Because of the tendency for cross-reactions between different chemical additives and contaminants of the diet and their ability to exert cumulative clinical effects in susceptible persons, somewhat different techniques are necessary to demonstrate these relationships. At least ten days may be required for a patient to recover from former exposures. Although an acute reaction may follow the first meal of purposely selected chemically contaminated foods in the highly susceptible person, at least two days of cumulative ingestion may be necessary before a relatively symptom-free patient manifests convincing evidence of a reaction.

These unsuspected uncommonly eaten commercially available foods are used for testing: raw apple, celery and lettuce; dietetic canned peaches, cherries, blueberries and pears; frozen broccoli, cauliflower, brussels sprouts and spinach; salmon, tuna and chicken canned in lined tins. These foods are selected because of their spray residues and their chemical contamination by means of phenolic resins employed in the manufacture of the linings of their metal cans — the two most important sources of the chemical contamination of the diet [9]. They are also selected because of their availability (to the writer) in chemically less contaminated form for use as controls for the purpose of ruling out the possibility of a specific food response *per se*.

Although the subject of the chemical contamination of the diet has been described in detail elsewhere [9], a few points will be reviewed briefly. Protein foods may be contaminated chemi-

cally by feeding livestock with forage or grain containing insecticide or weedkiller chemical residues; spraying or dipping animals for insect control; employing antibiotics and synthetic hormones as growth stimulants; washing dressed carcasses with detergents; dipping dressed fowl or fish in antibiotic solutions as a preservative and wrapping these foods in odorous wrapping materials or both. Many of these chemical contaminants are apparently concentrated in the fat portions. At least, cutting off the fats of meats prior to cooking tends to reduce the severity of reactions in patients presenting this clinical problem. Others may be maintained symptom-free only on a meat, fish and fowl intake of known cultural and processing pedigree [9].

Foods may also be contaminated by means of fumigants, fungicides, sulfur in various forms, artificial coloring, sweetening and ripening agents, protective waxes, impregnated containers, or when foods are allowed to stand in or are cooked in chemically contaminated water. Since certain less chemically contaminated foods are not readily available, it is necessary to maintain local and regional sources of supply for canning and freezing during seasons of availability.

When relatively symptom-free and at least 24 hours prior to discharge, patients dress in their formerly used synthetic clothing. Later, usually the same day, formerly used cosmetics are applied. If protheses, such as dentures, hearing aids, spectacles and other plastic devices are suspected, these will have been avoided for at least four days prior to test re-exposures. Checking the pulse rate prior to these re-exposures and at five-minute intervals for the first 30 minutes and at 60 and 90 minutes following is useful in interpreting borderline reactions. It may also be helpful to perform "sniff tests" for such inhaled materials as perfumes, tobacco smoke, odors of fresh newspapers, and others, similarly. But because of the extreme speed of these reactions to inhaled materials, the pulse should be recorded at minute intervals for the first five minutes and then at five-minute intervals for a half hour. In general, however, the pulse response is a far less reliable index of the existence of clinical susceptibility when testing for aspects of the chemical environment than when testing for specific foods *per se*.

SUSCEPTIBILITY TO FACTORS OF THE HOME AND OTHER ENVIRONMENTS

Then with the patient relatively symptom-free, having recovered from all previous test reactions and while receiving a compatible intake of test-negative materials he is returned successively to other former exposures. Upon first going home, he makes no other changes during the first two or three days. Then, one by one, he is returned to his former water supply, work, avocations and any other previously avoided routines. Of these the home exposures are by far the most important.

A recurrence of reactive symptoms during the first few hours or days after returning home most commonly suggests susceptibility to indoor chemical air pollutants, house dust, molds, animal danders, silk, odors from cooking foods or certain other home exposures or any combination of these. Since the possibility of outdoor chemical air pollution must also be considered, a record of wind direction and velocity is kept during this period in addition to the usual food diary and symptom record.

Of these home and neighborhood exposures, indoor chemical

air pollution is the most significant, the principal contributors being such home utilities as fuel-oil or gas space heaters, gas kitchen ranges, gas water heaters, gas refrigerators and gas clothes driers. Not only are the combustion products of fuel-oil and gas-burning devices located in the home noxious to highly susceptible persons, but the odors of uncombusted fuel-oil or utility gas also are major sources of exposure. Because of the primary importance of these hydrocarbons and their combustion products, the presence of reactive symptoms immediately upon returning home necessitates the evaluation of these factors before attempting to observe the effects of other home exposures. This usually entails checking the home for gas leaks and the temporary removal of at least the gas kitchen range — the number one exposure of houses in the North Central portion of this country.

After its removal from the living quarters for at least a week, the gas range is returned to the house, connected, used, and its clinical effect noted. However, if there is any doubt about the interpretation of these moves in respect to the patient's health and behavior, either the device or the patient is again removed temporarily and returned subsequently. If the patient is moved, he should be taken to quarters free of the major sources of chemical air pollution while continuing a compatible intake as previously outlined. On the basis of evidence obtained in this manner, several hundred gas ranges have been removed permanently from the homes of patients. Merely turning off the pilots, not using the stove, keeping the kitchen exhaust fan on or even turning off the gas supply to the premises do not constitute adequate tests [9]. The presence of an unused gas stove *in situ*, even though its gas supply has been turned off, emits sufficient fumes to perpetuate chronic symptoms in highly susceptible persons. If chronic manifestations persist after the range has been incriminated and removed, other gas-burning utilities are checked similarly.

The most difficult single source of indoor chemical air pollution to evaluate is the warm air furnace. This may be a major source of air contamination and chronic reactions during winter months, irrespective of whether gas, oil or coal are employed as fuels. This effect is best observed preliminarily after other sources of chemical indoor air pollution have been evaluated and removed if incriminated, by correlating reactive symptoms and weather conditions entailing operation of the furnace. It is confirmed by removing and returning the patient. The effects of sponge rubber, odorous plastics and synthetic textiles in the home are best appraised by placing these materials, one group at a time, in a tightly closed room for about a week. Although the patient may notice changes in symptoms following their removal, the key to the specific diagnosis depends upon what happens upon re-entering this room. Similarly, day-in-and-day-out chronic effects of exposure to insecticides, floor wax, perfumes, hair sprays, bleaches, cleansers containing bleach and household disinfectants and deodorants may not be suspected. However, the intermittency of some of these exposures induces acute readily apparent reactions. This is best exemplified by acute reactions associated with the inhalation of evaporating paints, varnishes, shellac and lacquers.

Determining the roles of house dust, animal danders, molds, silk, and certain other home exposures is usually aided by details of the history as well as noting the effects of massive exposures. The presence of positive skin tests with extracts of these materials may be helpful.

In the absence of a recurrence of reactive symptoms during the first few days after returning home and while still maintaining a compatible intake of food, effects of returning to the local water supply are noted. The patient is then observed as he returns to his work, avocations and other omitted past exposures. The diet is then enlarged gradually — no more than one food per meal — to include as wide a range of foods as possible, observing the effects of these additions. It is important to rotate and diversify the use of compatible foods, since this is the most effective known way of preventing the spread of specific food susceptibility [10]. Using fewer foods per meal and fewer food mixtures is helpful in this respect.

THERAPEUTIC ASPECTS OF COMPREHENSIVE ENVIRONMENTAL CONTROL

Phases of diagnosis and treatment of illnesses arising from specific susceptibility and maladaptation to environmental incitants are closely intertwined and impossible to separate. Indeed, treatment starts with the first day of this combined diagnostic-therapeutic regimen. Acute withdrawal effects may be partially alleviated by five gram doses of mixed alkali salts (2/3 sodium biocarbonate and 1/3 potassium bicarbonate) T.I.D., B.I.D. and once daily in water, respectively, the first, second and remaining days of the fasting period. Pure salt or potassium chloride have been permitted as desired and additional sodium chloride — orally or intravenously — has been helpful in combating nausea and vomiting. Care should be taken not to prescribe medications in tablet or capsule form during the entire period of observation, in view of the food-containing fillers of such formulations [18]. Alcoholic extracts or synthetic colors of pharmaceuticals, as well as the active chemical ingredients of such preparations, may also induce acute reactions [8, 11, 20, 21].

Acute test reactions resulting from the ingestion of foods or chemical contaminants of foods are most effectively treated by means of emptying the gastrointestinal tract as soon as possible by giving 10-15 grams of the above alkali salt mixture orally in a quart of spring water, a laxative dose of milk of magnesia, or a spring water enema. Following such an acute reaction, the patient is either fasted the next meal or fed test-compatible foods; otherwise, there may be an echo of either the clinical or pulse evidence of a positive reaction. Lesser grade food reactions and, especially, accidental inhalation reactions may sometimes be treated effectively by the alkali salt mixture in a non-laxative-inducing dose. Inhaled oxygen is also helpful.

Incriminated incitants are eliminated as detected. How to avoid corn, wheat, milk, eggs, certain other foods and incriminated chemical exposures [9, 10] is too detailed to be outlined here. Suffice it to say that complete avoidance of correctly identified specific exposures accomplishes several things. It not only tends to relieve chronic symptoms and the frequency of their infectious complications, but also gradually reduces the degree of specific susceptibility and the tendency of this process to spread to related materials. However, a relative tolerance gained as a result of prolonged avoidance must be preserved with care, as it is readily dissipated. After several months of avoiding a given exposure, an occasional dose may often be handled without apparent evidence of reaction. But a massive amount or frequently repeated dosage may reactivate specific susceptibility and thereafter each widely spaced amount is apt to induce an acute non-adapted response. Oft-repeated contacts are apt to be associated with adapted responses and a recurrence of chronic symptoms of unsuspected cause. The latter course of events usually occurs upon drifting back to former eating habits and other daily routines — the greatest single hazard to which the diagnosed patient is subjected. This constitutes an indication for omitting recently added items for several days prior to their single test re-exposure. If such a program does not provide an answer, other parts of the original investigation are to be repeated, for these circumstances are sometimes associated with the development of new susceptibilities.

SAFETY FACTORS

Initial complete food deprivation is a safe procedure as judged by the absence of complications in fasting over 1000 patients ranging in age between one and 80 years. Neither are there any untoward reactions following initial feedings, providing compatible foods are fed.

Although the clinical response to incompatible foods in individual food ingestion tests may be sufficiently severe to require treatment, deaths or irreversible complications have not been observed [10]. Neither has the technique of feeding cumulative menus of chemically contaminated commercially available foods, nor has returning patients to their home exposures after a period of avoidance been associated with hazardous reactions [9]. However, the deliberate exposure of patients to measured doses of given chemicals may be hazardous in view of the extreme range of susceptibility that may be involved [9].

SUGGESTION, ACCEPTANCE AND APPLICATION

The significance of suggestion is often raised in the interpretation of clinical reactions following test re-exposures to previously avoided potential incitants in the absence of camouflaging the identity of the test materials. But insofar as may be determined from a detailed study of individual cases, suggestion is not a major factor in the interpretation of these tests. This statement is based on the ability to induce acute reactions in susceptible persons when isolated doses of food are administered blindly by intubation and, conversely, the inability to precipitate reactions as a result of sham feedings in the presence of positive suggestion. Although such controls are not done routinely, they have been performed in a sufficient number of cases to reduce greatly the possibility of suggestion being a major error in this connection. Moreover, when several individual food ingestion tests are performed per patient under as near identical circumstances as possible to arrange, negative tests tend to control positive ones. Also, positive cause-and-effect relationships between a given material and a given symptom response are usually confirmed repeatedly by subsequent accidental exposures.

Moreover, the source of some test exposures may be traced only in retrospect, inasmuch as the quantity of the specific agent encountered had been below the threshold of perception. This is especially true of intermittent exposures to utility gas and certain other inhaled chemical and cooking fumes. Because of these relationships, such airborne exposures are referred to as fumes rather than odors.

As far as suggestion is concerned, chronically reacting patients are more apt to be negative to suggestions than acceptable to some new interpretation of their illnesses which might infringe upon their freedom. Even though a person may be intensely interested in learning the inciting causes of his symptoms, he is usually loath to accept an avoidance program as detailed as that associated with the elimination of corn, wheat, milk, egg or chemically contaminated foods, or as expensive as that entailed in the re-engineering of his home. Indeed, full acceptance of these cause-and-effect interpretations generally comes only after repeated demonstrations in which circumstances permit of no alternative interpretations.

Although the abstraction that chronic illness commonly results from daily exposures to which one is susceptible and maladapted may sound reasonable to the thinking person, the brain-fagged, confused, or depressed patient is apt to react negatively to such a suggestion. In fact, resistance to personal participation, even for a short period, is the major stumbling block to a wider dissemination of these views. Many patients are apt to be too tired to be attentive; too dull to grasp the continuity of what is said; too confused to read instructions comprehendingly; too embarrassed to ask questions and, most importantly, too stuck in their daily routines and too lacking in initiative to make any major changes. Such difficulties of instruction and acceptance of a program of action are compounded with advancement of the process. Too preoccupied with their own one-track recurring "thoughts" to comprehend, accept, decide or comply, it is far easier to drift along than to make upsetting changes, even though such "upsets" might demonstrate inciting causes of their illnesses.

Another obstacle to the acceptance and application of the ecologic principles involved in this work lies with the medical profession. The chief reason that physicians have been slow to develop an ecologically oriented program — in contrast to other biologists — is that the methods required to demonstrate cause-and-effect relationships in individual patients are not in the tradition of medicine. Physicians have long looked upon human illness as something to be treated, in contrast to medical scientists who regard disease as something to be observed. To observe the course of the untreated patient as his intake and surroundings are deliberately changed is essential if one is to have a sufficiently controlled experimental setting to demonstrate the inciting causes of illness — especially chronic illness. Not only must physicians train themselves to be better observers, but they must also encourage their patients to observe and record their symptom responses under different circumstances, rather than to discount and to minimize their symptoms. Indeed, ecologically oriented medicine is not to be carried out on, to, or even for the patient; it must be done with the patient.

Medical acceptance and application is further handicapped by the fact that these views have not been widely disseminated, in as much as training courses in these aspects of ecologically oriented medicine are not yet available.

Although altered bodily mechanisms may be responsible for the production of certain symptom syndromes, many times the findings of an analytical-bodily oriented medical investigation are nil or cannot be shown to bear directly on the presenting manifestations. Not having a workable approach to a patient's problem, physicians tend to treat the patient symptomatically or to turn to the psychiatrist for help. But neither approach is apt to render a satisfactory medical service if the illness in question is a chronic manifestation of the long-term impingement of unsuspected ordinarily "harmless" foods or other environmental agents whose impact is magnified by the subject's specific susceptibility. This is where the program of comprehensive environment control should be applied. Experience in its use after completion of the routine work-up and before resorting either to empiric therapy or seeking psychiatric consultation or both reveals its useful application in allergic and psychotic states [3, 8, 10] including borderline areas usually designated as neuroses. This approach is also applicable to a number of musculo-skeletal, neurologic and hematologic manifestations as well as to certain other chronic syndromes of poorly defined or idiopathic etiology. In fact, the over-all clinical application of this fourth technique of the medical investigation has not been delineated as yet.

This presentation has emphasized the role of demonstrable exogenous incitants of illness. But, obviously, both the external environment and the body's internal milieu are important in the etiology of illness. Also, both externally orientated and internally orientated investigative programs have their places in medicine. However, there are two points in this connection that bear emphasis: (1) Externally orientated investigative programs aimed toward demonstrating the exogenous incitants of illness have been relatively neglected. (2) Since the two programs do not mix — actually interfering with each other — they should not be attempted on the same patient at the same time. The principal reasons for this are that drug therapy often perpetuates and complicates chronic illness and significantly interferes with observations of its natural course.

DISCUSSION AND SUMMARY

Symptomatic therapy or other treatment which does not take into account environmental inciting causes of chronic illness are not sufficient. The net result of maintenance drug therapy for chronic illness (1) increases the load to which adaptation must be attempted; (2) permits specific susceptibility to spread by means of cross-reactions to related materials; and (3) favors the development of new susceptibilities, including adverse reactions to the therapeutic agents employed. Sooner or later, such a program either leads to advanced addictive phenomena or to depletion of bodily defenses (the stage of exhaustion of adaptation).

Maturity in health matters demands that medicine become more ecologically and dynamically orientated.

Somewhat at the risk of over-simplification, the following summarizing statements may be made: Ecologically orientated physicians are synthesizers (not analyzers) who observe (rather than treat) the dynamic course of illness in otherwise untreated patients under controlled conditions in respect to their intake and environment. Under these circumstances, cause-and-effect interpretations are either demonstrable or cannot be said to exist.

Comprehensive environmental control, followed by observations of the specific effects of test re-exposures — in keeping with the laws of specific adaptation — is the methodology of choice in demonstrating the inciting external causes of many chronic illnesses.

In the presence of high degrees of individual susceptibility, the stages of adaptation to specific environmental incitants are accelerated and exaggerated. These changes magnify the significance of minor dosage and result in ordinarily "harmless" agents becoming pathogenic for certain susceptible individuals. Under these circumstances, cumulative exposures of common external incitants of chronic illness are rarely suspected.

Diagnostically, potential incitants are eliminated on the basis of probability. Complete avoidance reverts adapted and partially adapted responses (in which causation is obscured) to nonadapted responses, in which an isolated exposure induces an immediate sharp reaction. This program, designated comprehensive environmental control, changes chronic illness to acute illness and demonstrates its causation.

Therapeutically, complete avoidance of incriminated incitants tends to decrease individual susceptibility and, later, may permit intermittent specific exposures in the absence of acute reactions. However, at any subsequent time, cumulative dosage may quickly enhance individual susceptability and lead to adapted and, later, maladapted responses again manifesting as chronic illness.

The common causes of chronic physical and mental illnesses — as demonstrated by this technique — are common foods and environmental chemical exposures, including synthetic drugs.

It is proposed that the program of comprehensive environmental control and the subsequent observation of the test effects of specific re-exposures be added to the other techniques of the clinical investigation.

REFERENCES

1. Randolph, T.G. and Mitchell, D.S.: Specific Ecology and Chronic Illness. J Lab & Clin Med 52:936, 58.
2. Randolph, T.G.: A Third Dimension of the Medical Investigation. Clin Physiol 2:42, 60.
3. Randolph, T.G.: Levels of Ecologic Mental Illness. Proc. Third World Congress of Psychiatry, June 4-10, 1961, Montreal, Canada.
4. Randolph, T.G.: Clinical Ecology as It Affects the Psychiatric Patient. Proc. First World Congress of Social Psychiatry, August 16-22, 1964, London, England.
5. Selye, H.: The General Adaptation Syndrome and the Diseases of Adaptation. J Allergy 17:231-247; 289-323; 358, 46.
6. Randolph, T.G.: The Specific Adaptation Syndrome. J Lab & Clin Med 48: 934, 56.
7. Randolph, T.G.: Significance of Specific Adaptation in Clinical Allergy, Program of the Fifth Internal. Congress of Allergology, October 10-16, 1964, Madrid, Spain.
8. Randolph, T.G.: Food Susceptibility (Food Allergy) H. Conn, Ed. Current Therapy, Phila., Saunders, pp. 418, 60.
9. Randolph, T.G.: Human Ecology and Susceptibility to the Chemical Environment. Ann Allergy 19:518; 657; 779; 908, 61; also Springfield, Illinois, Thomas, 1962.
10. Rinkel, H.J., Randolph, T.G. and Zeller, M.: Food Allergy, Springfield, Illinois, Thomas, 1951.
11. Randolph, T.G.: The Descriptive Features of Food Addiction; Addictive Eating and Drinking. Quart J of Studies on Alcohol 17:198, 56.
12. Smuts, J.C.: Holism and Evolution. New York, Macmillan, 1926.
13. Randolph, T.G.: The Ecologic Unit. Hospital Management 97:45-47, March, 1964 and 97:46, April, 1964.
14. Mitchell, D.S.: Personal Communication.

15. Coca, A.F.: Familial Nonreaginic Food Allergy, Springfield, Illinois, 1943.

16. Corwin, A.H., Hamburger, M. and Dukes-Dubos, F.N.: Bioassay of Food Allergens; I. Statistical Examination of Daily Ranges of the Human Heart Rate as Influenced by Individually Incompatible Foods. Ann Allergy 19:1300, 61.

17. Ettelson, L.N. and Tuft, L.: The Coca Pulse-Acceleration Method in Food Allergy. J Allergy 32:514, 61.

18. Rinkel, H.J., Lee, C.H., Brown, D.W., Jr., Willoughby, J.W. and Williams, J.M.: The Diagnosis of Food Allergy, AMA Archives of Otolaryng 79:71, 64.

19. Randolph, T.G. and Frauenberger, G.S.: Provocative and Neutralizing Skin Tests with Food Extracts. Program, 20th Annual Meeting, Amer Academy of Allergy, San Francisco, 1964.

20. Randolph, T.G.: Allergy to So-Called "Intert Ingredients" (Excipients) of Pharmaceutical Preparations. Ann Allergy 8:1, 50.

21. Lockey, S.D.: Allergic Reactions Due to F.D. and C Yellow No. 5 Tartrazine, An Analine Dye Used as a Coloring and Identifying Agent in Various Steroids. Ann Allergy 17:710, 59.

22
Cerebral Reactions in Allergic Patients*
Illustrative Case Histories and Comments

MARSHALL MANDELL

Ecologic mental illness is an important facet of man's total reaction to his natural and synthetic environment. This form of mental illness is often associated with many other types of often unrecognized hypersensitivity disorders as well as common allergies. The human brain may be viewed as a complex allergic shock tissue which is easily reached by inhaled and ingested excitants from the environment via its rich blood supply. No physician can render adequate care to any sick individual unless he acquires a thorough knowledge of ecologic disease.

INTRODUCTION

The author has employed various techniques of provocative testing in order to reproduce the presenting complaints of allergic subjects and, thereby, establish an exact etiologic diagnosis in each case. These procedures were initially applied to treatment-resistant respiratory and conjunctival diseases in an attempt to identify the specific allergens causing a specific symptom or syndrome in a particular individual. Valuable diagnostic information was acquired by observing the effects of deliberate experimental exposures to a wide variety of inhaled antigens: this data provided an accurate basis for the selection of appropriate extracts to be used in each patient's individualized hyposensitization program.

Provocative nasal inhalation tests induced numerous interesting reactions and combinations of allergic symptoms that gave the author a new understanding of chronic rhinitis, hay fever and asthma due to dusts, molds, danders and pollens. Occasionally, inhalation challenges with dry powdered allergens evoked responses which indicated that some soluble material had been absorbed from the respiratory mucosa and had been transported to the skin, muscles, gastrointestinal tract and the brain. These infrequently observed non-respiratory reactions were recorded for future reference but their full significance was not recognized at the time.

Provocative inhalation test data made it possible to obtain

*Second International Congress of Social Psychiatry, Section on Ecologic Mental Illness, London, August 8, 1969. Published by The New England Foundation for Allergic and Environmental Diseases, 160 East Ave., Norwalk, Connecticut.

clinical success in previous cases of failure and this experience eventually led the author to include provocative tests for food sensitivity and chemical susceptibility in his diagnostic studies. The reports of Lee, Randolph and Rinkel and their co-workers were carefully reviewed and the author has had the privilege and pleasure of associating with these modern medical pioneers in the field of clinical ecology. The author's original purpose in acquiring an orientation in clinical ecology was to achieve better results in patients whose therapy had been unsuccessful; a detailed knowledge of provocative food testing was desired. These expectations were fulfilled and an entirely new and fascinating perspective of human illness was gained.

No physician in any branch of medicine can be considered as an expert in his particular field until he becomes aware of the enormous scope of medical ecology. It is an illuminating and inspiring experience to revisit diseases and see them in a new light; the therapeutic possibilities which are opened by the ecologists' approach are almost limitless because they are concerned with the effects of all the possible incitants in man's total environment, natural and synthetic, on man's health.

With rare exception, most of the patients seen by the author had presenting complaints that were the traditional diseases of atopic hypersensitivity which all allergists treat. The cerebral reactions occurring in the sensitized brain tissue of allergic subjects were not unknown to this writer because he had read about them and they had been discussed by several colleagues in an academic fashion. In spite of the fact that cerebral reactions were not unknown, they appeared as a great surprise because they were provoked so often and unexpectedly. It was impossible to ignore mental symptoms of the magnitude that were frequently induced: emotional disorders and psychosomatic ailments were being reproduced in the patients who were suffering from neuro-allergies that could be relieved by simple measures. A working knowledge of the mental and physical manifestations of ecologic illness is essential to all who practice medicine and it is the author's hope that this monograph will stimulate an active interest in this most important area of medicine.

To the uninitiated, the case histories and laboratory findings reported herein may seem to be unusual and the results of treatment little short of miraculous: this is not true. Cases like these are present in large numbers in the daily practice of every physician but he does not yet know how to recognize them. The author and his technicians have performed approximately 125,000 provocative tests of various types and the office files are a treasure house of exciting findings which include thousands of reactions of great significance.

Comments and discussion of various subjects will accompany the case presentations because they enhance the teaching value of the clinical data. Motion picture films taken in the office will also be demonstrated as visual evidence of adverse reactions to common environmental substances.

C.S. is a 10 year old girl under treatment for asthma, hay fever and hypersensitivity to stinging insects. The peculiar hieroglyphic-like symbols and disorganized linear "numbers" and the "alphabet" which appear on the inside and back cover were drawn while she was reacting to a provocative test for chemical susceptibility. The test material was synthetic ethyl alcohol (ethanol) which was given intracutaneously according to Randolph's method. During her reaction, of three hours' duration, this patient became hyperactive, extremely irritable, disoriented, silly, regressed to infantile behavior with screaming and biting and did not recognize her mother who was sitting next to her. She believed that her mother, wearing a white blouse and green sweater, was a former male teacher whose class she had been in two years previously; the man (her mother) was wearing a blue shirt and an orange sport jacket. She was not able to identify any colors correctly; she could not spell three-letter words, when asked to count she jumbled numbers out of sequence and mixed them with a confused alphabet. This reaction is documented by a tape recording and motion picture film.

As her reaction to petroleum ethanol progressed, she saw purple spots floating on a yellow background, did not remember where she lived and did not recognize her physician. She became hysterical when addressed by her given name and insisted on being called by her middle name which was never used. She was unable to read a comic book aloud and played a game with office equipment in which she cooked matches (tongue depressors), peas (cotton balls), tomatoes (flashlight bulbs) and carrots (marking pencils) on the stove (floor).

Upon recovery following a relieving treatment dose of ethanol, she had complete amnesia for the entire reaction but she did recall becoming dizzy and sleepy shortly after receiving an injection. Some of her cerebral reactions to chemical pollutants of indoor and outdoor air were quite severe; she had often become disoriented following exposure to the exhaust fumes of automobile engines and the combustion products of the natural gas fuel used in her kitchen. The volatile solvent (xylene) from a permanent felt tip marker made her very irritable, caused a headache and confusion which resulted in her destroying the poster she had been working on in art class. A freshly mimeographed paper that was passed out in school produced nausea, dizziness, headache and inability to concentrate; visits to the front office were also associated with these symptoms when the duplicator was being operated — the solvent was methyl alcohol. A pine oil lavatory disinfectant/deodorant caused a severe episode of confusion and bizarre behavior followed by amnesia; several of her classmates had complained of mild headaches and nausea in the same lavatory and this solution was eventually eliminated from the school at the author's suggestion.

In addition to receiving hyposensitization therapy, she was placed on a modified program of environmental control which consisted of removing the gas range and oven from her home and eliminating numerous household cleaning products whose volatile components contributed to the indoor chemical pollution of the air in her home. This environmental change was immediately beneficial; she no longer was dizzy and tired in the morning and there was a striking improvement in her school work.

F.D. is a 38 year old man with a history of childhood asthma and hives who believed that milk had been responsible for past headaches. This is one of the few cases referred to the author for an allergic evaluation of an "emotional problem." He was sent by his wife whose case is reported in another publication; her multifaceted illness is extremely interesting and is briefly presented here:

The patient's wife was seen for respiratory allergy and was subsequently shown to have numerous unsuspected ecologic disorders including colitis, headaches, mental depression, irritability, fatigue, tension/anxiety, tachycardia, palpitations, generalized itching, urinary frequency, a "lump" in her throat and claustrophobia. A gastroenterologist had diagnosed emotional spastic colitis and ordered a milk and dairy diet which was of no benefit; her provocative test for milk allergy brought on an anxiety attack with many of her familiar symptoms which terminated with an acute episode of severe colitis. Her diet therapy was perpetuating the digestive tract ailment that was due to milk and its complete removal from her diet cleared a long term illness of "psychologic origin". Space limitation does not permit the inclusion of the other details in this complex but successfully treated case.

This man complained of severe fatigue, mental confusion, nervous tension and frequent "virus infections" characterized by respiratory symptoms and the usual systemic accompaniments. A psychiatric consultant had concluded that emotional stress was the underlying cause of the recurrent and disabling illness; he informed the patient that his poor health was due to lowered resistance which, in turn, was the consequence of unresolved mental problems that required a psychotherapeutic approach.

In view of his past history of classical atopic diseases and the nature of his presenting illness, a series of provocative food tests were performed to demonstrate the presence of allergic sensitivity to dietary factors. Fifteen of these tests were positive and 6 foods did not elicit any reactions. Subcutaneous injections of aqueous food extracts were given in various concentrations and it was readily shown that his entire problem was a food allergy syndrome that could be provoked and neutralized (relieved) by appropriate dilutions of certain food extracts. Some of his food tests are reported below:

WHEAT — restless, tense, yawning and unable to concentrate; nasal burning, desire to sneeze, drawing sensation in occiput, increased peristalsis with loud abdominal rumbling.

COFFEE — lightheaded, visual blurring, yawned and became very tired; postnasal drip, belched, pulsating supraorbital headache that radiated to the occipit, tension in posterior nuchal muscles.

Comment: The above symptoms were elicited on his first day of testing and he was advised to stop drinking coffee and drastically reduce his intake of wheat. Three days later his chronic state of fatigue had lessened considerably.

MILK — "nervous", generalized headache, yawned, tired, dizzy, confused; sneezed, sore throat, postnasal secretion, felt very warm, "blocked" ears, retrobulbar soreness and pressure in the frontal and ethmoidal sinus areas. A familiar vascular phenomenon was noted; the dorsal surface of his fingers became red and the fingertips were cold and white.

CHICKEN — irritable, nervous, sleepy, felt as if he were going to faint; nasal obstruction, eyes sore, stiffness of posterior neck muscles.

EGG — yawning, intermittent fatigue, nervous, unable to concentrate: sneezed, cleared throat, right ear full, heavy sensation in lower forehead, perspiring and felt "like I was getting a cold."

PEA — yawned, tired, headache, nervous: flushed face, burning throat and palate, ears blocked, "feels like a cold": itching hands, "stomach rumbling like crazy".

CORN — tense, irritable, yawned, very tired: coughed, felt like sneezing, nasal discharge, ears full; face flushed, frontal headache, intermittent dizziness, generalized malaise, periorbital and retrobulbar pain "like the virus"; aches and soreness in upper back, shoulders, right elbow and wrist; face felt "puffy".

Comments: From the above reactions to food tests it is clearly evident that the patient's physical and mental symptoms can be duplicated by provocative exposure to a number of foods. His illness was not of psychic origin and his recurrent misdiagnosed syndrome could not possibly be successfully treated by therapy based on psychiatric concepts. He has been well for one year without any medication or allergy treatment: he avoids the major test-incriminated foods and restricts his intake of minor offenders. Occasional lapses in dietary control do not often cause significant illness and the flare-ups that do occur are understood by the patient: it has been possible to break the distressing cycle of allergic reactions inducing allergic mental symptoms which formerly evoked psychologic responses that aggravated the original cerebral hypersensitivity reaction. Patients learn a very reassuring lesson from their provocative food test reactions; they have experienced mental symptoms that are not due to emotional causes and they search for offenders rather than worry about their inferior nervous systems that are unwilling victims of psychic trauma — alleged, postulated, assumed, presumed etc. but unproven.

J.W. is a 20 year old woman with a past history of hives and asthma who was seen for grass and weed pollen hay fever. After ingesting a small amount of any alcoholic beverage she always had visual blurring and a headache: her family believed that this was a "psychological reaction" because it took such a small quantity of alcohol to bring on her symptoms.

Comment: Most alcoholic beverages are prepared by yeast fermentation of cereal grains which happen to be members of the grass family. This patient has recently been tested by provocative nasal inhalation with many species of undefatted dry grass pollens and showed a high degree of sensitivity to grasses. Her studies are incomplete at this time but her reactions to cereal grains are:

CORN — frontal headache, visual blurring, fatigue, flushed face and moist hands.

RYE — frontal headache, visual blurring, eyes felt "heavy", tired and lightheaded.

RICE — frontal headache, heavy sensation in left eye.

WHEAT — frontal headache, visual blurring, nasal discharge, sneezing and lacrimation.

Comments: Her wheat test was indistinguishable from an attack of hay fever in most respects; each cereal grain tested was shown capable of reproducing her familiar alcohol-induced symptoms. The clinical significance of adverse reactions to potable alcohol have been thoroughly studied by Randolph who concluded that immediate or delayed (hangover) reactions to small amounts of grain alcohol are evidence of sensitivity to either yeast or cereal grain since beverages contain rapidly absorbed substances derived from their source materials. The above reported reactions support Randolph's conclusions: alcohol related symptoms were produced by the basic fermentable ingredients in the absence of alcohol. Her response to pollen hyposensitization might not be satisfactory if particular attention is not given to the wheat problem: she might not be able to tolerate dietary wheat during the period of pollen exposure and hyposensitization or elimination might be necessary to remove the effects of this cereal.

M.S. is a 32 year old housewife with asthma, hay fever, gastrointestinal disturbances, urinary frequency, fatigue, depression and irritability. The clinical application of provocative food test data made it possible for this patient to be happy and comfortable after years of poor health. Her excellent response from the elimination of test-postive foods which were identified during the early phase of her investigation made further studies unnecessary. Some of her important reactions to injected food extracts are:

POTATO — felt "peculiar," lightheaded, weak, lights seemed to be too bright; became depressed, put her head down on the desk and began to cry. This was followed by an interesting period of irritability during which she became sarcastic and wished that her husband were present because she does not care for him at such times and she wanted to argue with him and aggravate him; she had no control over these feelings and could not explain their sudden appearance. The reaction was treated with a neutralizing dose (.1cc of 1-300,000) of potato extract to preserve family harmony; the symptoms disappeared promptly.

TEA — nausea, throbbing frontal headache, tired and leaning back with head against the wall, heavy sensation in limbs. A neutralizing treatment cleared the headache in less than 3 minutes and the fatigue was gone within 5 minutes.

Comment: This patient drank tea frequently throughout the day and had undoubtedly become sensitized by her heavy exposure. Three weeks after discontinuing tea drinking she had a cup of tea with a neighbor and fell asleep in her chair shortly thereafter — she woke up about two hours later. Her reaction was a manifestation of the hyperacute state of sensitivity that follows abstinence from an offending ingestant; a low grade chronic symptom is converted to an acute diagnostic flare and this is the basis for Rinkel's deliberate oral test.

MILK — irritable, restless, sharp abdominal cramps and bloating with visible distention; her slacks suddenly became too tight and she had to loosen them. All of the symptoms, including bloating, were relieved by a neutralizing dose of milk extract (.1cc of 1-60,000).

WHEAT — nausea, abdominal pain and headache; quickly relieved by .1cc of 1-300,000 wheat extract.

Comments: She regularly took a cold wheat cereal with milk each evening at 10:00 P.M. after arriving home from work. By

10:15 P.M. she was always uncomfortable and irritable but she had never associated her "nerves" with this habitual snack of wheat and milk. Her religious adviser and family physician had suggested that the bitter arguments that she had with her husband every nite were due to the physical and emotional stress of her very long day which included household duties, the care of four children and a part time job each evening. She was urged to give up her job in order to "give her nerves a rest". Instead of giving up her work, she gave up her usual nightly snack and reduced her wheat ingestion starting on the day that the wheat provocative test was performed. On the following morning she arrived at the office with renewed vigor, an almost radiant smile and her eyes were shining. For the first time in over a year she awoke without her usual morning "hangover" and did not have to start the day with her customary two aspirin tablets. She had been reluctant to admit that it was not possible for her to face the new day without medication for her hangover; if she had not been embarrassed about this symptom it would have been possible to evaluate and relieve her condition many months sooner.

J.B. is a 10 month old boy with gastrointestinal, respiratory and cerebral sensitivities that were diagnosed and managed by the use of Rinkel's Diversified Rotary Diet. No provocative food tests with parenteral extracts were performed because the author wished to spare an already irritable infant any additional discomfort and relieve the mother of her apprehension regarding her son's reaction to a series of injections.

Gastrointestinal symptoms began at age two days and persisted until he was seven months old; his major reactions were vomiting and diarrhea associated with restlessness, perianal dermatitis, irritability and crying with his knees drawn up. There were numerous formula changes and diet adjustment measures; every change appeared to be beneficial for 2 or 3 days and then ceased to help. He was unable to tolerate a majority of the foods offered him and all formulas caused frequent and loose stools. Rashes occasionally appeared on his face and trunk. At age 10 months his diet was limited to 7 foods that did not disturb him as far as his mother could determine.

Respiratory symptoms appeared at age 3 months and became progressively worse as he grew older; they began with a deep throaty cough and nasal discharge that varied in intensity but never cleared completely. At 7 months he had a prolonged episode of asthmatic bronchitis which subsided very slowly; there were audible and palpable ronchi in his chest for one month and a cough persisted from the onset of this infection, being present when he was seen in consultation at age 10 months. Microscopic examination of stained nasal secretion revealed the presence of a moderate number of eosinophiles which is a finding that is accepted as evidence of an allergic state.

The author's initial diagnosis was gastrointestinal allergy to foods which caused vomiting, diarrhea and abdominal distress: it was believed that these symptoms led to a state of irritability and restlessness — his behavioral symptoms were assumed to be consequences of the pains arising in a reacting allergic digestive tract. The respiratory symptoms, which began at age 3 months, were thought to be due to foods and/or inhalants.

The Rotary Diversified Diet, a technique devised by Rinkel, was employed to evaluate the etiologic role of foods in this case. A 5-day 15-food diet, arranged in five groups of three foods each,

was designed for this patient. A different group of foods was eaten every day for 5 days and, on the sixth day, the diet sequence was repeated by starting with the first group again.

He was given 3 test feedings daily: at 4 to 6 hour intervals one of the three foods was given alone in order to observe its effects. This program of testing presented the patient with 15 individual dietary challenges in rotation over a 5 day period and each food ingestion test result, positive or negative, was critically reviewed every 5 days as the rotation of foods was repeated. It should be recalled that a food-sensitive individual will develop a hyper-reactive state to an offender if it is completely eliminated from the diet for a period of 4 days; when eaten on or after the fifth day of abstinence, an acute exacerbation of symptoms due to this particular food will be noted. On the second rotation of a diet consisting of commonly eaten foods, each meal constitutes a provocative exposure to a potential unrecognized allergenic substance which is taken in its usual form through its normal portal of entry.

Very often, an allergic individual's tolerance to a food is a variable condition which depends upon the quantity of this particular food that is eaten or the frequency of exposure to the same substance; at times, the reaction is modified by the presence of another food that is ingested concurrently. Each of the aforementioned modifying factors can be employed for the patient's benefit if normal size portions makes it possible for food-sensitive individuals to include many dietary offenders in their menu because their reactivity to specific foods is cyclic or variable. Naturally, this technique will not be effective when the food allergy is a fixed condition and will not respond to prolonged abstinence from an offending food to which this type of sensitivity exists. It is a relatively simple matter to plan and follow such a diet and the rewards can be spectacular.

A remarkable clinical success was achieved in this infant by application of the rotary diet: invaluable diagnostic information was obtained. The patient's mother and the author plan to report this case in depth in a future publication; our major findings in this cooperative effort are briefly presented here.

A large part of the following information is based on a long series of telephone calls which were conducted twice a week with the patient's mother.

There were amazing and predictable changes in the infant's behavior that were not associated with gastrointestinal disturbances. Initially, it had been the author's impression that the patient's state of irritability was due to abdominal pains of allergic origin. Behavioral manifestations were precipitated by foods that had no demonstrable effect on the digestive tract; no reactions were accepted as valid clinical evidence until they had been repeatedly provoked by a minimum of three oral challenges. The test-negative foods were retained in his diet and have been given at least 10 times at the time of this presentation; most of the positive tests were repeated 5 to 7 times. His reactions to testing were:

SWEET POTATO — diarrhea consistently produced in 10 to 16 hours without any other symptoms.

BEEF — nasal stuffiness present about one hour after eating this food on five occasions; "a miserable disposition for the rest of the day" associated with anorexia.

RICE — extreme irritability, nasal discharge and minimal regurgitation.

WHEAT — no reactions noted except for a change in the appearance of his stools. About 24 hours after taking a wheat cereal his movements "looked very much like the cereal".

Comment: Wheat was not responsible for any discomfort, behavioral changes or respiratory symptoms after being ingested once in five days but it is quite possible that he might react significantly if it were eaten with greater frequency. A major benefit of the rotary diet is the preservation of tolerance to a food that an allergic subject has a variable (cyclic) sensitivity to.

OAT — oatmeal eaten in the morning caused extreme irritability that persisted throughout the day; he also developed nasal discharge and obstruction between one and two hours after taking this cereal.

By dietary manipulation, this 10 month old baby's mental state and behavior were controlled in a predictable manner; it was clearly established that his disposition was a function of his hypersensitivity to foods. This permits one to speculate over a wide range of "emotional problems" which involve a variety of postulated maternal responses to infants we have come to accept as facts although they are unproven hypotheses. An emotionally healthy woman, with a miserable allergic baby that has an unrecognized cerebral hypersensitivity, has difficulty in accepting the fact that, despite her excellent adjustment (to marriage, housekeeping, social life; no obvious or urgent problems and a deep sense of contentment with her new maternal role), a specialist in pediatrics, internal medicine or psychiatry has concluded that her infant's behavior is evidence that she is rejecting the baby she loves or she is emotionally immature. She knows that she loves the infant she has waited for so long and she can not understand that her excellent adjustment to many life situations had been accomplished by an immature woman who apparently was mature until her recent motherhood. Her baby is uncomfortable from his allergies and she is concerned, worried, anxious and tense; she may become irritable or depressed by this situation but these are normal reactions of a frightened and loving mother. Her response to this unhappy situation may aggravate the problem but she did not originally contribute to its genesis.

A simple diagnostic technique has shown that physical symptoms, localized in the respiratory and gastrointestinal tracts, and behavioral responses are this infant's manifestations of previously unrecognized food allergy. His irritability and restlessness are a form of *infantile ecologic mental illness*. A reproducible cause-and-effect relationship between symptoms and specific dietary excitants has been clearly established in this case with excellent results following clinical application of observations made during oral testing.

W.R. is a 19 year old asthmatic male who came with two diagnoses for the same complex of presenting symptoms. Discussion of his numerous localized and systemic food allergies is omitted in this report which is confined to his problem of chemical susceptibility which was diagnosed as hypoglycemia in one clinic and as a psychiatric disturbance involving his relationship with his mother at another world-famous clinic. The medical staffs of these clinics were not familiar with ecologic diseases or they never would have overlooked the obvious diagnostic clues that were elicited from a properly oriented history.

The results of provocative testing which was conducted in the office were subsequently confirmed in the hospital when this patient was placed on a program of comprehensive environmental control. He was fasted in an environment where chemical pollution of the air was kept to a minimum and his intake was restricted to spring water and sea salt. At the termination of his five day fast he was started on a rotary diet of organic foods which were free of insecticides, herbicides, artificial fertilizer, coloring, waxes, fungicides, preservatives etc. At the end of the rotary diet he was given commercially raised foods that contained all of the additives and contaminants that modern chemical technology has made possible. Food allergy and chemical susceptibility were established as the etiologic factors in this case and he is presently living a normal active life after years of illness. The hospital program of comprehensive environmental control was developed by Randolph who combined Rinkel's rotary diet with the therapeutic fast devised by Mitchell.

His test with petroleum-derived ethyl alcohol induced a group of symptoms which duplicated either the "hypoglycemic" episodes or the expression of his mother-centered "psychic conflict," depending upon which of the presenting diagnoses one had accepted prior to the ethanol provocation. A .05cc injection of dilute alcohol containing traces of many petroleum hydrocarbons caused dizziness, headache, mental confusion, nausea, fatigue, pallor and profuse perspiration. The patient immediately recognized his familiar syndrome and then recalled the fact that these symptoms usually appeared when he was driving his sport car which had a defect in the exhaust system and a leak in the floor. He knew that fuel combustion products entered the car but he had not realized that these petroleum fumes were making him ill. There was a tear in the flexible mask at the base of the gear shift: repairs were suggested.

Another aspect of his chemical susceptibility problem is of considerable interest. In the past he would have claustrophobia and an exacerbation of his asthma when he entered the kitchen if the oven or several burners of the gas range were in operation. He also would develop a headache and fatigue and go to his room and rest. Not aware of the existence of chemical susceptibility or the serious effects of an exposure to volatile petroleum compounds, his family had concluded that his kitchen syndrome was a psychosomatic disorder and they tried to keep him in the room to confront and overcome his supposed emotional problem. The longer he remained in the gas polluted air of the kitchen, the worse he became; this was accepted as evidence of the psychological nature of his difficulty.

I.S. is a 25 year old woman who suffered from "neurotic symptoms" for four years and had been in group therapy for one and one-half years under the care of a psychologist who had diagnosed emotional immaturity. Her many ailments included colitis, fatigue on awakening each morning, tension, fainting spells, depression, lightheadedness, anxiety states approaching panic and periods of visual impairment 3 to 5 times a day "with everything becoming grey and dark". Repeated examinations and laboratory studies, including an EEG, were negative.

Exposure to chemically polluted indoor and outdoor air caused a variety of respiratory and cerebral symptoms and she was aware of a number of untoward reactions to certain foods and alcoholic beverages. Specific foods were known to produce heartburn, diarrhea or urinary frequency. Potable alcohol evoked respiratory, gastrointestinal, urinary bladder and cerebral reactions.

Symptoms from small amounts of alcoholic beverages, as previously mentioned, indicate a probable sensitivity to alcohol soluble factors derived from brewer's yeast and/or the fermentable sugars from cereal grains, fruits and vegetables from which the offending beverage has been prepared. The patient made several interesting comments regarding her experiences with different drinks: they are most suggestive and are quoted herein. "One drink and I am drunk. I am in a world of my own. I feel rotten the next day." At times she had a sense of unreality feeling detached from her surroundings and was unable to comprehend the content of conversations although she could hear each word distinctly. Alcohol often caused severe headaches, lightheadedness and her typical attacks of loss of vision. Wheat, corn and rye tests provoked episodes of visual blurring that were similar to her usual complaint; all of these grains are used in the manufacture of alcoholic beverages.

Provocative tests with food extracts duplicated and, therefore, explained many of her recurring symptoms. She had a number of unusual mental, visual and somatic reactions to house dust and a number of molds. Her responses to ethanol, cigarette tobacco and tobacco smoke extracts were prolonged and of clinical significance because they shed much light on her alleged "emotional immaturity" and provided etiologic data which was subsequently applied in the treatment of her ecologic disorder.

Her reactions following recent exposures to cigarette smoke and a liquid floor wax are especially interesting. She smoked a single cigarette after discontinuing this habit for three weeks; immediately after taking the first few puffs of smoke there was a change in her personality. She became lightheaded, irritable and restless; she had been in excellent spirits the entire day before inhaling cigarette smoke. Suddenly, she "felt mad at the world" and a companion was very puzzled by this unexpected change that seemed to "come from out of nowhere." Smoking was continued intermittently from that day on and she was uncomfortable for three weeks noting that she "did not have a good day since she resumed smoking."

For an unexplained reason this patient was "always miserable after waxing her wood floors." Her ecologic orientation led her to suspect some agent in the waxing compound and she carefully observed the events related to, what proved to be, her final exposure to this product. Within five minutes after she began to wax the floor, she became very "aggravated" and the muscles of her upper and lower extremities felt tense. She was unable to control an unprovoked state of anger that became progressively more intense; she described herself as "getting madder and madder." During past episodes of this nature, she had become very concerned because she could not understand why she should be feeling tense and angry when she was working quietly, alone in the house, and not thinking about anything in particular. She was very pleased that she had been able to identify one of her major offenders and had experienced a typical attack that she was now in a position to prevent.

When individuals having cerebral hypersensitivity to chemical incitants are not aware of the nature of their illness, each unexplained episode of ecologic mental illness is interpreted as evidence of a psychiatric disturbance. This woman was suffering from an environmental disease that her doctors were not aware of and the only diagnostic possibilities that they considered were those in which the causes were related to emotional stress.

S.T. is an 8 year old allergic boy who regularly developed late afternoon fatigue associated with a lack of interest in his surroundings and poor scholastic performance near the end of each school day. This situation was brought to the author's attention because an afternoon teacher had suggested that his "daydreaming" might, somehow, be related to the stinging insect hyposensitization treatments that he was being given. Another daily syndrome that made its appearance between 9:00 A.M. and 10:00 A.M. had been overlooked by his morning teacher; at this time he became quite restless, had a dry cough and a severe degree of itching in both eyes.

The predictable appearance of cerebral involvement between 1:00 P.M. and 2:00 P.M. every day indicated that his fatigue and mental changes were probably due to regular contact with some exogenous factor present in his diet or the air in his school. The logical starting points were his luncheon menu and possible air pollutants in his afternoon classrooms. Similarly, his recurring morning reactions suggested the possibility of cerebral, conjunctival and pharyngeal sensitivity to (1) a regularly eaten breakfast food, (2) a delayed, or withdrawal, effect from a food ingested on the previous day, (3) a chemical exposure on his way to school, and (4) a chemical pollutant of the air in his morning class.

A constant and prominent feature of his school lunch were a group of chocolate flavored foods. He always had chocolate milk and chocolate ice cream; in addition, he alternated between chocolate cupcakes and chocolate chip cookies. He was very fond of a cold breakfast cereal prepared from oat flour and he usually had at least two bowls of it every morning. Throughout the day, he was frequently seen "in and out of the kitchen" taking handfuls of his favorite snack.

His eating habits are characteristic behavior for cases of *chronic food addiction*; they are very common. Food-addicted individuals like, love or crave their unsuspected dietary offenders because they provide temporary relief from the unrecognized or misunderstood withdrawal (hangover) symptoms that result from the ingestion of foods to which such addiction has occured. The various discomforts experienced by such individuals when they miss, or are late for, a meal are well known to all; irritability, fatigue, headache, tension, nausea etc. are often encountered but rarely diagnosed correctly — hypoglycemia is a currently popular misinterpretation of food withdrawal symptoms. Middle of the night or early morning reactions in any body system are very often withdrawal symptoms; likewise, headache and fatigue on arising also belong in this category.

Food-addicted persons usually realize that they, somehow, feel better after eating an addicting allergen and they explain the salutary effects of their favorite addictive ingestants in terms of their elegant nutritional properties or their assumed antihypoglycemic effects. This self-perpetuating cycle of withdrawal cravings and their temporary satisfaction may continue for many years without coming to the attention of the individuals in whom this problem exists; they eat the food they desire in the quantities that are required at the times when the withdrawal state induces "hunger" of a specific type.

The suspected diagnosis of food allergy of the chronic addictive type proved to be correct in this case. Chocolate was identified by an oral challenge and oats were incriminated by a provocative test with oat extract given subcutaneously. Chocolate intolerance was dramatically verified by Rinkel's test which, incidently, was partially described by Hippocrates who observed that foods taken after a fast would often cause severe reactions in the allergic ancient Greeks. After four chocolate-free days, he was tested with this food and an acute exacerbation of his chocolate sensitivity was demonstrated: he drank two cups of cocoa and ate two bars of chocolate for "lunch" of the fifth day of abstinence. Within an hour he developed generalized hives and became moderately tired; there was considerable mental confusion during this reaction. Lee's provocative test with aqueous extract of oats confirmed the diagnostic suspicion obtained from his dietary habit history; the morning syndrome of restlessness, coughing and itching eyes was promptly duplicated within a few minutes. Elimination of chocolate and oats from his diet has given complete relief from two serious allergic problems which had made this child uncomfortable, changed his personality and interfered with his school work.

B.B. is a 42 year old woman with a four year history of gall bladder attacks whose referring physician suspected food allergy in view of a negative series of x-ray studies and a history of colitis for 24 years. Her right upper abdominal pains had been so severe that she had begged her doctor to have this organ removed. She suffered from a daily morning syndrome characterized by fatigue, dizzy spells, headache and episodes of mental confusion. She also had chronic rhinitis, joint and muscle pains, extrasystoles and dysuria. Hypoglycemia had been suspected because of her craving for pie, cookies and graham crackers. Her reactions to alcoholic beverages were clinically significant; limited social drinking was poorly tolerated. Small quantities of alcohol made her very irritable and she often developed "a nasty disposition" which offended other guests. Irritability usually progressed to a state of depression and most of her reactions were followed by very severe hangovers.

Chemical Susceptibility was manifested by nausea and "an awful sensation that I can't breathe" when she entered textile stores; she vomited after exposure to certain perfumes. Many volatile substances caused headaches after she inhaled their fumes; she reacted in this manner to paint, turpentine, new odorous plastic articles, freshly manufactured rubber products and chlorine laundry bleach. She liked the odor of gasoline fumes and she liked to travel on or near freshly tarred roads; somehow, she felt better after exposure to gasoline and tar. In addition, she found mothballs to have a pleasant odor and a nice effect on her. Chemical exposures that produce beneficial effects have acted as treatments for chemical sensitivities that are actively present in subjects who are not aware of the fact that they have a health problem due to these materials. Likes, dislikes and an ability to readily detect chemical odors have been shown to be important evidence in cases of adverse reactions to the chemical environment.

This patient was seen eight times during a period of two months and her progress was very gratifying. Many tests for major dietary offenders were never performed because she felt so well after eliminating important excitants immediately upon their discovery by provocative food testing. Her total "allergic load" was greatly reduced early in the course of her evaluation and this gave a degree of relief that was sufficient for us to discontinue testing after relatively few studies had been completed.

Some of her reactions to provocative food tests with aller-

genic extracts were confirmed by ingestion tests which reproduced many of her chronic ailments. The true nature of her complaints had not been understood in the past and, consequently, had not been treated appropriately; a variety of medications had been employed to relieve symptoms because the causes of her disorders were not known. The results of many of her parenteral tests had been very convincing and she saw no need to repeat them by oral challenges, especially when it was apparent that avoidance of the test-positive foods was accompanied by a welcome remission from her chronic symptoms. Some of her reactions to foods were:

COFFEE — stabbing pains in left knee and leg, muscle cramps in forearms, neck, upper back and right shoulder; headache, nausea, dizzy, unable to concentrate and diminished vision with inability to read the print she had been reading before the test. She felt "fuzzy and vague" and said, "My center of gravity is shot." She stood up but was not steady and doubted her ability to walk safely without assistance.

Comment: Coffee was immediately eliminated and her headaches were greatly reduced in number and intensity. All of the coffee-induced symptoms were familiar to the patient.

PORK — unilateral headache, brief sharp knee pain, generalized muscular soreness.

WHEAT — sudden severe shooting pain in right thigh and upper leg that caused her to get up from the chair to obtain relief by a change of position; muscle spasm and pain of posterior neck and lower back. The back pain was referred to as "colon spasm" in the past.

CHOCOLATE — tired, nervous and restless: an attack of acute biliary colic with RUQ abdominal pain radiating to the infrascapular area: suprapubic pain, LLQ abdominal pain identified as a "spasm"; aches in knees, elbows, wrists and fingers: severe muscle pain in forearms.

Note: In the past the author and his colleagues often combined the extracts of related foods in a single injection as a time saving screening measure: this method of testing is no longer employed here.

ORANGE & GRAPEFRUIT — gall bladder attack, right earache, soreness of elbows, wrists and fingers.

EGG & CHICKEN — epigastric pain, nausea, weakness, pallor, chill, hands shaking, tightness of the nuchal area and hunger; mental confusion, poor motor control with difficult walking, unable to fix eyes on an object without pain and had to look away. She had difficulty completing sentences and was unable to answer questions; she could not state her husband's occupation. Quotations: "It feels like I'm going to fall off the chair" ... "like hypoglycemia" ... "I am afraid that I might get lost somewhere." "Boy, does my head feel funny!" "I can sit on the chair now." "This was a beautiful attack!"

POTATO & TOMATO — headache, restless, uncomfortable, yawning, tired, unable to read with comprehension; a few sharp gall bladder pains, lower abdominal pain, soreness of upper and lower back, aching shoulders and thighs.

Oral tests for chicken and egg were performed after the usual four day period of elimination. After eating two hard boiled eggs she had a reaction that persisted for six hours; there was nausea, dizziness and a sensation that she was falling. Her response to chicken consisted of fatigue, mental confusion, a "floating sensation" and her usual, and reasonable, fear of driving her car or engaging in any potentially dangerous activity.

It is of particular interest to note that this patient was in her third year of psychiatric therapy which had been unsuccessful for obvious reasons. Demonstrable and reproducible cerebral hypersensitivity reactions to foods and environmental chemicals can not be relieved by the application of any form of therapy that does not interfere with the external non-personal environmental substances; psychiatric treatment is of no value in hypersensitivity and medications only suppress manifestations while the disease continues and leads to irreversible changes. Cerebral food allergy was responsible for a group of incapacitating ailments which had made this woman miserable and often confined her to bed when she was afraid to expose herself to physical danger at times when she could not control her body or her contact with her surroundings was impaired.

G.I. is a 36 year old woman with joint pains, headaches and "emotional problems" who was referred by one of the author's patients who suspected that her friend was an unrecognized case of "allergy." She had been receiving private and group psychotherapy for six years; she frequently had distressing, and unexplained, symptoms which are best described in her own words below.

"I have frequent crying spells for no apparent reasons; feelings of anger and depression . . . I would be feeling fine and suddenly be triggered to behave in a way that I did not understand. I have attacks with distorted vision, lack of concentration; numbness on the left side of my body which is followed by a terrific headache. During the past year I had three difficult sessions where it almost reached the point that I should be hospitalized for my emotional problems. I felt that I was weird and the future was hopeless; I was afraid that I would always have to live in this uncomfortable manner."

The patient had never been satisfied with the various interpretations which had been offered to explain her illness. She could not bring herself to accept the fact that, for psychological reasons which were completely unknown to her, she could become so miserable. She questioned the sudden appearance of symptoms that would be noted when there positively were no identifiable emotionally provoking circumstances and wondered why past or present problems that she was totally unaware of should be causing intense symptoms during tranquil periods. In reviewing her past life experiences, she was unable to distinguish any remarkable psychic trauma and believed that she had led a normal life. She had searched her conscience and probed her innermost feelings to no avail; there did not seem to be sufficient evidence that childhood trauma or past and present emotional stresses were the cause of her disability. She did not believe that it was possible to be completely ignorant of psychic and social factors of the magnitude that she felt would be required to produce such profound delayed effects on her physical and mental health. The patient came to the author "out of desperation and not convinced that any help might be available . . ."

The first hour of our initial consultation was not a pleasant experience for the author because the patient was unhappy, irritable and suspicious; she projected an aura of hostility and made it very clear that she doubted, very much, the author's qualifications, "theories" and intentions. With little hope of success, she had come with reluctance and was afraid to trust another physician and be disappointed.

Fortunately, there were several very suggestive diagnostic leads in her history and, before concluding the first visit, she was informed that her problem appeared to be similar to the difficulties experienced by other "allergic" individuals who had been helped in our office. Her hostile attitude persisted and she made some sarcastic remarks which were mildly insulting; her skepticism was not concealed by tact or good manners. It must be emphasized that such attitudes and conduct may be cerebral manifestations of neuroallergic hypersensitivity and an inexperienced physician may be the innocent recepient of unwarranted behavior of a reacting patient. One may have to resist the understandable temptation to immediately withdraw from a case when the prospective patient seems to offer no opportunity to develop the proper rapport, exhibits a lack of confidence in the consultant and openly questions his ability in addition to voicing doubts concerning his professional or personal integrity.

She became restless and stated that she could not remain in the office any longer and, as she was preparing to leave, the patient mentioned that she was going to buy a milk chocolate candy bar on her way home — and, she had to have it immediately! This was a most fortunate incident because it immediately suggested the possibility of chocolate addiction or a chronic allergic addictive sensitivity to one of the components of this confection and, it was possible that her conduct in the office might be a withdrawal phenomenon. (This reminds the author of a coffee sensitive patient who would stop her car every 10 to 15 minutes to get a cup of coffee for relief of her frequently occurring coffee withdrawal symptoms. The coffee addict never realized the significance of her past reactions to this beverage which caused immediate severe symptoms every time it was taken during each pregnancy; it was well tolerated soon after each delivery and she would drink coffee in increasing amounts and re-establish her addiction.)

The chocolate-craving patient was persuaded to remain at the office for just a few minutes in order to have a "preliminary test" in preparation for her next visit. Without informing her of the identity of the test materials or the purpose of the procedure, sublingual neutralization with chocolate extract was attempted. The first dose was 0.1cc of a 1-300,000 solution (Rinkel #6): this dose often is effective in relieving symptoms but on this occasion, and in this particular subject, the #6 solution was too strong and it acted as a provoking test for chocolate sensitivity. She experienced a sudden wave of generalized warmth which was followed by a chill: next, her speech was affected and she spoke slowly with slurring of words. She complained that her fingers were cold and she felt sleepy, dizzy and confused. A very severe headache, which she described as "sharp and horrible," localized in the frontal area: it lasted for a period of four minutes. Eight minutes after the sublingual administration of two drops of a dilute solution of chocolate extract she developed acute anxiety and depression: she was "very cold" and said that she was "fearful and anxious" and she felt "like I am going to cry."

She was given 0.1cc of 1-1, 500,000 extract by the sublingual route and, within a few minutes all of the test-induced symptoms had disappeared and she no longer craved chocolate. Twenty minutes after her sublingual neutralization, there was a notable change in her personality: all of us were very pleased to see her smiling for the first time and she was amazed to actually feel "cheerful." At the conclusion of this visit she was told that there had been a test and treatment for chocolate sensitivity and this confection was prohibited henceforth. With optimism, she was informed that her condition was the type of disorder that should be carefully studied for other evidence of reversible sensitivity to dietary factors she could eliminate or be treated for.

Some critical readers may conclude that the aforementioned reactions to chocolate were psychological in origin and suggest that we are concerned with a hopeful and strongly motivated patient who was extremely suggestible and unstable. Furthermore, it might be argued that she had been profoundly influenced by the positive attitude and expectations of the ecologist and his technician even though the test had been conducted with unidentified materials. Some colleagues have taken this situation and attitude even one step further and credit the author's success in such cases to some imagined qualities of personality which appear to approach the achievements of animal magnetism. Being absolùtely void of such highly desirable clinical assets, the author modestly, with humility, reluctantly denies any claims to such attributes and acknowledges his indebtedness to his co-workers in clinical ecology whose work he has pursued with vigor and diligence.

There is no doubt that this patient was desperately searching for help and this was a new approach to her difficulties by a physician who was interested in symptoms like the ones she had complained of for years. In addition, she had never accepted the opinions of her other professional consultants who had concluded that her symptoms were of psychic and/or social causation and, at last, was being seen by a doctor whose beliefs in externally caused "allergies" were acceptable to her. One could say that she had deeply rooted problems of an emotional nature and suppressed their surfacing because she was not able to face the trauma of dealing with the unpleasant emotions that a confrontation would release. The complaints she had, it would be argued, were far less dangerous to her than the violence and pain that was locked up in her subconscious mind and were periodically released in the form of physical and mental symptoms. A protective mechanism was, supposedly, shielding her from the discomfort of recalling past emotional trauma which, it was alleged, had an enormous effect on her emotional development and was responsible for her present difficulties.

The above explanations of her initial tests with chocolate extracts are completely wrong as shown by subsequent developments in this case. Currently accepted psychiatric interpretations of her original symptoms and her test responses are interesting, but clinically harmful, speculations that can serve no useful purpose. An extraordinary clinical success was accomplished within a few months as the etiologic agents in this case were painstakingly identified and subsequently eliminated or controlled.

First, it must be mentioned that the chocolate sensitivity test was repeated as an unknown to both the author and the patient; a technician performed this test and did not indicate that it was being carried on at the time. Concentrated (stock) extract of chocolate (provided by Hollister-Stier Laboratories for this study) was given subcutaneously without the patient seeing the color of the contents of the syringe. Sublingual testing was avoided because the foods can be identified at times when the concentrated extracts reach the taste buds. 0.2cc of this material in a 1-10 dilution as supplied by the manufacturing chemist was rapidly effective in provoking a reaction; she developed a familiar "arthritis pain" in her right elbow, had nasal itching and began to yawn. This was followed by fatigue and depression. She said, "I'm too tired to feel anything." Shortly thereafter, looking quite weary, she stated that she had begun to feel "very angry and nasty". When this reaction to chocolate is compared to her previous response, it will be noted that the test-evoked symptoms were not identical each time the procedure was carried out but the essential feature of each reaction was demonstrated to be an emotional response — ecologic mental illness due to a common ingestant that she frequently craved. The strength of the provoking doses was different, 1-300,000 the first time and 1-10 the second time, and she had not eaten any chocolate since her first visit. In addition, she had many allergic food sensitivities whose combined effects would vary from day to day and have important effects on the overall state of her reactive nervous system shock tissues.

Testing revealed dust and mold allergy, food sensitivity and chemical susceptibility. It is not possible to report all of her reactions to provocative testing in this paper and only a few will be briefly given.

CORN — sore throat, brief sharp pains in the mid-sternal area, aching in the left elbow and fingers of the left hand, frontal headache, intermittent LLQ abdominal pain: unable to concentrate, visual difficulty, "irritable and miserable", unable to stop crying; gall bladder attack and urinary urgency and frequency.

Comment: There are acute non-surgical allergic gall bladder attacks which are not often recognized although patients are often advised to avoid certain foods because of their fat content. If the particular individual happens to be allergic to pork or eggs or milk, etc., the avoidance will be beneficial. It is well known that some patients who have had their gall bladders removed will continue to have attacks; this is due to allergic effects on the remaining structures. Foods that cause spasm of the duct will be responsible for postoperative colic in the RUQ; the allergens must be identified and eliminated. The author has cleared up a number of chronic urinary bladder problems that were the result of allergic hypersensitivity to foods; the cases were previously diagnosed as infections and had been frequently treated with anti-infectious medications and studied by x-ray and endoscopy without benefit. Many individuals have experienced urgency and frequency as a response to provocative tests and this includes a woman who was told that she had an "immature bladder"; periodic non-infectious urgency and frequency is often misdiagnosed as a psychosomatic disorder.

EGG — lacrimation, nasal itching, coughing, shooting and burning pains in the left upper extremity, generalized itching; nausea, yawning, fatigue, detached and indifferent to her surroundings.

LEMON — confused, unable to concentrate, visual blurring, very tired, depressed, headache.

PEA — "miserable in general", tired, unable to concentrate, lacrimation.

ALTERNARIA — unable to concentrate, had to squint to see reading material clearly, itching scalp, postnasal discharge.

FUSARIUM — fatigue, coughing, postnasal drip.

HORMODENDRUM — mood swings, depressed, itching eyes, desire to sneeze.

HOUSE DUST (Endo Laboratories) — visual blurring, brief

period of mental confusion, appeared to be dazed, felt that she was becoming numb, brief sharp headache, foreign body sensation in eyes; found it necessary to close her eyes because the light in the room was "blinding." The foreign body sensation felt like tickling and usually precedes her episodes of extreme photophobia. The test was performed with 0.1cc of a 1-4000 solution which was given sublingually. Reaction subsided in 15 minutes.

TOBACCO SMOKE (Direct exposure) — Shortly after guests in her home begin to smoke she immediately becomes very tired. With effort she can remain awake but she is mentally sluggish and is "not herself for about a week" after each exposure. During this time she feels detached from her family. She is vaguely uncomfortable when she picks up and cleans ash trays and she is very much aware of the odor present. She avoids smoke exposures whenever possible but when she is in a smoke containing environment she experiences a craving to smoke.

Her case report ends with quotations from a letter she wrote to her internist who kindly forwarded a copy to this office. ". . . for the first time in my life I am coping with daily problems beautifully. I have not had one crying spell for the past five weeks which is a miracle. . . . I am not taking any tranquilizers and feel no need for them. . . . I do not feel tense. . . . I am now using a rotating diet, eliminating the foods I know bother me. The only time I now experience discomfort is when I go off the diet. . . . I can only say that I have never felt better in my life and my husband is raving about the new me and how well I function. . . . I have had remarkable changes in my personality as well as physically . . ."

23
Maladaptive Reactions to Frequently Used Foods and Commonly Met Chemicals as Precipitating Factors in Many Chronic Physical and Chronic Emotional Illnesses

WILLIAM H. PHILPOTT

INTRODUCTION

As man scientifically examined his environment, he began to discover sources of environmentally produced illness. From this ecologically oriented information the areas of bacteriology, virology, toxicology, and so forth, developed many useful public health measures and effective medical treatments. The specialty of allergy came from the findings of these ecological discoveries. Before these ecological values had been fully integrated into a medical practice, a competitor was developing which was body-centered. A particular representative of this viewpoint is pharmacology. In this body-centered orientation, the physician does something to the patient which favorably alters the state of illness from within, rather than keeping something from the patient such as a toxin, an infectious agent, or an allergen which favorably influences the course of the disease. So today medicine has its aspirin for fever, tranquilizers for nervousness, antidepressants for depression, antibiotics for infections and even adrenal cortical hormones and histamines for allergies, numerous headache agents, and so forth.

At this stage of medicine, there is rightfully occurring a challenge as to which is most important – the information coming from ecological sources or the body-centered sources. The question is being asked: what is the most useful, the most efficient, and in what combinations should we use these two systems. The promise of quick relief of symptoms has tended to overshadow overall efficiency of methodology. To wit, the large number of headache remedies modern medicine has invented. Sometimes the allergic headache may leave quickly with such a medicine, while it would take a four-day fast and several days of meals of individual foods to discover the incriminated food. So the cause of the headache never gets discovered, and the disastrous consequences of long-term allergy goes on, blossoming into chronic physical and mental disease. So our promise of relief of a headache in five minutes ends up reducing our efficiency of diagnosis and treatment and leads to chronic illness; whereas, the ecologically oriented system would have solved our problem of headache and chronic illness. The specialty of allergy takes its cues from the overwhelming, ever-increasing promises coming from the anthropocentric information. Any field of medicine we mention is only partially making use of the possibilities of ecologic diagnosis and treatment. Typically, it is thought of last, if at all, even though it is the greatest of all masqueraders [1, 2].

The first allergic reaction described was anaphylactic shock in 1902 [3], which involved among other things a reaction of the central nervous system. Here and there through the years allergists or neurologists observed allergic and allergic-like reactions occurring to the central nervous system. These observations never materially influenced the specialties of neurology and psychiatry. The specialty of psychiatry has done many anthropocentric things to the nervous system, such as shocking it, tranquilizing it, giving it antidepressants, feeding it nutrients. One useful ecologically oriented viewpoint which we can now from our vantage point see has been overrated, and that is how one person influences another. Now, psychiatry is in the dilemma of being warned about the side effects of its tranquilizers and antidepressants and left with a load of patients in a poorly functioning, tranquilized state, all of which have helped little in discovering the cause of the illness. It is time for a reassessment. This paper is an attempt at such a reassessment.

Methodology

With increasing insistence, allergists are telling us they have much to offer the practice of medicine in general and the central nervous system reactions in particular [4, 15]. They also tell us the field of allergy is larger than the immunologists have cut out for it [16]. There are many maladaptive, allergic-like reactions not manifesting antibody formation and, therefore, not fitting the immunologists' definition of allergy. Clinical ecology is a more inclusive term and would include all maladaptive reactions occurring on exposure to a substance, whether this be (a) allergic with antibody formation, (b) idiosyncratic-toxic in which small amounts of toxins not affecting the majority produce toxic reactions in these susceptible persons and (c) deficiency-type reactions which include nutritional deficiencies and metabolic errors.

To test these claims I set up an experiment in which the patient was fasted for four days and fed his commonly used foods by single meals, while observing for mental changes occurring during the fast and during the exposure to test meals. This was supplemented by a less effective method of sublingually placed extracts of foods and chemicals. I participated in a double-blind study on the sublingual method of testing [17].

Test Observations

1. Sixty four percent of schizophrenics manifested symptom formation on exposure to wheat (hard data on 53 schizophrenic patients).

2. Fifty one percent of schizophrenics manifested symptom formation on exposure to mature corn products (hard data on 51 schizophrenic patients).

3. Fifty percent of schizophrenics manifested symptom formation on exposure to pasteurized whole cow's milk (hard data on 56 schizophrenic patients).

4. About 75 percent manifested symptom formation to tobacco, mostly minor symptoms such as dizziness, nausea, headache, blurred vision, and so forth. However, 10 percent of the schizophrenics became grossly psychotic on exposure to tobacco. A paranoid reaction is the most common type of reaction in tobacco psychosis. The tobacco psychotics also developed psychosis on exposure to several other items.

5. About 30 percent of schizophrenics developed symptoms on exposure to petrochemical hydrocarbons such as found in petroleum products and the combustion of such products. Some reactions were so severe as to precipitate suicidal attempts, and in others delusions developed. Marked weakness was common.

6. There was an average of ten items reacted to with symptom formation in schizophrenics.

7. Over 92 percent of schizophrenics reacted with symptom formation (hard data on 53 patients).

8. The symptoms ranged from minor central nervous system symptoms such as weakness, dizziness, blurred vision, anxiety, depression, and gross psychotic symptoms such as catatonia, dissociation, paranoid delusions, visual and auditory hallucinations, and so forth. There likely is no schizophrenic symptom that has been described in the literature that was left out of the 150 patients tested. Gross psychotic symptoms occurred in a high percentage. Wheat was the most common evoker of paranoid reactions.

9. Symptoms of schizophrenia commonly occur as withdrawal phase symptoms of food addiction. These food addictions are to the patient's favorite foods, which are frequently eaten for partial and temporary relief of symptoms. A four-day fast interrupts the state of addiction, and when exposed on the fifth day or therabouts, there is manifested an allergic or similar maladaptive response occurring within minutes. Thus, the former delayed reaction (withdrawal phase reaction) now can be read as an immediate reaction, thus providing convincing evidence of the relationship between the food and symptoms.

10. Each symptom can have, and often does have, multiple-evoking causes. A symptom can have several foods, chemicals or inhalants that evoke the same symptom, and also there can be an assortment of conflictual, interpersonal or cued situations that evoke the same symptom. All such symptom-evoking causes need to be determined and treated simultaneously.

11. Some responses relate to neurological symptoms unrelated to learned responses, while a majority give evidence of facilitating existing learned responses. A patient may hate a parent for a real or fancied mistreatment which usually does not grossly interfere with his social function. Under the facilitating effect of this learned response provided by central nervous system allergic (or similar maladaptive) reaction, this can be activated into a socially paralyzing response of psychotic proportions.

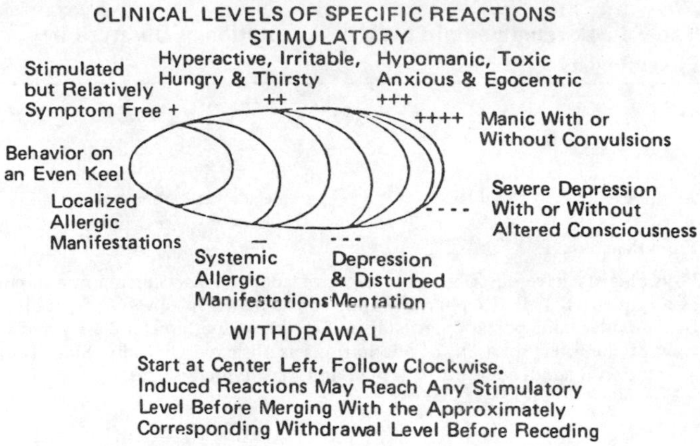

CLINICAL LEVELS OF SPECIFIC REACTIONS

Fig. 1

12. There evidently are multiple causes for these maladaptive responses such as immunological, metabolic inborn error, nutritional deficiency, toxic, and so forth. Some patients could be returned to the foods without symptom formation after a period of nutritional supplementation based on findings of deficiency on a chemical survey of vitamins and minerals, while others could only return to a four-day rotation of the symptom-producing foods. If such a patient ate these foods even two days in a row, symptoms would develop. Dohan found 21 percent of schizophrenics to have antibodies to wheat gliadin [18, 19]. In our series 64 percent reacted to wheat. Twenty-one percent of these with reactions can be accepted as explainable on an immunilogical basis, while 43 percent likely have other than immunilogical causes. There needs to be a biochemical investigation into the causes of these non-immunological reactions.

Physical reactions were being equally observed with that of emotional reactions. The physical reactions were numerous, and such as headache, dizziness, unsteadiness, inability to read or write, numbness, neuritis, myalgia, arthralgia, tension, weakness, sleepiness, insomnia, tachycardia, bradycardia, gastritis, diarrhea, colitis, constipation, hypertension, hypotension, hyperglycemia, hypoglycemia, itching, hives, psoriasis, seborrhea, and many, many others.

These chronic physical and mental illnesses were observed to fade in intensity and often even completely disappear on a four-day fast, and emerge as acute reactions on exposure to test meals to foods, provocative food tests, and provocative chemical tests. With each case studied one is impressed with the evidence of having performed a truly scientific experiment of turning off an illness and knowing why, and turning on the illness and again knowing why because of the controlled conditions under which the study is being done and again turning off the illness and maintaining the symptom-free state and knowing why. These test results tell us much good will come from avoidance of these incriminated substances, and so it does. The values of avoidance are superior, more sure, and more lasting than a pain relieving pill, an adrenal cortical supportive or replacing hormone, or a host of other anthropocentric remedies.

DIAGNOSIS AND TREATMENT OF FOOD ADDICTION

This statement is made for (a) those who have undergone an ecological diagnosis in an environmental control unit by a physician, and who are ready to continue the process of diagnosis and

Table 1. Developmental Levels of Adaptation as Observed by Physiologists

Stage I.		Stage II.		Stage III.
Preadaptive		Adapted		Postadapted
(Nonadapted)	II. a		II. b	(Nonadapted)
Alarm reaction	Adapted		Maladapted	Stage of exhaustion

From Randolph.

Physiologists have described the stages of adaptation occurring in animals as a sequential I, II, III phenomenon, consisting, respectively, of preadaptive, adapted and postadapted stages. For the sake of greater clarity and in view of the interpretations of adaptations as observed clinically, Stage II of adaptation is subdivided into adapted and maladapted phases.

treatment at home; (b) those who, under the supervision of a physician, will do the ecological diagnosis and treatment in the home environment; (c) those who wish to make a self-diagnosis and treatment in the home environment.

Diagnosing and treating food addiction is not always an easy job. Some lose their motivation to try or to stay by the task until the job is satisfactorily completed. Some are discouraged or lose their judgment with the emergence of symptoms during the first two days of the fast. Others have such severe reactions during the testing as to have an interference with judgment and, therefore, abandon the program. After the diagnosis of food addiction has been made, there still is the tendency to return to the addictive substance, since it has been used for so long as a favorite reliever of symptoms.

Sources of Food Addiction

Rinkel, Randolph and Zeller [20] observed what they called "masked food sensitization." The various stages of sensitization and tolerance of foods to which the subject was allergic were worked out. The value of a four-day fast with food testing starting on the fifth day was described. Later, Randolph, [21, 22] observing the relieving aspect of frequently eaten foods to which maladaptive reactions were made, called this "food addiction." Addiction has been defined as relating to substances frequently used for relief (or partial relief) of symptoms, while the same substances produce symptoms on withdrawal of the substance. Many food reactions clearly fit this definition of addiction, the same as tobacco, alcohol or narcotic addiction does.

Maladaptive reactions to foods can be caused by (a) addiction caused by food and chemical allergies with typical antibody reaction and nutritional deficiencies; (b) metabolic errors such as phenylketonuria [23], galactosemia, lactase deficiency and vitamin dependent states. A few metabolic errors have been clearly understood, but it is suspected there are many yet to be discovered. In the metabolic error reactions there is lacking the addictive quality of relief when the substance is contacted, but rather there is an immediate production of symptoms; (c) idiosyncratic toxic reactions such as reactions to chlorine, fluorine, food additives, food coloring, insecticide residues — all of these occurring at levels below that which causes reactions in the majority of people. In any event there is a common denominator in all of these reactions (allergic, deficiency, metabolic error and toxic), and that is that symptoms are reduced by avoidance of these specific incriminated substances.

Reverting Addictions to Immediate Maladaptive Reactions

A four-day (or sometimes up to six) abstinence from food to which a person is addicted reverts the addictive state to that of immediate symptom production rather than the delayed addictive withdrawal symptoms. This is best achieved by a four-day fast. It can also be achieved if foods to which the person is not maladaptively reacting are used during this four-day pretest period. When the testing produces symptoms then all possible causes for symptoms must be considered, such as: allergic; nutritional deficiency; metabolic error; or idiosyncratic toxic reaction. The reaction on a test does not in itself tell us the cause of the reaction.

Comprehensive Environmental Control [24]

The purpose of environmental control is to isolate the person from all substances to which he may be reacting. There will include feeding of foods, fumes, animals, cosmetics, hair conditioners, and so forth. Homes are notoriously filled with fumes from such as gas stoves, hot air oil- or gas-fired furnaces, spray fresheners, moth balls, and so forth. It is easier to arrange for an adequate environmental control in a hospital setting where such a unit has been especially set up, and in some cases this is an absolute necessity. If during the fourth or fifth day of the fast the pulse still remains high or there still remains ongoing common symptoms, then it is likely due to a lack of proper environmental control, and in this case the environment must be reexamined to

Table 2. Stages of Specific Adaptation in the Presence of Individual Susceptibility as Observed by Clinicians

Stage I.		Stage II.		Stage III.
Nonaddicted		Addicted		Nonaddicted
(Nonadapted)	II. a		II. b	(Nonadapted)
Test reaction	Adapted		Maladapted	Stage of exhaustion
(Alarm reaction)				
Clinically, this is employed diagnostically		Onset of the present illness		Clinically, this is more often approached than actually reached
Acute postexposure effects from intermitten exposure	Relatively symptom-free		Chronic manifestations	Acute postexposure effects from cumulative exposures

Physicians do not ordinarily have the opportunity to observe the sequential development of adaptation as described by physiologists and as outlined in Figure 1.

Instead, their patients are already adapting (see Stage II.a) or, more commonly, maladapting (see Stage II.b) to nonidentified material(s) when first seeking medical advice. The point is, this transition between State II.a and II.b, when the reacting individual is no longer able to maintain his accustomed stimulatory responses by dint of his own routines and relatively uncontrolled withdrawals predominate, is usually regarded by all concerned as the "onset of the present illness."

In clinical medicine, especially when dealing with responses to specific foods, the nonaddicted Stage III or stage of exhaustion is more apt to be approached than actually reached. A common exception to this statement occurs in advanced stages of alcoholism when each drink of alcoholic beverage is followed by an immediate acute and severe reaction.

Reversion to nonaddicted Stage I or test reaction (also referred to by some physiologists as the alarm reaction) may occur either accidentally or by design, as a result of (a) avoidance of specific exposure(s) until recovery from the effects of the last amount of the same substance has subsided or (b) result of a massive dose which breaks through adapting or maladapting responses. In either instance, it is characterized by an acute immediate and convincing test response. Its deliberate induction is employed diagnostically to demonstrate specific etiology.

see if there is some agent to which the person is reacting, and the fast continues for another two or three days until the major symptoms have subsided. Especially the pulse should be normal, that is, below 85, before testing begins.

Considerations During a Four-day Fast

During the first two to three days of a fast, symptoms often emerge due to the fact of passing through the addictive withdrawal phase of symptom production. This emergence of symptoms is not due to a starving need for nutrients, but to the withdrawal phase symptoms of an addiction. A person without food addictions will not have an emergence of symptoms on a fast. Usually by the fourth day of the fast, symptoms have materially subsided, or even disappeared. If symptoms have not subsided by the fourth day of the fast, then the fast should be extended one, two, or three more days to see if symptoms will further subside. If there is not adequate environmental control, symptoms may continue because of the exposure to a substance to which the person is reacting. In some cases, such as a chronic paranoid state, symptoms may not subside while on a brief fast. This appears to be due to the severity of the chronic reaction to foods. Some severe and long depressive states also will not clear on a fast, which again is apparently an indication of the severity of the reaction that has been occurring to foods.

The following should be considered:

1. Asthmatics. On withdrawal of food, as well as reentry of foods as test meals, asthmatic attacks can be evoked in susceptible persons.
2. Epileptics. On withdrawal of foods, as well as test meals of foods, seizures may occur.
3. Diabetics on insulin.
4. A markedly debilitated state.

The cases of asthmatics, epileptics, diabetics on insulin, and markedly debilitated cases should be tested and treated under direct medical supervision. Emotional reactions in food-sensitive persons during the fast and also during the food testing can range from mild reactions such as tension, fatigue, headache, dizziness, and so forth, to marked psychotic and insightless states involving depression with a wish to die, hallucinations, delusions and illogical aggression. When fasting and testing an emotionally disturbed person, an objective observer needs to be available so that medical emergency help can be obtained if indicated. It helps to realize that the symptoms occurring during the food testing are likely to subside in one, two or three hours, although in some cases it may be as much as five hours. In rare instances, severe reactions may last up to three days. In these more severe, prolonged reactions, medical assistance is indicated to stop the reaction. However, this can be done by simply waiting until the symptoms subside before proceeding with further testing. Characteristically, symptoms will subside, and three to four test meals a day can be used.

Method of Four- to Six-day Fast

Water not chemically treated, such as spring, well or filtered water, is used since some people are known to react to chlorine and/or fluorine. There is to be no smoking during the fast days or the subsequent test days. If symptom-free by the fourth day of the fast, tobacco can be tested if desired. This is achieved by chain smoking as fast as possible a maximum of six cigarettes. The test ends as soon as symptoms develop. Dizziness, nausea and weakness are common minor symptoms of tobacco allergy, but in a few (about 10 percent of schizophrenics) frank psychosis develops, especially of a paranoid type, including delusions and hallucinations. After the tobacco test, it may be necessary in severely reacting cases to continue the fast another day or two or three for symptoms to clear. There is the danger during the tobacco test of judgment being affected and, therefore, the program being abandoned. If the person will agree to stop smoking without such a test, this is the better plan. But if he has to be convinced that he is tobacco-allergic, then do the test. Many people will remember the symptoms that developed when they smoked their first cigarette. When they are informed that this is evidence of allergy to tobacco, it is sufficiently convincing for many people to stop smoking.

Four days on a fast is not enough for symptoms to clear in some cases. In these cases, the fast can be extended up to seven days. In some chronically depressed and some severely paranoid patients, symptoms will not clear even on a seven-day fast. If this occurs it is an indication that they need special help from a psychiatrist to receive treatment which will stimulate a return of function. This may need to occur even before definitive food testing can be done or completed. These are characteristically found to be highly reactive to a number of substances. The evidence would indicate that the reaction has been so severe and so prolonged that the fast alone does not produce a chemical rebound to normal and that this reinstatement of normal chemical function can only occur due to stimulation of the brain.

Four Days Off Food Without a Fast

This is a less desirable method than a fast, but since some will prefer it, it is described. The foods used during these four days before food testing must of necessity be foods to which the person is not maladaptively reacting. These nonmaladaptive foods will be foods that are rarely eaten by that person. A fruit, vegetable, meat, fish, or nut should all be tested beforehand. Be sure this food has not been eaten for more than a week before using it as a single meal taken between meals, such as 11 A.M., 3 P.M. or 8 P.M. If no symptoms develop within a two hour period, then you may assume that no maladaptive reaction exists. These foods are tested as single meals. Unfortunately, some of these foods turn out to be maladaptive reactors after they have been loaded for the four days. This is why the fast is the best method.

Another method is to drink all you want of alfalfa or comfrey tea during the four-day period, if found not to be maladaptively reacting on the test dose. Vitamin C powder one to two teaspoons (4 gm per teaspoon) plus baking soda (½ baking soda to vitamin C powder) three times per day can be used for symptom reduction. Rarely, a patient highly sensitive to corn will react to vitamin C due to a corn residual in the vitamin C, this having been manufactured through enzymatic action on corn sugar.

Selection of Foods for Testing

If a person maladaptively reacts to a food when occasionally eaten he is aware of this, and for this reason does not like this food. Such reactions to infrequently eaten foods are rare and obviously are not producing the chronic addictive state. A food has to be eaten two or more times a week to be addicting. The more frequently a food is eaten, the more likely it is to be incriminated in addiction. Even though a food is infrequently eaten it may belong to a family, a member of which is frequently eaten, such as legumes, squash-melon-cucumber, dairy products, gluten-bearing cereal grains such as wheat-rye-oats-barley-corn, and so forth. One member of a family eaten frequently sometimes predisposes a person to maladaptive reactions to other members of the same family, even if infrequently eaten.

A choice has to be made as to the types of food to be tested: (a) foods grown without insecticides, (b) market-grown foods which will contain insecticide residues, (c) raw foods, (d) cooked foods and (e) foods with preservatives and colors added. Theoretically, each of these categories needs to be tested separately. Sometimes, a raw food can be eaten when it cannot be eaten cooked, or vice versa. Sometimes, foods without spray residues can be eaten without a reaction. Sometimes, there are reactions to food colors and food preservatives. The most practical way is to start with the foods as usually eaten, which are market-grown fruits, vegetables and meats, and the food eaten in the usual form, such as either cooked or raw. Definitive testing can then be done on those foods in which reactions occur. Colors and preservatives are left out of the initial food testing.

Food and Symptom Diary

Give the day and the exact time of each item listed in the diary.

Describe all symptoms occurring during the night.

Describe any physical or mental symptoms occurring upon arising in the morning.

List each food and approximate amount eaten for breakfast.

Between breakfast and noon, list and record the time of appearance of any symptoms that occur, and record the time and amounts of any snacks that may be eaten, drinks or smokes.

List the noon meal.

List any symptoms or snacks, smokes, etc., between the noon meal and the evening meal.

List all foods eaten at the evening meal.

After the evening meal until bedtime, list all symptoms, snacks, smokes, and so forth.

Also during the day, note any undue exposure to dusts, pets, molds, pollens, chemical fumes or odors. Also list where you went, what you did, anything that agreed with you, made you feel good or better, anything that upset you or made you ill or worse, etc.

A food-symptom diary is kept a week or two before the fast begins. A symptom dairy is kept during the fast days. Symptoms usually emerge during the first three days and subside on the fourth day of the fast. Continue the fast during and after the test meals.

Methods of Deliberate Food Testing

Foods can be accurately tested for 10 days with a maximum of 12 days after the fast, after which a refractory reactive state may set in for some foods.

Each meal is a single food, raw, boiled, or baked, with nothing other than pure salt (preferably sea salt) added. Any water used in cooking should be the same water that is not chemically treated as used during the fast and as being used during the test days. Usually four test meals a day can be done by arranging an 8:30 P.M. meal (usually fruit). It is best that the first day of food testing be foods not suspected as maladaptive reactors. These are foods that are eaten no more than twice a week. When starting to test one member of the family it is preferable to test all members of that family consecutively, or another possible method is to wait four days between members of the family for testing.

On the morning of the second day of testing, start with the cereal grain family and proceed consecutively with wheat, mature corn, fresh corn, oats and rice. Wheat is tested as cooked Ralston, salted to taste, with two or more bowls initially and, if no reaction, another bowl at one hour. Wheat continues to be tested until there is evidence of a reaction even if it takes four meals a day for three days. This testing is done this way due to the poor absorption rate of wheat. Sometimes, the more severe reactions occur on the second or third day after the intestinal mucosa has been injured by the initial test meals. If it is necessary to continue the wheat testing more than the one meal, then other forms of wheat could be used for variety such as puffed wheat, Cream of Wheat, or Shredded Wheat biscuit. Mature corn is tested as corn meal mush with dark Karo syrup, salted to taste. Two or more bowls of corn meal mush with Karo syrup are given, and if there is no reaction, another bowl in one hour. If there is no reaction then eat a second test meal of mature corn. Oats is tested as two or more bowls of oatmeal, salted to taste, with another bowl in one hour if no reaction occurs. Only one test meal of oats is necessary. Rice is tested as cooked rice, salted to taste, with two bowls or more as the test meal, and if no reaction one bowl in one hour. Rice is tested as one meal. Rye is not tested simply because it is so much like wheat. Also, wheat and rye are always mixed grains as they come from the fields. Wheat is permitted to have 10 percent rye. Rye also contains wheat. These grains grow together and are not entirely separated as they grow in the fields. Therefore, if there is a reaction to wheat, it is assumed there is a reaction to rye. Besides, there is no way for these to be separated in the processing of foods. Barley is a grain very closely related to wheat and rye and is not usually tested unless there is a particular reason that this person has been using the barley, such as an alcoholic drink or food substance containing barley. It is assumed that if wheat and rye are reactive, so is barley. Barley can be tested by cooking the grains into a cereal. Rice is not gluten-bearing; therefore, there are less reactions to rice than gluten-bearing cereal grains. However, there are common molds on all of the cereal grains, and for this reason there may be a reaction to all of the cereal grains.

Dairy products are then introduced by starting with pasteurized cow's milk. It is preferred to obtain this in glass containers rather than either plastic or wax-corn cartons, since there may be a reaction to the wax-corn plastic. However, this is not always possible, and the milk is therefore tested in the container from which it usually comes. Two glasses or more of milk are given at the beginning of the test meal and if no reaction another glass at one hour. A second test of dairy products is powdered skim milk. There are two or more glasses of powdered skim milk to begin with, and if no symptoms, another glass or two in one hour. Then cheeses are tested. Usually, American cheese and cheddar cheese are given separate test meals. If there are other cheeses that are used commonly, then they also are given a separate test meal. In testing cheese, the person eats all he wants. Each dairy product is tested separately simply because the processing makes a difference in whether reactions will occur or not. The molds on the cheese can determine whether there is a reaction to a particular cheese or not. If cottage cheese is tested, it should be tested as dry cottage cheese without cream unless it has already been demonstrated that there was no reaction to pasteurized cow's milk or powdered skim milk. Then it could be tested with the cream present. If buttermilk is used, it should be given a separate test. It is often true that cow's butter can be used when pasteurized cow's milk or powdered skim milk or the cheeses are reactive. This can be determined by a separate test, but often the testing is not done and the butter is introduced into the diet later when the testing is over. In this way, it is determined if there is a reaction to butter.

Dairy products deserve some special mention. There are many people who were known to be reactive to milk as infants and children but who in later years are using milk and assume they have outgrown their allergic reaction to milk. This usually proves to be a mistake, and they are now highly reactive and addicted to dairy products. Dairy products pose three problems: allergic and allergic-like reactions; galactosemic reactions in those in which galactosemia has been demonstrated to be present, which is one out of five of schizophrenics; lactase deficiency, which is reportedly 70 percent in blacks and 10 percent in whites. Those with gastrointestinal cereal grain reactions run very high in lactase deficiency because of the damage that has occurred to the upper intestinal tract. The classic reaction occurring on a deliberate food test of dairy products due to lactase deficiency is gastrointestinal pain, diarrhea and anxiety attacks occurring at about one to two hours. The anxiety attack occurs because in the face of low lactase, lactose ferments, producing lactic acid, which is absorbed into the blood, the flood of lactic acid tying up calcium and magnesium. All dairy products other than cheddar cheese contain lactose. The amount of galactose in butter is negligible. In cheeses and yogurt it is concentrated. Galactosemia is a condition in which the liver sometimes on an inherited basis, at other times on a developmental basis, is unable to adequately change galactose (a relatively nonuseable and if in high enough amount, toxic, sugar) into glucose. The first step in the metabolism of lactose is to split lactose into glucose and galactose. The second step must change the galactose into glucose. Therefore, galactosemic subjects should not use milk as a beverage or cheeses other than cheddar cheese. If the subject is not otherwise reactive to cheddar cheese, it is a suitable food for the galactosemic.

Meats, fish, vegetables and fruits can usually be adequately determined on a one-test-meal basis. Fruits are usually placed in the 8:00 to 8:30 evening meal.

If on introducing a supposedly test-compatible food into the diet there is a suspicion of a reaction, then this food should be submitted to a retest. The second test should follow this sequence:

While using test compatible foods, introduce into this diet a food to be tested or a suspected reactive food, taking this food three times a day. If within the three days or less there is a reaction, then it is known that this food is maladaptive. However, if there is no reaction, then this food can continue to be eaten a minimum of once a day along with the other test-compatible foods, and another food introduced on a three-times-a-day basis. Do this until all of the foods have been added into the diet and eaten for at least a week before going on a fast, and then retesting by single meals all the foods that have not been known to be producing a reaction.

Adaptive Food Schedule

The goal is to avoid maladaptive food reactions and avoid the development of food addictions. The principle is to avoid the demonstrated maladaptive foods until the refractory phase develops after a few days, weeks or months. The refractory phase begins at about three weeks and is usually well established in three months of complete avoidance. These maladaptive reactive foods can then be introduced on a once-in-four-day basis. If this is satisfactory over a period of time, then try on a twice-in-four-day basis, always eating the two meals consecutively, such as twice on the fourth day of a four-day rotation. Some can do this without symptoms occurring, and others cannot, or it may apply to one food and not another. A food-symptom diary should be kept at all times so that maladaptive reactions can be spotted and related to the foods being eaten.

A problem of addiction sometimes develops in frequently eaten foods, even though these foods were test-normal on the original testing. The stress of frequently eating the food creates this addictive state. If and when this happens, then these foods are removed for a period of time before again reintroducing them, this time once or twice on a four-day rotation basis.

The most reliable method is a diversified rotation diet, eating the food once or twice on the fourth day of a four-day rotation of foods. This involves all foods eaten in family groups in which there has been a reaction. The entire family of foods is kept on the four-day rotation basis. One member of the family is eaten on the fourth day of the rotation; that is, other members of the family cannot be eaten on other days of the rotation than on the fourth day. If one chooses, several members of the same family can be eaten at the same meal, or if on the two-meal rotation, twice on the fourth day of the rotation, if eaten consecutively.

No food addictions will develop on a four-day rotation basis. On this program of necessity there will be a wide assortment of foods eaten. This is useful because this wide assortment of foods provides a more adequate intake of nutrients than a smaller number of foods would provide.

Provocative Food Testing

This can only be performed under medical supervision. Two methods are to inject an aqueous extract of a food sufficiently deep into the skin so as to be circulated by blood to all tissues of the body and to place drops of varied dilutions of aqueous food extracts under the tongue for quick absorption by the mucous membrane of the mouth, providing for quick absorption with the bloodstream carrying the extract to all tissues of the body. These extracts are in serial dilution, and the person need not be exposed to any greater amount than causes the minimal evidence of reaction. These food extracts have the disadvantage of being aqueous in source, and therefore not carrying all of the qualities of reaction of a complete test food. There is an estimated 80 percent value of comparison between deliberate food tests and provocative food tests.

Provocative Testing of Chemicals

Extracts of chemicals are prepared for sublingual testing the same as in provocative food testing. Cat, dog, dust, molds, pollens, trees, and so forth, can be tested by this method.

Sniff Test

Some items are best tested by a sniff test, such as magic marker. Many items can be tested this way, such as cats, dogs, dust, pollens, and so forth.

Home Testing of Chemicals

Food colors can be tested by placing certified food coloring in a glass of water and taking this as a test meal. The following colors should be tested: red, yellow, blue. Green need not be tested because it is a combination of yellow and blue, and if the person reacts to either yellow or blue, he will react to green. Pets such as cats, dogs, and so forth can be held close to the nose for sniff testing for three to five minutes. Dust can be determined by vacuuming the house and seeing if there is a reaction during the process. A gas stove can be tested by lighting the burners and being near the stove for five or more minutes. This often is determined by the fact that symptoms develop during the preparation of a meal while cooking over a gas stove. It must also be considered that fumes from the food being cooked are also a possible cause of symptoms, and these must be differentiated. Another way to test for petrochemical hydrocarbons is to stand behind a running automobile for three to five minutes to see if symptoms develop. Candles can be sniffed, waxes sniffed, decorative kerosene lamps can be sniffed, magic markers can be sniffed. There are numerous items in any home that are manufactured from petroleum products. All these are potential hazards for the petrochemical hydrocarbon reactor. Plastics are made from hydrocarbons, and some people are known to react to foods stored in plastic containers or in plastic bags. Cosmetics and hair conditioners should be sniff tested. Clothes could be sniff tested after being bleached or the subject exposed to the laundry room during the bleaching process to determine a possible reaction to chlorine. Food preservatives and additives can be tested by introducing these foods in prepared forms after having demonstrated that the foods were test normal without the preservatives.

As near as possible all chemicals should be tested after a four-day abstinence from these contacts, the same as the foods, although these do not always carry the same addictive quality as foods because some of these are idiosyncratic toxic reactions. However, the reaction to petrochemical hydrocarbons may carry the same quality of addiction as that of foods; therefore, a period of abstinence of four days should occur before exposure. Reactions to petrochemical hydrocarbons can be just as serious as reactions to foods. Likely the most dangerous instrument in the home is the gas kitchen stove. Many people are chronically sick, either mentally or physically, due to exposure to fumes from a gas stove or a gas- or oil-fired hot air heating system. Some have been known to react seriously to fumes from a newspaper or recently printed book. This is due to the hydrocarbons in the ink. Fumes of magic markers are particularly prone to give petrochemical hydrocarbon reactions. Chap sticks have petrochemical hydrocarbon petroleum bases, as do many hair conditioners, and so forth. The entire home should be surveyed for possible chemical contacts. After demonstrating a reaction to petrochemical hydrocarbons, such as a gas stove or magic marker, waxes or paints, there is no particular reason to continue the search for reactions. It is best to remove as near as possible the petrochemical hydrocarbon contacts and keep these as minimal in amount and frequency as possible. Plastics do need to be tested separately from other petrochemical hydrocarbons simply because the more flexible plastics diffuse more easily than the hard plastics, and there is not a complete crossover between a gas stove and a pine panel door or a Christmas tree. Pine scented cleaners are particularly known for their production of serious reactions in susceptible persons.

TRAINING OUT PHOBIAS

Oft-repeated symptoms, no matter how they are evoked, even if it be because of a disturbed biology, tend to become overlearned and evoked by cues. The heightened excitement of the central nervous system occurring during the stimulatory phase of an addictive reaction to foods or chemicals drives the person to obsessive-compulsive thinking and acting. The uncomfortable withdrawal level state of the maladaptive addictive state and the continuous discomfort of the maladaptive state activate the avoidance areas of the brain. The person is uncomfortable from within and thus has uncomfortable responses to environmental stimuli. Under these circumstances, phobias train in rapidly. Correcting the biological driving forces is only part of the therapy needed, since these phobias need to be trained out after achieving the biologically normal state. This occurs either by a chance meeting of favorable life circumstances or by therapeutic design. Therapeutic design is the most efficient.

The most efficient training technique for phobias I have discovered is that of preparing the patient for the reexposure to the aversive stimuli by adrenal cortical/pituitary normalization. The treatment is suitable for all classes of patients, neurotic or psychotic, who may have phobias. It is suitable for both hospital and office practice. In the majority of cases, the time spent for training out phobias ranges from three to ten minutes per symptom. All phobias and all other symptoms are treated at the same time.

The symptoms are gathered by having the patient fill out the fear inventory [25], the Hoffer-Osmond Diagnostic Test and, if a psychologist is helping, then give a word association test and a battery of psychological tests. All symptoms of any type gathered from these sources, as well as the initial interview with the patient, are dictated onto a cassette tape (usually 30 minutes in length is sufficient). The best way to proceed is to record an interview with the patient in which a symptom is read to the patient who amplifies the significance of that symptom and thus enlarges the number of cues either evoking or relating to that particular symptom. This taped interview can be prepared by the doctor, nurse, psychologist or any professional worker assigned to the task. This is played back to the patient for an hour or more each session after he has been prepared by adrenal-pituitary normalization so that he will not make any unadaptive responses while listening to the tape. An earphone is used so that no one else can hear the taped message. The treatment proceeds with the patient lying comfortably on a bed. Several patients can be in the same room, since each is hearing his own message.

The patient is taught to judge his response to each stimulus by closing his eyes and thinking of the fear, tension, obsessional thinking, depression, and so forth, that occur when he places in his mind a particular stimulus. On the scale 0 is equated to no symptoms at all; 100 represents being overwhelmed by symptoms and responding to the stimuli, even against better judgment; 30 represents the beginning awareness of symptoms; and below 30 is increasing comfort, above 30 is increasing discomfort. The patient is asked to close his eyes and concentrate on whatever bothers him most. He is then asked to place himself on the scale, above or below 30.

Using a "butterfly," an intravenous injection is given.

1. Vitamin C diluted with 50 percent normal saline, 7.5 gm (range 4 to 10 gm). If electing to exceed 10 gm give 10 cc calcium gluconate or 10 cc Calphosan before 10 gm is exceeded. This is to prevent the symptoms of calcium deficiency which may occur beyond 10 gm of vitamin C. Have the patient restate where he is on the scale when thinking of whatever bothers him most. Vitamin C usually reduces the symptoms to about half of the original. Rarely, it is adequate to reduce the symptoms below 30. Vitamin C has an antistress and detoxifying value and reduces the use of adrenal cortical hormones to about half. Whenever the patient reaches 30 or below, the desensitization practice is ready to begin.

2. Adrenal cortical extract (standardized at 200 µg of Hydrocortisone per cc) is given. Give 10 cc intravenously, wait two to three minutes and have the patient grade himself on the scale. Keep giving 10 cc increments until the patient is below 30 on the scale. It may take 10-150 cc to achieve this goal; 30-60 cc is a common amount needed at the beginning of the therapy sessions. As the therapy sessions progress, the need subsides so that later sessions require less and you can finally go to the place where the patient lies down, relaxes, and is below 30 on the scale without medication, listening to the tape without symptom formation. You should proceed to this achievement. It usually takes five one-hour sessions but it may require up to ten one-hour sessions.

Synthetic glucocorticoids have been successfully used in the place of adrenal cortical extract without noting adrenal cortical suppressive side effects. The use of these hormones is sufficiently brief that adrenal cortical suppression is not present as observed in chronic use of glucocorticoids.

3. Additional possibilities.

A. Those deficient in calcium may need 10 cc of calcium gluconate or 10 cc of Calphosan added to the program in order to produce a symptom-free state. Consider adding this

if more than 30 cc of adrenal cortical extract is needed.

B. Some are deficient in magnesium and need magnesium sulfate 1-2 gm IV added to the program. Consider adding this if calcium has not materially reduced the symptoms.

C. If vitamin C plus adrenal cortical extract plus calcium plus magnesium has not adequately prepared the patient, then add 1000 mg of pyridoxine IV and proceed to 3000 mg if needed. In an occasional patient pyridoxine is the key to symptom reduction more than any of the other vitamins or minerals.

4. Complications.

A. Rarely, a patient has adversely reacted to vitamin C. If so, he will complain of marked burning of the veins. There are two possible reasons:

   1. Reaction to the preservatives. If this is the case, vitamin C can be purchased without preservatives, but under CO_2 pressure.

Table 3.

DIRECTIONS:	Start at zero (0) Read up for predominantly Stimulatory Levels Read down for predominantly Withdrawal Levels
++++ MANIC WITH OR WITHOUT CONVULSIONS	Distraught, excited, agitated, enraged and circuitous or one-track thoughts, muscle twitching and jerking of extremities, convulsive seizures and altered consciousness may develop.
+++ HYPOMANIC, TOXIC, ANXIOUS AND EGOCENTRIC	Aggressive, loquacious, clumsy (ataxic), anxious fearful and apprehensive; alternating chills and flushing, ravenous hunger, excessive thirst.
++ HYPERACTIVE, IRRITABLE, HUNGRY AND THIRSTY	Tense, jittery, hopped up, talkative, argumentative, sensitive, overly responsive, self-centered, hungry and thirsty, flushing, sweating and chilling may occur as well as insomnia, alcoholism, and obesity.
+ STIMULATED BUT RELATIVELY SYMPTOM-FREE (SUBCLINICAL)	Active, alert, lively, responsive and enthusiastic with unimpaired ambition, energy, initiative and wit. Considerate of the views and actions of others. This usually comes to be regarded as "normal" behavior.
0 BEHAVIOR ON AN EVEN KEEL AS IN HOMEOSTASIS	Children expect this from their parents and teachers. Parents and teachers expect this from their children. We all expect this from our associates.
LOCALIZED ALERGIC	Running or stuffy nose, clearing throat, coughing, wheezing (asthma), itching (eczema or hives), gas, diarrhea, constipation (colitis), urgency and frequency of urination and various eye and ear syndromes.
SYSTEMIC ALLERGIC MANIFESTATIONS	Tired, dopey, somnolent, mildly depressed, edematous with painful syndromes (headache, neckache, backache, neuralgia, myalgia, myositis, arthralgia, arthritis, arteritis, chest pain) and cardiovascular effects.*
DEPRESSION AND DISTURBED	Confused, indecisive, moody, sad, sullen, withdrawn or apathetic. Emotional instability and impaired attention, concentration, comprehension and thought processes (aphasia, mental lapse and blackouts).
SEVERE DEPRESSION WITH OR WITHOUT ALTERED CONSCIOUSNESS	Nonresponsive, lethargic, stuporous, disoriented, melancholic, incontinent, regressive thinking, paranoid orientations, delusions, hallucinations, sometimes amnesia and, finally, comatose.

*Marked pulse changes or skipped beats may occur at any level.

From Randolph.

2. Some corn-sensitive persons react to synthetic vitamin C, which has been manufactured from corn glucose.

B. Rarely, adrenal cortical extract has produced reactions which are allergic in nature, likely due to beef allergies, pork allergy or a response to the preservatives.

C. Rarely, a patient will complain of pyridoxine burning veins.

The therapeutic cassette tape should contain all the patient's symptoms whether phobic, obsessional, depression, delusional, hallucinations, perceptual distortions, and so forth. People learn to respond to the verbal cues of their symptoms, and therefore, these need to be desensitized. Low impact is made on obsessions and compulsions by this method unless anxiety is driving the symptom.

CONSIDERATIONS OF COMPLETENESS

Though it is beyond the scope of this presentation it should be clearly understood that these maladaptive reactions (allergic and otherwise) relate in a large way to the general physical homeostasis of the person and in a smaller way to his psychological homeostasis [26-28]. The stress of every metabolic error diagnosed should be honored (especially note galactosemia and lactase deficiency as mentioned earlier). The stress of every demonstrated nutritional deficiency and imbalance should be corrected (consider results of laboratory tests for folic acid, B_{12}, B_3, B_6 thiamine, vitamin A, essential amino acids and essential minerals). The stress of every demonstrated infection should be corrected. In the psychological realm phobias, obsessions and compulsions are trained out and new adaptive responses trained in by behavioral techniques.

It would be well if general practitioners, internists and pediatricians would employ behavior therapists such as psychologists, sociologists, psychiatric nurses, psychiatric social workers and medical assistants to work with the corrective behavioral training of their patients. The doctor has the role of diagnostician and medical therapist for organic factors underlying the illness, and the behavior therapist has the role under the doctor's supervision of training out the complications of overly learned unadaptive responses resulting from the illness. Fortunately for some, life's circumstances are sufficiently favorable so as to train out the unadaptive responses without professional help. After the correction of the biological driving effect, the symptoms are more easily

Symptoms To Look For During Testing of Foods and Chemicals

JOINTS
  Ache – Pain
  Stiff
  Swelling
  Erythema – Warmth – Redness

SKIN
  Itching Local – General
  Scratching
  Moist – Sweating
  Flushing – Hives
  Pallor – White or Ghostly

HEAD PAIN
  Headache, Mild – Moderate
  Severe Migraine
  Ache – Pressure
  Tight – Explode
  Throbbing – Stabbing

FATIGUE
  Tired
  Generalized Heaviness
  Sleepy – Yawning
  Exhausted
  Fall Asleep

GENERALIZED
  Dizzy – Lightheaded
  Imbalance – Staggering
  Vertigo – Blackout
  Going to Faint
  Chilly – Cold
  Warmth – Hot Flashes

DEPRESSED
  Withdrawn – Listless
  Vacant – Dull Facies
  Negative – Indifferent
  Confused – Dazed
  Depressed
  Crying – Sobbing

STIMULATED
  Silly – Intoxicated
  Grimacing
  More Altert – Talkative
  Hyperactive
  Tense – Restless
  Anxious – Apprehensive
  Fear – Panic
  Irritable – Angry

SPEECH COMPREHENSION
  Mentally Sluggish
  Concentration Poor
  Memory Loss (Acute)
  Speech Slurred
  Stammering – Stuttering
  Speech Paralysis – Loss of
  Reads Aloud Poorly
  Reads s Comprehension
  Hears s Comprehension
  Math – Spelling Errors

MUSCLE
  Muscle Tremor – Jerking
  Muscle Cramps – Spasms
  Pseudoparalysis – Weak

CONTACT
  Poor Contact
  Surroundings Unreal
  Disoriented – Catatonic –
    Stuporous
  False Belief – Delusion –
    Hallucination – to wander
    in mind; false perception
  Suicidal – feel like hurting self
  Maniacal – Very highly disturbed

NASAL
  Sneezed – Urge to
  Itching – Rubbing
  Obstruction
  Discharge
  Post-nasal Drip
  Sinus Discomfort
  Stuffy Feeling

THROAT, MOUTH
  Itching
  Sore – Tight – Swollen
  Dysphagia – Difficulty in
    Swallowing – Choking
  Weak Voice – Hoarse
  Salivation – Mucus
  Bad, Metallic Taste

EARS
  Itching
  Full – Blocked
  Erythema of Pinna (reddening)
  Tinnitis – Ringing in Ears
  Earache
  Hearing Loss
  Hyperacusis – Abnormal
    Sensitivity to Sound

LUNGS – HEART
  Coughing
  Wheezing
  Reduced Air Flow
  Retracting – Sob
  Heavy – Tight
  Not Enough Air
  Hyperventilation – Rapid
    Breathing
  Chest Pain
  Tachycardia – Rapid Pulse
  Palpitations – Rapid, vilent
    or throbbing pulses
  PVC

EYES
  Itch – Burn – Pain
  Lacrimation – Tearing
  Injected – F B Sens.
  Allergic Shiners
  Feel Heavy

VISION
  Blurring
  Acuity decreased
  Spots – Flashes
  Darker – Vision Loss
  Photophobia – Brighter
  Diptopia – Double Vision
  Dyslexia – Difficulty reading –
    Transposition of simila letters
    Letters or words becoming
      small or large
    Words moving around

G-U
  Voided – Mild Urge
  Frequency
  Urgency – Pressure
  Painful or Difficult Urination
  Dysuria – Genital Itch

G-I – ABDOMEN
  Nausea
  Belching
  Full – Bloated
  Vomiting
  Pressure – Pain – Cramps
  Flatus – Rumbling
  B M – Diarrhea
  Gall Bladder Symptoms
  Hunger – Thirst
  Hyperacidity

MUSCLES
  Tight – Stiff
  Ache – Sore – Pain
  Neck – Trapezius
  Upper Lower Back
  Upper-Lower Extremities

trained out by behavioral treatment. The maximum therapeutic value is to be found in the combined biobehavioral therapy.

SUMMARY

The latter part of the nineteenth century and the early part of the twentieth century brought to medicine a significant array of ecologic facts which led to some valuable present-day public health measures and especially such as bacteriology and allergy. Before the ecologic orientation had made its full contribution, such bodily centered areas as pathology and pharmacology were giving promise of rapid cure or rapid symptom relief. This promise of rapid relief has tended to eclipse the significance of ecologic facts. Recently, a resurgence of interest in ecologic contribution has been occurring due to a forced consciousness as to how increasing pollution of our environment is adversely influencing man. Another factor is also the increasing evidence that frequently eaten foods and commonly met chemicals are capable of adversely altering central nervous sytem function.

The method of comprehensive environmental control provides for avoidance of possible incriminated substances which in many instances turn off by the fourth to the sixth day the chronic physical or mental illness. The illness is turned back on by precipitating an acute reaction on an exposure to a single substance. Thus induction evidence of symptom causes is demonstrated. Under these circumstances, we can at least believe what we see. This evidence leads to the conclusion that basic organic driving forces behind many chronic physical and chronic mental illnesses are from addictive reactions to frequently eaten foods and commonly met chemicals and/or idiosyncratic reactions to small amounts of toxic substances. Recognizable symptoms, called an "illness," develop when the relative symptom-free adaptive addictive state is decompensating into a maladaptive symptom-producing addictive state. The adaptive addictive state is one of precariously poor physical and mental homeostatic function much like walking a tight rope, with any number of things capable of precipitating a fall. The stress of the addictive treadmill invariably leads to chronic symptom production. Many factors can aid in shifting the relatively symptom-free adaptive addictive state to a symptom-producing maladaptive addictive state. All possible stresses must be considered as adversely affecting the addicted or idosyncratic toxic state, such as: (1.) Overload of addictive substances; (2.) Overload of allergens, such as seasonal pollens, and so forth; (3.) Overload of toxic substances; (4.) Physical stresses such as: (a.) Extreme or prolonged cold; (b.) Extreme of heat; (c.) Fatigue; (5.) Stress of malnutrition; (6.) Stress of infection; (7.) Emotional stress. Correcting these items without correcting the addictive or idosyncratic-toxic state can cause a shift toward the adaptive addictive state, which still remains a delicately precarious state, only slightly removed from symptoms, and all set for failure again. Treating the addicted state and/or the idiosyncratic-toxic state, plus the other stressful factors, provides a broad based strong physical and emotional homeostasis able to handle the commonly met physical and emotional stresses.

The most effective therapy handles simultaneously (a) the addictive state; (b) the idiosyncratic-toxic state; (c) all stressors, physical and emotional; and (d) trains out maladaptive responses occurring from the illness or from life experience and now serving as stressors, and trains in adaptive replacements. The most critical and significant fact should be understood — that the order of priority of treatment is to handle first and foremost the addictive state, since this is the strongest of the forces driving toward symptom production. To leave this addictive state untreated is to leave the person subject to symptom production by every little wind of stress that blows.

Schizophrenia appears to represent the ultimate of possibilities of metabolic disorders as far as emotional reactions are concerned. Significant variations from normal are observed in a significant percentage in many areas — carbohydrate metabolism, mineral metabolism, vitamin metabolism (deficiencies and dependencies), endocrine function, lipid metabolism [29], metabolic errors, eosinophilia and lack of eosinophils, excessive lymphocytes and atypical lymphocytes, disorder of immune mechanism and likely disorder of auto-immune mechanism. No one disorder can be taken as the cause. The illness represents the focus of the numerous disorders. The maladaptive reactions to foods and chemicals represent the focal clinical expression of these numerous disorders. The most immediate and observable precipitating factor in symptom production in schizophrenics occurs on exposure to substances maladaptively handled by the subject. Therefore, the most profitable starting point for therapy in the schizophrenic is to handle these maladaptive reactions by avoidance. The second step in treatment is to treat all demonstrable metabolic defects. The third step is to train out unadaptive responses and train in corrections.

REFERENCES

1. Crook, W.G.: "Allergy . . . the great masquerader," in *Pediatric Basics*, Gerber, 1973.
2. Crook, W.G.: "A practicing pediatrician looks at allergy," in *Pediatric Basics*, Gerber, 1973.
3. Richet, C.: Anaphylaxis in general and anaphylaxis to mytilocongestine in particular. *Ann. Inst. Pasteur*, 21:497, 1907.
4. Speer, F.: Allergic diagnosis and treatment, in *Allergy of the Nervous System*, Springfield: Charles C Thomas Company, 1970, p. 228.
5. Crook, W.G., Harrison, W.W., Crawford, S.E. et al: Systemic manifestations due to allergy. *Pediatrics*, 27 (pt. 1), 1961.
6. Mandell, M.: May emotional reactions be precipitated by allergens? *Conn. Med.*, vol. 32, 1968.
7. Mandell, M.: Cerebral manifestations of hypersensitivity to the chemical environment: Susceptibility to indoor and outdoor pollution. *Rev. Allergy*, 22:, 1968.
8. Mandell, M.: Cerebral reactions in allergic patients. Published by the New England Foundation for Allergic and Environmental Diseases, Norwalk, Connecticut, 1969.
9. Mandell, M.: Allergies alleged to be the cause of pyschosis. New England Foundation for Allergic and Environmental Diseases, Norwalk, Connecticut, January, 1970.
10. Mandell, M.: Central nervous system hypersensitivity to house dust, molds, and foods. *Rev. Allerg.*, vol. 24, 1970.
11. Randolph, T.G. and Rollins, J.P.: Beet sensitivity: Allergic reactions from ingestion of beet sugar (sucrose) and monosodium glutamate of beet origin. *J. Lab. Clin. Med.*, 36:407-415, 1950.

12. Randolph, T.G.: Allergic factors in the etiology of certain mental symptoms, abstracted. *J. Lab. Clin. Med.*, 36:77, 1950.

13. Randolph, T.G.: Ecologic mental illness — levels of central nervous system reactions. *Proc. Third World Congress of Psychiatry*, Vol. 1. Montreal, Canada: University of Toronto Press, 1961, pp. 379-384.

14. Randolph, T.G.: *Human Ecology and Susceptibility to the Chemical Environment.* Springfield: Thomas, 1962.

15. Randolph, T.G.: Domiciliary chemical air pollution in the etiology of ecologic mental illness. *Int. J. Soc. Psychiat.*, 16:243-265, 1970.

16. Randolph, T.G.: Ecologically Oriented Medicine: Its need, I. Comparison with Anthropocentric Medicine, II. The Roles of Specific Adaptation and Individual Susceptibility in Chronic Illness, III. Stimulatory and Withdrawal Manifestations of Specific Reactions. 1973.

17. Klotz, S., Philpott, W.H. and von Hilsheimer, G.: Double-blind study on provocative testing with sublingual food and chemical extracts. Speech delivered at the International College of Psychosomatic Medicine, Amsterdam, Holland, June 21, 1973.

18. Dohan, F.C., Martin, L., Grasberger, J.D. et al: "Antibodies to Wheat Gliadin in Blood of Psychiatric Patients: Possible Role of Emotional Factors." In *Biological Psychiatry*, Vol. 5, No. 2. (1972) Plenum Publishing Corporation, New York, N.Y.

19. Dohan, F.C. and Grasberger, J.D.: Relapsed schizophrenics: Earlier discharge from the hospital after cereal-free, milk-free diet. *Amer. J. Psychiat.*, 130:6, 1973.

20. Rinkel, H.J., Randolph, T.G., and Zeller, M.: *Food Allergy.* Springfield: Charles C. Thomas, Publishers, 1951, pp 58-102, 130.

21. Randolph, T.G.: Food allergy and food addiction. 9th Ann. Congress, Amer. College of Allergists, Chicago, Illinois, April, 1953 (Exhibit).

22. Randolph, T.G.: Descriptive features of food addiction: Addictive eating and drinking. *Quat. J. Stud. Alcohol.*, 17:198-224, 1956.

23. Perry, L., Hansen, S., Tischler, B. et al: Unrecognized adult phenylketonuria: Implications for obstetrics and psychiatry. *New Eng. J. Med.*, 289: 1973.

24. Randolph, T.G.: The ecologic unit, part I and part II. *Hosp. Manage.*, March and April, 1964.

25. Wolpe, J.: *The Practice of Behavior Therapy.* New York: Pergamon Press, 1969, pp. 91-149.

26. Philpott, W.H.: "Biobehavioral psychiatry and learning disabilities. In *The Child with Learning Disabilities: His Right to Learn.* San Rafael: Academic Therapy Publications, 1971.

27. Philpott, W.H.: Chemical defects, allergic and toxic states as causes and/or facilitating factors of emotional reactions, dyslexia, hyperkinesis, and learning problems. *J. Int. Acad. Metabol.*, 2:58-69, 1973.

28. Philpott, W.H., Mandell, M. and Shammas, E.: The significance of the chemical/allergic-ecologic survey in schizophrenia, emotional disorders, and alcoholism. *J. Int. Acad. Metabol.*, 2:17-28, 1973.

29. Fleischman, A.I., Philpott, W.H. and von Hilsheimer, G.: Lipid Chemistry and the Psychiatric Patient. Speech given at the International College of Psychosomatic Medicine, Amsterdam, Holland, June 21, 1973.

24
Immunological Deficiency in Schizophrenia
Schizophrenia as a Variant Syndrome
in the Nutritional Deficiency
Addiction — Diabetes Mellitus — Infection Disease Process*

WILLIAM H. PHILPOTT

The fact that central nervous system maladaptive reactions which are allergic or allergic-like in origin occur has been documented by several observers (Speer, 1970; Randolph, 1961; Weiss, 1971; Dohan, 1972). These reactions range from minor central nervous system reactions such as headaches, dizziness, blurred vision, dyslexia, hyperkinesis, phobias, obsessions, compulsions, and so forth to major reactions such as hallucinations, delusions, time distortion, disorientation, gross perceptual distortions, catatonia, epileptic seizures, and so forth. What is the cause or varied causes for these reactions?

REAGIN VERSUS NONREAGIN REACTIONS

It has long been recognized that reagins do occur in the central nervous system, however their frequency and importance have not been considered great. There are several reasons for this state of affairs such as: 1) Allergists rely on evidence from reactions from skin testing, and skin testing reveals no cause and effect relationship to central nervous system reactions. 2) Allergists are not taught usually to systematically observe central nervous system reactions by a convincing symptom induction method. 3) Psychiatrists and neurologists are not taught to place reagin type reactions in their differential diagnosis and are not taught methods of testing for allergic central nervous system reactions.

There is good evidence that the majority of central nervous system maladaptive reactions to foods, chemicals, and inhalants are nonreaginic in origin. The immunologist Arthur F. Coca (1953) recognized there are numerous reactions of a nonreaginic origin. F.C. Dohan (1972) determined antibody reaction to wheat gliadin as being 3.1 percent in the non-ill population, 20.6 percent in the hospitalized nonschizophrenic psychiatric patients and 20.1 percent in the schizophrenic patients. My observations are that better than 60 percent of schizophrenics are symptom reactive to wheat. Comparing Dohan's and my observations would indicate schizophrenics do have significant reaginic reactions to wheat, but almost two-thirds of the reactions observed during symptom induction food testing are nonreagin in origin.

*Canadian Schizophrenia Foundation, Fifth Annual Meeting, Winnipeg, Manitoba, Canada, June 6, 1976

ACUTE NUTRITIONAL DEFICIENCY REACTIONS

Testing varying doses of various nutrients given intravenously reveals evidence that Pyridoxine in doses of approximately 1000 mg. is the central nutrient in relieving maladaptive reactions to foods and chemicals. This was determined under the circumstances of doing deliberate exposure symptom induction testing after a four to six day period of avoidance. The B6 supporting nutrients, Vitamin C and Magnesium, improve the percentage and quality of correction of evoked responses. Responses can be prevented by giving these nutrients intravenously ahead of the test. Giving the nutrients orally one and one half hours ahead of the test reduces or may even completely prevent the reaction from occurring. This occurred with single test meals, but could not be completely maintained on serial test meals.

A chronic state of nutritional deficiency (starvation) has the characteristics of edema. Also, when food is supplied to the starved person acute edema occurs, and therefore a starved person is fed small frequent feedings to prevent the development of acute edema. Acute nutritional deficiency reactions also have the characteristics of edema which is usually local, likely revealing evidence of the most nutritionally deficient tissues. In a marginally nutritionally deficient state there are no symptoms unless the person's chemical state is challenged by a stress such as a food or chemical which makes demands for essential chemistry which is in low supply. When the tissues swell symptoms occur. The symptoms are dependent on the specific tissues involved.

THE ROLE OF CHRONIC INFECTION

Physicians are taught to understand and treat acute infections producing such as fever, acute symptoms, and acute tissue damage. However, chronic infections are by and large ignored and undiagnosed or even unsuspected.

Acute nutritional deficiency reactions or true allergic reactions produce a fertile medium for opportunist organisms to flourish. Each time edema with its local reduction in oxygen supply to tissues occurs, there exists a favorable biological state for a flare up of infection. Each time this favorable condition occurs latent organisms quickly multiply and become toxic producing. Acute nutritional deficiency reactions even more than

151

true allergic reactions invite infectious invasion due to its inherent low level immunological defense. Antibodies against the infectious agents cannot be made unless nutrition is adequate. This is especially true of B$_6$ deficiency (Axelrod, 1973).

Schizophrenics, like other organically ill patients harbor multiple infectious agents. My experience is that it is common to culture ten to fifteen types of infections from schizophrenics. In one very ill schizophrenic I cultured twenty-nine infections including bacteria and fungi. I have found that fungi such as Candida albicans, Altenaria, Aspergillus and so forth are important infecting agents.

It is not only important that these infectious agents are present but it is also important that mental symptoms can at times be produced by re-exposure to these infectious agents. A twenty year old catatonic schizophrenic developed catatonia on sublingual exposure to Candida albicans. She had a history of episodic Candida albicans vaginal infection. A paranoid schizophrenic with a nasal Staphylococcus infection became paranoid as well as having a stuffy nose when sublingually tested with Staphylococcus vaccine. The patient with twenty-nine infections when sublingually tested for her group of infections from her autogenous vaccine became so weak and generally ill that of necessity she spent several hours in my office before she sufficiently recovered to be able to leave. One patient when given his first intramuscular autogenous vaccine dose of multiple bacteria became so weak that he could barely stand with support. Also, severe chest pains occurred as well as a phobia of impending death and the activation of several other phobias. These symptoms of chest pain, impending death and numerous phobias were presenting symptoms and had subsided when symptom reactive foods and chemicals were withdrawn. One gets the impression that in his case and likely all cases the reactions to foods and chemicals and the activation of chronic infections are synergistic in symptom production. Logically both should be adequately treated.

In spite of numerous infections cultured from schizophrenics there is only one organism that has been observed as characteristically being present in all cases. That organism is Progenitor cryptocides. The consistent presence of Progenitor cryptocides in schizophrenia is a common denominator with cancer which also reveals one hundred percent presence of Progenitor cryptocides. Dark field studies of the blood reveal morphologically no difference between the schizophrenic and cancer patient's infection with Progenitor cryptocides. Progenitor cryptocides fits James Papez' description (1951, 1952) of the pleomorphic microbe consistently found in brain cultures from schizophrenics. He also observed in schizophrenics, as Virginia Livingston has in cancer and in schizophrenia, the characteristics of parasitized red blood cells. Papez described viral size inclusion bodies in neurons from which the pleomorphic microbe grew.

Progenitor cryptocides is a fungus origin type pleomorphic microbe with viral size bodies, several bacterial types, fungal types and colonies. The infection is as common to the human race as athlete's foot and it infects approximately four-fifths of the population. However in cancer and schizophrenia the difference from healthy people is that it is in a proliferative, red cell invasive and pleomorphic state. With successful treatment it loses these characteristics. Progenitor cryptocides culture has a fetid odor. Cancer and schizophrenic patients characteristically have the same fetid odor.

TREATMENT OF INFECTIONS

The following combination of treatments favorably builds defenses against infections.

1. Avoidance of symptom evoking foods, chemicals, and inhalants.
2. Supernutrition.
3. Autogenous and stock vaccines.

Avoidance of symptom evoking substances is of prime importance since it provides an immediate improvement in the health of tissues. The normal oxygen content of human tissue is a natural barrier to infection, whereas edema with its low oxygen supply to tissues invites infection.

Pyridoxine and Pantothenic Acid are necessary for immunological defense since antibodies cannot be formed when these are deficient. These central vitamins of course require adequate support with other nutrients especially Riboflavin, Zinc, Magnesium, and Manganese. Vitamin C in adequate supply is known to suppress infectious invasion. Virginia Livingston states Vitamin A suppresses Progenitor cryptocides.

Vaccines can be made from the infections cultured from skin, ear, nose, throat, and mouth, arm pits, external genitalia, cervix, prostate, feet, urine, and feces. These autogenous vaccines are the most appropriate for each patient. Two stock vaccines of importance are BCG and Maruyama. BCG is from Mycobacterium tuberculosis and Maruyama is from Mycobacterium leprae. Both of these vaccines have a cross antigenicity with Progenitor cryptocides since they all belong to the order Actinmycetales. Other stock vaccines that have varying degrees of usefulness in stimulating immunologic defenses are such as Sheep Cell — spleen and erythrocytes (Pantogen), Flu vaccine, Poison Ivy-Oak-Sumac, and stock respiratory bacterial vaccine.

RESEARCH CONSIDERATIONS (Newbold, 1975; Plesch, 1947)

Another possible autogenous vaccine comes from the observation that in schizophrenia bacterial substances can be isolated from the urine (Frujita, 1961; Chapman, 1961, 1962). These substances can be used as autogenous vaccines. Giving the patient the conjugating substance, Glucuronolactone, theoretically will produce toxoids out of the toxins. Thus, autotoxoid therapy can be used. The system can be on this order:

1. Feed a meal of symptom evoking foods.
2. Provide Glucuronolactone with the meal.
3. Collect the urine two to three hours after the meal of incriminated foods.
4. Sterilize the urine by passage through size .45 μm and .22 μm filters.
5. Combine 10 cc. of sterilized urine with 2 cc. of two percent Procaine and inject intramuscularly.
6. Treat once or twice a week for an unlimited number of times. Eight such injections are suggested as minimal.
7. Patients should be informed that autogenous toxin (toxoid if Preltran is used) therapy is experimental and a statement should be signed that they know it is an

experiment, and no claim of cure is being made. Also all stock vaccines should have such a disclaimer since they are being used for their nonspecific immunologic effect rather than the specific treatment values for which they are allowed to be marketed by the FDA.

A twenty-two year old schizophrenic with an illness of five years duration consisting of morbid depression, weakness, and perceptual distortions, remained ill after electroshock therapy, tranquilizers and an ample trial of megavitamin therapy. I studied her reactions to foods and chemicals revealing numerous reactions but she still remained depressed, weak, and frequently complained to me of her plight. A dark field study of her blood and supernutrition were provided. She still kept complaining. I sent her to Carl L. Eckhardt, M.D., who gave her eight autogenous injections at weekly intervals. Before each injection she ate symptom reactive foods and collected the urine for injection two hours after eating the meal. By the eighth injection her depression was gone, and her strength had returned and she had little to no reaction to her foods. At this stage no one knows how frequently this success could be repeated. I point out this possibility of autotoxin (or autotoxoid) therapy because it appears worthy of definitive study.

One of my patients is an 18 year old schizophrenic with autistic features. His illness was first noted at age four when normal speech failed to develop. Amphetamines were tried without success. Mellaril initially produced minimal improvement with side effects of weakness and sleepiness. Chronic fatigue, odd compulsive movements of hands and neck, periods of silence, perseveration and episodes of irritability were major features of his illness. Major symptoms disappeared on a four day fast and reemerged during specific food and chemical tests. Induction testing revealed 21 foods or chemicals to which he reacted and 79 items to which he did not react. Six foods evoked a blood sugar beyond 160 mg.%, the highest being that of cane sugar at 220 mg.%. The infectious survey cultured eight chronic infections. The hair test revealed six mineral deficiencies and two excesses. Figlu test indicated Folic Acid deficiency.

The food and chemical testing required one month. Twice a week for a total of four weeks he was given autotoxoid injections which consisted of 10 cc. of urine with 2 cc. of 2 percent Procaine given intramuscularly. The injections were begun one month after the end of food testing. The urine was filtered through 0.45 μm and 0.22 μm filters. The urine was collected two hours after eating a meal of symptom incriminated foods and exposure to symptom incriminated chemicals. At the time of this exposure he also took orally 335 mg. of Preltron (Glucuronolactone).

His initial induction test for raisins had produced sleepiness, irritability, and a blood sugar of 210 mg.% at one hour post test meal. After the completion of the eight autoxoid injections he ate raisins three times a day with his meals for three days without evidence of symptoms occurring. On the fourth day he ate a single post test meal blood sugar of 75 mg.%. During the period of receiving the autotoxoid injections he also was in the process of receiving meganutrients, Sheep Cell Spleen and Erythrocyte Vaccine, Flu A and B Vaccine, Poison Ivy-Oak-Sumac Vaccine and autogenous vaccines for all bacteria cultured from him.

This system involving multiple factors has not revealed to us clearly the significance of the component parts but has clearly indicated the value of the total treatment. Each aspect of treatment is logically calculated to favorably influence the disordered metabolism. These factors are: 1. The two months of avoidance before retesting would reduce the reaction rate; 2. Appropriate individualized supernutrition with emphasis on B_6 would reduce the reaction rate and encourage the development of an immunological defence; 3. Stock vaccines of Sheep Cell, Ivy-Oak-Sumac and Flu would strengthen the immunological defenses. Three days of use three times a day of raisins was calculated to so stress the chemistry as to reinstate the reaction if the chemistry would permit it. The normal blood sugar and lack of symptoms during the retest establishes evidence that the therapy has prevented a reinstatement of the maladaptive reaction.

The preferred method of administering autotoxoid therapy is as follows: 1. Eat small portions of all foods reacted to and arranged for exposure to all chemicals and other inhalants reacted to; 2. Empty urinary bladder before eating above meal and again empty bladder two hours after eating meal. 3. Filter 10 cc. of this two-hour-after meal urine through a 0.45 μm Millex filter; 4. In a 20 cc. syringe draw up 5 cc. of Preltron (1250 mg. Sodium Glucuronate) and pour in 5 cc. of the urine. Prepare two of these. 5. Attach a 0.22 μm Millex filter to these 10 cc. syringes with filtered urine and Preltron. Attach a one inch needle and inject intramuscularly. The final filtration is achieved by filtering through the 0.22 μm filter during the step of injection. Five cc Preltron mixed with the urine conjugates toxins making toxoids. The intramuscular injection of combined Preltron and urine is not painful and no Procaine is necessary to eliminate pain. An alternative is mix 10 cc. of urine with 2 cc. Preltron which can then be given in one injection. This will not be as comfortable as the 50-50 mixture. To establish evidence as to whether the autotoxoid therapy had a value or not follow this method. 1. Eat single or multiple incriminated foods or chemical exposure three times a day for three days and monitor for symptoms. 2. A single meal exposure of the incriminated substance on the fourth day. 3. Also monitor blood sugar before and one hour after the test if it was abnormal on the original test. A further even more convincing method would be to sustain an exposure for two to three weeks followed by four days of avoidance and then test with a single exposure monitoring for symptoms and blood sugar abnormality. Theoretically maximum value of autotoxoid therapy could only be achieved in the presence of optimum nutrition especially B_6 and Pantothenic Acid which are required for antibody production.

SUMMARY

Out of my research and clinic experience, I have developed the formulation that although schizophrenia has multiple causes, a frequent central cause is observed to be that of being a variant of the basic disease process which leads to several chronic degenerative diseases. The diseases are named according to the tissues impaired, the secondary invading organisms, the endocrine disorders produced or the autoimmune reactions evoked. The basic features of this disease process are:

1. Marginal nutritional deficiency with the consequences of . . .

2. Addiction as an adaptive mechanism which develops into the . . .
3. Chemical Diabetes mellitus state, which includes such as hyperglycemia (as reaction state), hypoglycemia (as addictive withdrawal state) and hyperinsulinism.
4. Infectious invasion.

For many the metabolic state remains at the addictive-chemical diabetes state, the stress of which injures tissues giving rise to various diseases indicating the altered tissue function. Schizophrenia represents one of the variants of the basic disease process in which the cerebral tissues are central reactive tissues. Each type of tissue has its distinctive nutritional needs; and whenever these metabolic needs are not met, for whatever reason, these tissues become reactive due to acute nutritional deficiency, thus evoking symptoms by stressors which make specific metabolic demands (for such as enzymes and hormones) such as foods, toxins, inhalants, or infections, and so forth. It has long been understood that adult onset Diabetes mellitus has a set of associated complications involving specific tissues especially such as eyes, kidneys, the vascular system, and the central nervous system. What has not been widely appreciated is that the Chemical Diabetes mellitus state is a precursor to many chronic diseases, and these diseases can be characterized as associated complications of this Diabetes mellitus process.

Another viewpoint that is likely more central is to characterize the disease process as adaptive addictive adjustment to frequent contact with foods and chemicals for which the person is too nutritionally deficient to metabolically handle without reactions. Characteristic of the addictive adjustment are:

1. Carbohydrate interference producing episodes of acute metabolic acidosis, and
2. Chemical Diabetes states of hyperglycemia, hypoglycemia, and hyperinsulinism. The presence of a chemical diabetes can be demonstrated by monitoring glucose and insulin metabolism (Brambilla, 1976) and is best demonstrated by monitoring blood sugar before and one hour after induction food tests.

Characteristic of this deficiency-addiction-diabetes state is low resistance to infectious invasion. Usually infections are multiple. However, a consistent invader in this disease process is the pleomorphic microbe Progenitor cryptocides. Some strains of Progenitor cryptocides produce Chorionic gonadotropin (Livingston, 1975) and others do not. Also some cultures producing Chorionic gonadotropin lose this characteristic under certain conditions (Minjarich, 1976). Chorionic gonadotropin encourages cellular division, and thus presumably can encourage the development of cancer. Schizophrenics are not cancer prone even though a comparative dark field study of the blood of schizophrenics and cancer patients reveals a comparable degree of ploriferation, invasion, and pleomorphism of Progenitor cryptocides. The following should be considered as possible reasons for the low cancer incidence in schizophrenia:

1. The strain of Progenitor cryptocides involved in schizophrenia may not be Chorionic gonadotropin producing.
2. Perhaps schizophrenia's chemical state discourages the production of Chorionic gonadotropin by Progenitor cryptocides.

3. A successful immunological defense against tumor formation may occur in schizophrenia but not against the microbe itself.

Since schizophrenics are immunologically deficient, one aspect of treatment should involve maximum reinforcement of immunologic defenses or reinstatement of immunologic defenses. This can be achieved by stock and autogenous vaccines under the favorable circumstances of optimum supernutrition. Vaccines can be made from the bacterial bodies provided from killed bacteria or from toxins or toxoids of the infectious agents. B_6 and Pantothenic Acid with their supportive nutrients are central in the process of building immunologic defenses and therefore need to be provided while the patient is undergoing vaccine therapy.

Under test conditions autogenous microbes can be demonstrated to be equally symptom producing as are foods, chemicals, and inhalants. Therefore the infections the patient is harboring should be a part of the differential diagnosis as to causes of symptoms. Also we should consider the probability that the final deteriorating process in organic diseases is one of microbial invasion with its tissue damage and toxins interfering with the patient's hormonal and enzymatic systems. All humans suffer from microbes attempting to eat them alive, and in the final state they will either be killed by these microbes, or if killed by some other cause, the microbes will consume their remains.

The work of James Papez would lead us to conclude that the final organic deteriorating process of schizophrenia is a microbial one with neurons invaded by Progenitor cryptocides and with flare ups of infection destroying neurons, in which metabolic shifts allow this to occur.

In order is an experiment determining the amount of ingested Sodium Glucuronate needed to conjugate bacterial toxins to toxoids, or determining if the best method is to mix injectable Glucuronic Acid with the urine.

It is likely true that in the urinary spillage is found the maximum concentration of microbial toxins. Unfortunately there is a universal phobia about urine being unclean which tends to hold even when the urine has been sterilized. On the other hand, the autogenous vaccine for Progenitor cryptocides is cultured from the urine, and why should we consider these microbes from the urine more acceptable than their toxins in the urine. It would be of clinical value to find a method of separating the toxins from the urine, thus giving the autotoxoid therapy more aesthetic acceptance.

Although we do see mental reactions as manifestations of hypersensitivity to the bodies of bacteria and fungi as tested by vaccines, it can be assumed as true that the most serious reactions are to the products of the organisms poisoning vital metabolic processes. This is certainly true of acute infections, and therefore should be true of chronic infections. A form of autotoxoid vaccine therapy would appear to be as much in order as vaccine treatment with the bodies of dead pathogenic microorganisms.

REFERENCES

Axelrod, A.E.: Nutrition in Relation to Acquired Immunity, pp 493-505. *Modern Nutrition in Health and Disease.* Goodhart, Robert S., and Shild, Maurice E. (Eds.). Lea & Febiger, Philadelphia, 1973.

Brambilla, F.: Guerrini, A.; Riggi, F.; Rovere, C.; Zanoboni, A.;

and Zanoboni-Muciaccia, W.: Glucose-Insulin Metabolism in Chronic Schizophrenia. Dis Nerv Sys, Vol. 37, No. 2, February, 1976.

Chapman, George H.: Microbial Origin of the Gummy Substance of Fujita and Ging, Trans NY Acad Sc 11, 25:1, pp 66-69, 1962.

Chapman, George H.: Personal Communication to Laverne, Albert, M.D., Editor of Behavioral Neuropsychiatry, July 21, 1961.

Coca, Arthur F.: *Familial Nonreagenic Food Allergy*. Third edition, Springfield, Thomas, 1953.

Dohan, F.C., and Grasberger, J.C.: Relapsed Schizophrenics: Earlier Discharge from the Hospital after Cereal-Free, Milk-Free Diet. Am J Psy, 130:6, 1973.

Dohan, F.C., and Grasberger, J.C.; Boehme, C.; and Cattrell, J.C.: Antibodies to Wheat Gliadin in Blood of Psychiatric Patients. Possible Role of Emotional Factors. Biological Psychiatry, Vol. 5, No. 2, 1972. Plenum Publishing Corporation, 227 West 17th Street, New York, NY 10011.

Fujita, S., and Ging, N.S.: Science, 134:1687, 1961.

Livingston, Virginia Wuerthele-Caspe, and Livingston, Afton Munk: Some Cultural, Immunological and Biochemical Properties of Progenitor Cryptocides. Trans NY Acad Sc, Vol, 36, No. 6, pp 569-582. June 1974.

Minjarich, John: Personal Communication to Philpott, 1975. 1115 East Pike Street, Seattle, Washington 98122.

Newbold, H.L.: *Mega-Nutrients For Your Nerves*. Peter H. Wyden Publisher, New York, NY, 1975. pp 65-69.

Papez, James W., and Bateman, J.F.: Changes in Nervous Tissues and Study of Living Organisms in Mental Disease. J Nerv Men Dis, 114:5, 1951.

Papez, James W.: Form of Living Organisms in Psychotic Patients, J Nerv Men Dis, 116:5, 1952.

Papez, James W.: Living Organisms in Nerve Cells as Seen Under Dark Contrast, Phase Microscope. Trans Amer Neur Assoc, 1952.

Philpott, William H.: Progenitor Cryptocides in Cancerous and Schizophrenic Patients. Editorial Comment, International Acad Meta, Vol. 5, No. 1, March 1976.

Plesch, Johan: Urine Therapy. The Medical Press, London, England. 1947.

Randolph, Theron G.: Ecological Mental Illness — Levels of Central Nervous System Reactions. Proc. Third World Congress of Psychiatry, Vol. 1, 379-384. Montreal, Canada, University of Toronto Press, June 1961.

Speer, Frederick: *Allergy of the Nervous System*. Springfield, Thomas, 1970.

Weiss, Jules M., and Kaufman, Herbert S.: A Subtle Organic Component in Some Cases of Mental Illness. Arch Gen Psy, Vol. 25, July 1971.

PACKAGE INFORMATION

1. Virginia Livingston, M.D., cultures Progenitor cryptocides from which autogenous vaccines are made. 3232 Duke Street, San Diego, CA 92110.
2. John Minjarich, Ph.D., Bacteriologist. Provides Maruyama vaccine. Cultures Progenitor cryptocides for autogenous vaccines. 1115 East Pike Street, Seattle, WA 98122.
3. Millex Disposable Filter units. Purchases from Millipore, Bedford, MA. a) 0.45 μm SLHA 0250S in packages of 50. b) 0.22 μm SLGS 0250S in packages of 50.
4. Preltron. Pasadena Research Labs, Inc. Pasadena, CA 91107. Preltron/oral. Glucuronolactone 335mg. Preltron/Injection. Sodium Glucuronate 250 mg/cc in 10 cc vials.
5. The following may be contacted for guidance in BCG Vaccine research:
   a) Ray G. Crispen, Ph.D., Director, ITR Biomedical Research, University of Illinois at the Medical Center, 904 W. Adams Street, Chicago, IL 60607.
   b) National Cancer Institute, Bethesda, MD 20014. There is a book available from this agency entitled, "Conference on the Use of BCG Vaccine in Therapy of Cancer." This is the HEW Publication No. NIH-74-511. Cost is approximately $7.
6. Eleanor Alexander-Jackson, Ph.D. 390 Riverside Drive, New York, NY 10025. She cultures Progenitor cryptocides for autogenous vaccines.
7. For Stock Bacteria Vaccine: Hollister-Stier Laboratories, Box 3145 TA, Spokane, WA 99220.

25
Hypoglycemia: The End of Your Sweet Life

WILLIAM CURRIER, JOHN BARON, DWIGHT K. KALITA

Hypoglycemia is not a disease. Neither is it an infection nor a response to an invading virus. Succinctly stated, hypoglycemia is LOW BLOOD SUGAR. More technically, it is an abnormality of metabolism that results in a precipitous drop or a flat curve in normal blood sugar levels. In spite of the fact that the low blood sugar condition was discovered in 1924 by Dr. Seale Harris, M.D., who 25 years later received the Distinguished Service Medal for his research from the American Medical Association, it is still difficult to find a physician who has a thorough understanding of this problem. For more than 35 years only one book was available for the public on hypoglycemia, but in the last couple of years about 10 more books have been published. This developing interest in the subject is occasioned, I believe, by the rapid increase in the numbers of Americans suffering from low blood sugar. Roberts and Hurdle estimate that over 50 million Americans have hypoglycemia in varying degrees of severity [1]. "There is probably no illness today which causes such widespread suffering, so much inefficiency and loss of time, so many accidents, so many family break-ups, and so many suicides, as that of hypoglycemia." This startling statement was made in 1957 to a meeting of the American ·Medical Association by Dr. S.P. Gyland. Ironically, and tragically, over twenty years later we now have an American hypoglycemia epidemic!

The proper maintenance of constant and adequate glucose (blood sugar) levels in the body is one of the most important functions of our biochemical being. Your brain needs glucose in order to think clearly; your muscles need glucose for strength and action; in fact, your entire body needs glucose to maintain life. A delicately regulated process of the body insures us that we have proper levels of glucose in our blood. The anterior pituitary gland, which produces hormones that elevate blood sugar, the adrenal medulla, which produces epinephrine (adrenalin) that stimulates the breakdown of stored glycogen (carbohydrate stored in the liver), and the adrenal cortex, which produces a number of hormones called glucosteroids that are necessary for the metabolism of all carbohydrates, simultaneously act like instruments in a harmonious and complex symphony of metabolism just so an adequate level of glucose can be supplied to the body. The pancreas, in turn, produces insulin in order to reduce the level of blood sugar and thus avoid diabetes.

For several reasons, the precision and beauty of this delicately tuned symphonic metabolism can become all jazzed up.

Modern man, for one example, has been eating for too long a time a vitamin depleted diet which is over-loaded with processed carbohydrates (sugar, white flour, processed foods of convenience, etc.). The pancreas has no other alternative than to over-react to this refined carbohydrate feast. As a result of this continued abuse to the pancreas — and other endrocrine glands of course — an overdose of insulin continues to flow into the bloodstream and the result is a drop in blood sugar to below normal levels. To add fuel to the fire, alcohol, coffee, tea, cola drinks and tobacco all interfere with the proper function of the adrenal glands by overworking them to produce adrenalin secretion which increases blood sugar. This continued dietary challenge to endocrine functions throws off the body's inherent balancing mechanism, and the metabolic disaster which results is becoming as common as the previously mentioned stimulants. In short, hypoglycemia is, as Dr. Nathan Pritikin, Director of the Longevity Research Institute, Santa Barbara, California suggests, a problem that is intimately related to a patient's diet, and more specifically, to his or her overconsumption of *refined* and/or processed carbohydrates. On the other hand, if the patient eats a diet high in *complex* carbohydrates (i.e., "foods as grown in nature without any processing") rather than refined carbohydrates, Dr. Pritikin has discovered that hypoglycemic symptoms can be eliminated. Since complex·carbohydrates take from 4 to 10 hours of digestion time, they provide, reasons Dr. Pritikin, a more constant flow of glucose to the body over a 24 hour period than do the more quickly absorbed simple, processed or refined carbohydrates. With the complex ҳarbohydrates, the endocrine balancing mechanism, therefore, is not over-worked as it is with simple carbohydrates, and thus, the glands are less likely to fail in their functions. It is as simple as this: if you continue to challenge your endocrine system with the wrong quantity and quality of foods, those glands will someday challenge you in an abnormality called hypoglycemia.

There are other Orthomolecular physicians who have discovered that low blood sugar can be evoked in a person who has ingested any food or has come in contact with any chemical to which he is allergic. As Dr. William Philpott, M.D., has said: "Broad spectrum food and chemical symptom induction testing with blood sugar and pH monitored before and after the test reveals the surprising evidence that hypoglycemia and hyperglycemia can be evoked by foods of all types whether fats, carbohydrates or proteins, and that chemicals also such as tobacco, petro-chemical hydrocarbons and so forth equally evoke hypoglycemia and hyperglycemia in susceptible persons . . . There is strong evidence that hyperglycemia as well as hypoglycemia reactions are usually caused by an assortment of reactions to foods, chemicals and inhalants. The foods causing these reactions are specific for each person. Carbohydrates predominate as symptom precipitating factors, but the reactions are not limited to carbohydrates. These reactions can be caused by any substance to which the person reacts maladaptively (allergic, allergic-like and addictive) [2] ." In short, Dr. Philpott and others believe that hypoglycemia is caused by specific allergic like reactions to specific substances. These substances must always be individually diagnosed for each person by provocative food testing. Surprisingly enough, Dr. Philpott has clinically observed low blood sugar in response to pasteurized cow's milk, cream cheese, hydrocarbons and many other non-carbohydrate substances. This is not to say that milk will cause low blood sugar in all people, but it does point to the fact that hypoglycemia should not be considered strictly as a carbohydrate metabolism dysfunction. Rather, clinically suspected incriminating substances of all kinds must be seen in the light of allergic biochemical individuality and treated accordingly.

There are various symptoms which may or may not occur when there is a rapid fall in the blood sugar level.

MENTAL SYMPTOMS: confusion, forgetfulness, difficulty in concentrating, the mind goes blank.

EMOTIONAL SYMPTOMS: emotional instability, strong temper, impatient and irritable, depression, uncontrollable crying spells, loss of a sense of meaning and purpose in life.

BODILY SYMPTOMS:
Vision: vision is blurred, see double, sensitivity to light.

Fatigue: Very tired and weak most of the time, dizziness, insomnia, cold sweats, fainting spells, feel strong after eating candy, cakes, coffee, or alcohol but later on the previously mentioned symptoms become worse.

Pains: headaches, joints ache and muscles twitch, weakness, irritability and mental confusion after physical stress or emotional stress.

Related Illness: allergies or asthma, alcoholism, very susceptible to infectious diseases, emotional instability (i.e., "neurotic").

Time of Symptoms: feelings of weakness and irritability in the morning before breakfast, other symptoms can occur generally two or more hours after eating or after exhausting physical or emotional stress.

The previously mentioned symptoms are reported to physicians many times during the year by countless numbers of patients. What is most appalling is that doctors often misdiagnose hypoglycemia and treat it symptomatically as an "emotional problem," as a "psychosomatic illness," or as the favorite phrase has it, "Your problem is nerves." Let us assure you: hypoglycemia is none of these. It is a physical problem that relates to

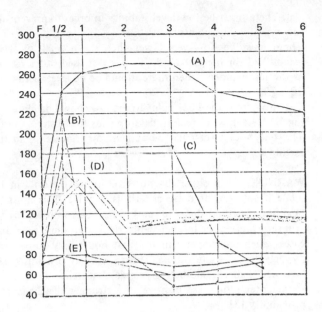

Fig. 1   Abnormal Glucose Tolerance Tests

body and mind. Certainly, it can and does cause all kinds of emotional symptoms. And why shouldn't it? The thalamic area of the brain (i.e., the emotional center) needs proper glucose levels to maintain emotional health. So do all areas of the brain. If this particular area called the emotional center is starved for glucose — as it most certainly is in some forms of hypoglycemia — then all kinds of anti-social emotional symptoms can ensue. But the symptoms are not the root problem. The real problem is in a glandular dysfunction with the most important deficit being in the pituitary-adrenal-liver-pancreas endocrine axis.

Figure 1 illustrates varying degrees of abnormal blood sugar levels. Line A is diabetes in which there is not a sufficient amount of insulin in the blood. The sugar level is obviously too high. Line B shows a very sudden drop from 220 to 80 after the first 1/2 hour. The speed of the drop is a very important diagnostic tool. Line C illustrates a late hypoglycemia that occurs in the 3-4th hour. Line D is called functional hypoglycemia. Line E represents a flat curve hypoglycemia. There are other terms for the other various forms of hypoglycemia. What is important to realize, however, is that any variation from the solid "normal" pattern in Figure 1 should be considered as a sign of hypoglycemia and thus worthy of investigation, diagnosis and proper treatment. These abnormal curves (i.e., "symptoms" of hypoglycemia) can be evoked by either a 5-6 hour seven sample glucose tolerance test or by provocative food allergy testing in which specific allergens are eaten or inhaled by the patient and sugar levels are simultaneously monitored.

Dr. Alan Nittler, M.D., has listed five criteria for the interpretation of the five hour, seven specimen test. They are:

1. The blood glucose level must rise to the half hour and on up to the one hour level. In other words, there must be at least one hour of increased energy because of the glucose intake.
2. The percentage differential between the fasting and the lowest sugar levels must not exceed twenty percent differen-

tial. There must be low level stability in order to prevent the low symptomatic points.

3. There must be no levels lower than the normal low level established for the test used. If your test used states 70-110 as the normal range, then there should be no levels below the 70 mg.%.

4. The drop from the high point to the low should be about 50 mg.%. A steep and precipitous drop adds to the stress of life.

5. The one hour level must be at least 50% greater than the fasting level.

WARNING: A positive diagnosis of hypoglycemia can be made if any one of these criteria is positive. This must be qualified since a diabetic curve can be positive in #3 criterium and not be hypoglycemia. However, there are many cases which are diabetic in the first hours only to become hypoglycemia in later hours. This type of dysinsulinism can be called diabetogenic hypoglycemia. Naturally, the more of these criteria that are positive, the stronger the diagnostic probability [3].

An individually determined proper diet is the cornerstone of all hypoglycemia therapy. In order to determine specific nutritional needs in their patients, many Orthomolecular Physicians run a computerized diet survey. It is a simple computerized test of questions and answers that relate to the individual's entire nutritional-dietary habits. It points out deficiencies of all kinds (i.e., vitamins, minerals, trace elements, bulk & fiber, amino acids, calories, cholesterol, sugar, polyunsaturates, protein-fat-carbohydrates, etc.), and gives a very accurate nutritional foundation from which to treat metabolic disorders.

When studying the patient's dietary habits, allergic reactions, of course, have to be taken into consideration. Fasting, together with sublingual and/or provocative food allergy testing is one very accurate — although time consuming — way to test for specific maladaptive allergic reactions. The Lopapa "R.A.S.P." (Radio Allergen Sorben Principle) blood allergy test, which is based on the reaction between an antigen (allergen) coupled on to solid particles in confrontation with specific reagenic immunoglobulins present in the patient's serum, is a relatively new method of evaluation of allergies (food and otherwise) and is proving to be the most accurate anti-body type test of its kind we have ever had for specific allergic reactions. It must be kept in mind that not all allergic like reactions will produce anti-bodies, and this is true especially for the cerebral allergic reactions.

It has been clinically demonstrated that in some hypoglycemia people, the use of tobacco, sugar, alcoholic beverages, certain individually diagnosed chemicals and foods, and particularly the grains, have to be permanently abandoned. Many other foods in the carbohydrate family will, of course, have to be eliminated, but specific biochemically related allergic reactions to particular proteins, fats and carbohydrates should first be determined.

Allergic reactions to certain foods are dependent to some degree on nutritional and hormonal deficiencies, and metabolic errors in tolerating specific food families. Frequently eaten foods to which a person is allergic often cause the most severe maladaptive reactions. For these reasons, and based on clinical findings, it has been demonstrated that after a period of 6 to 12 weeks in which the patient faithfully avoids all diagnosed aller-

gens — a period in which metabolic normalization is achieved via megavitamin-mineral and hormone supplementation — a limited infrequent exposure to the incriminating foods will not usually evoke the symptoms of low blood sugar. After this period of achieving metabolic homeostasis, the patient can often (not always) space his exposure to previously determined food allergens as frequent as every fourth day, since it takes approximately four days for a single food to be entirely eliminated from the body.

Foods should always be avoided and then rotated every fourth day in families since there may be cross allergic reactions between family members. For example, tomatoes, potatoes, bell peppers and tobacco are all of the same food family. If low blood sugar symptoms are evoked by this entire family of foods — then each food within this family should be first avoided for 6 to 12 weeks and then rotated on a four day basis. More specifically, this means that if I eat tomatoes on Monday, I should not eat potatoes, bell peppers or tomatoes until Friday of that same week. In rotating one's diet, a wide variety of food should be used. It is important to realize that this plan not only reduces allergic type reactions, but it also increases one's exposure to a greater number of different foods, and thus, of course, one's nutritional needs have a better chance of being met by the broader spectrum of nutrients now being encountered.

Optimum protection against maladaptive allergic food reactions occurs when megavitamin-mineral and hormone supplementation (details discussed later on in the article) plus a diversified rotation diet are combined. For an even greater enhancement of protection, all necessary nutrients should be taken about one hour to 1½ hours before meals. This procedure adds to the body's enzyme priming effect.

A small number of patients have, and a minority of foods are, fixed food allergies. These are easy to diagnose because each time the patient eats the specific allergen, symptoms develop. As previously mentioned, such foods as coffee, tea, alcohol, sugar and the grain family should be avoided permanently and rotation is not advised. Chemical, hydrocarbon and tobacco allergic reactions usually fall into the "fixed allergy" classification and should also be avoided as much as possible. People who react to petrochemical hydrocarbons usually also react to one or more of the certified food colorings. Many prepared food contain food colors, preservatives, and other substances to which people can maladaptively react. Even fluorinated water can be a problem. The following case history provides a good example of the severity of any fixed food allergy.

A case history of a four day fast, provocative food allergy test resulting in severe hypoglycemia is given in full by Dr. Philpott. Clinical treatment is also presented in detail:

A thirty year old man presents as a manic depressive reaction, depressive type with episodic psychotic degrees of depression including a suicide attempt, dissociated episodes during which time he went places and did things for which he has no memory and a characterological change of not being truthful. As an infant he was diagnosed as having a milk allergy and of necessity used soy milk instead of cow's milk. As an adult he assumed he had outgrown his milk allergy and daily used dairy products in large quantities.

He was symptom free by the fourth day of the

fast using non-chemically treated water only. A test meal of pasteurized cow's milk plunged him into the depth of a depression. Blood sugar was normal before and after the test. His symptoms were relieved by the following intravenous nutrients: Vitamin C 12.5 grams, B₆ 1000 mgs., Calcium Gluconate 10cc, Magnesium Sulfate 2 grams, Adrenal Cortical Extract 20 cc (double strength). Powdered Skim Milk, Cheddar Cheese, and American Cheese gave no symptoms. With Swiss Cream Cheese he was cold and sweaty. Dairy Butter evoked a severe depression. Cream Cheese was a favorite food which he frequently used. He loved and frequently used a Blue Cheese dressing containing Cream Cheese. Before the test for Cream Cheese began he was symptom free. Within fifteen minutes of the test meal for Cream Cheese symptoms began to develop. At first he felt like withdrawing from other people due to a contemplative and depressive feeling. Within another fifteen minutes he was severly depressed and withdrew from the hospital parlor to the seclusion of his room. He was overly reacting to sounds and sights and would cringe as if afraid of being attacked. At this point of one half hour after the test meal he was dissociated and had no memory of what happened around him. At two hours after the test meal he was fluctuating between extreme fright of environmental stimuli with no verbal communication and a comatose state of no response to sight and sound stimuli. His pulse was 123 and his blood pressure 170/110 and fluctuating with a pulse of 50 and blood pressure of 114/50. *At this point his blood sugar was 20 mg.%.* It was difficult to believe this and so the test was run four times. He was given Vitamin C 12.5 grams, B₆ 1000 mg., Calcium Gluconate 10cc, Magnesium Sulfate 2 grams, Adrenal Cortical Extract 20 cc (double strength). With this he awakened, was communicative, understood and was not frightened by environmental stimuli. He was too weak to stand. He had a pounding headache. His pulse was 80 and blood pressure 130/84. He was given 50 mEq. of Sodium Bicarbonate intravenously and his headache left. He still was too weak to stand and he complained of spots and indistinct vision. *His blood sugar was again taken and found to be 30mg.%.* He was given six teaspoons of beet sugar, a glass of pineapple juice, and several bites of chocolate cake. Prior testing had demonstrated him not be symptom reactive to cereal grains, beet or pineapple. Within thirty minutes his blood sugar was 160 mg.% and he was symptom free other than an apprehension for several hours that the symptom state could suddenly return . . .

The above described hypoglycemia occurring in response to a food test is the most severe and most prolonged I have observed. The assumption that these disordered carbohydrate reactions will be in response to carbohydrate only is not valid. Testing reveals that they occur to any type of food and that the central cause is that of being allergic to or allergic in a specific way to a specific food whether fat, protein or carbohydrate. In this case, the hypoglycemia response was Cream Cheese which is largely a protein and fat food [4].

Some interesting studies have shown the need of vitamin and/or megavitamin supplementation for hypoglycemia [5]. Experimentally induced pantothenic acid and Vitamin C deficiencies has led to a rapid disturbance in corticosteroid metabolism and ultimately to symptoms of adrenal insufficiency. And, of course, if there is adrenal dysfunction, proper blood sugar levels can be dramatically altered. The adrenal glands contain large amounts of vitamin A, but experiments to establish its place in adrenocortical function have been inconclusive.

It is important to realize that any vitamin supplementation for hypoglycemia must always be tailored to individual biochemical needs. The following daily amounts of vitamins have been suggested for hypoglycemia treatment. These requirements vary greatly among individuals:

Vitamin C	1 gram (3 times daily)
Vitamin A	25,000 IU (3 times daily)
Vitamin E	100 IU (3 times daily)
Vitamin B₁	10 mg. (3 times daily)
Vitamin B₂	10 mg. (3 times daily)
Vitamin B₃	100-150 mg. (3 times daily)
Vitamin B₆	20 mg. (3 times daily)
Choline	300 mg. (3 times daily)
Inositol	90 mg. (3 times daily)
Bioflavonoids	350 mg. (3 times daily)
Panthothenic Acid	100 mg. (3 times daily)
Folic Acid	.800 mcg. (3 times daily)
Hydroxycobalamin (B₁₂)	Weekly shots (1 cc: IM)

(Note: all vitamins should be taken 1 hour before meals)

Some Orthomolecular Physicians suggest that methionine be included in the list of nutritional supplements. In the computerized diet survey, practically all hypoglycemic patients are low in this nutrient. It is a methylater and one which is essential for the production of hormones, including adrenal cortical hormones.

A urine Diagnex Text should also be given to determine achlorhydria. If the patient has a deficiency of hydrochloric acid secretion, it is important to correct the disorder immediately, since the hypometabolic factors that have caused the hydrochloric acid secreting glands to atrophy and fail to function no doubt will also adversely affect other digestive enzyme secretions to a significant degree, which as we know, are necessary for the proper utilization and absorption of all nutrients.

Most Orthomolecular physicians will want to take a hair and/or blood analysis in order to determine the amounts of minerals that are synergistically working with vitamins and other nutrients inside the tissue cell. It is necessary for all the nutritional elements of the cell to be supplied for maximum efficiency and health. It is one thing to eat good food and take a lot of vitamins, but we also need all the essential minerals so that proper absorption and utilization of our other nutrients is accomplished. The hair analysis involves a couple of tablespoons of hair taken from the nape of the neck and sent to a laboratory. When properly interpreted, it gives the doctor information about deficiencies in important minerals or excessive amounts of harmful toxic elements like lead or mercury.

Adrenal Cortical Extract (ACE), 10-20 cc intra-muscular injection is also given to hypoglycemics once or twice each week for a period of time until improvement is noted. For the IM injection, most Orthomolecular Physicians use Lipo-Ace/1cc/IM. The IM injection is not as potent, but it tends to last longer. Since the adrenal gland produces hormones which are necessary for the metabolism of carbohydrates and for the raising of blood sugar levels, ACE, which is a natural extract of hormones taken from young calves' adrenals, has proven to be a useful "tool" for hypoglycemia treatment. ACE is not cortisone! The latter is a synthetically made hormone and represents only one cortical hormone of the adrenal gland. But over 50 different steroids have been identified from the adrenal cortex. If you give only one of the 50, you upset the natural balance among the various hormones. This threat to the hormonal homeostasis usually results in rather severe clinical contraindications. ACE treatment, on the other hand, contains all the naturally occurring corticosteroids; the hormone balance nature intended, therefore, is not altered in anyway by this form of Orthomolecular therapy. Accordingly, ACE contains none of the dangerous side effects so commonly produced by synthetic adrenal steroids. The theory behind the use of ACE is simply stated: It gives the adrenal glands a 4-8 hour rest in which time they can "recuperate" so to speak and thus regain their normal sugar metabolizing functions. Some Orthomolecular physicians also think that it is helpful to give their patients desiccated gland powder and/or tablets consisting of adrenal, liver, pituitary, pancreas and others. These glandular supplements act directly on all the patient's poorly functioning glands in a recuperative fashion.

It is frightening to think of the numbers of people suffering from undiagnosed hypoglycemia today. Due to many factors — environment, allergic, genetic, etc. — some people's ability to properly metabolize certain foods has been impaired. If their treatment is along the lines of symptomatic relief (i.e., shock, psychoanalysis, drugs), they are doomed to a miserable life. We cannot repress hypoglycemia with traditional methods: that is, we cannot tranquilize it, shock it, punish it, ignore it, and we most certainly cannot talk it down with cliches like "psychosomatic" or "nerves."

Today a few brave scientists are emerging who know that our human biochemical mechanism is an extremely complex delicately balanced dynamism of millions upon millions of chemical reactions. They also know that man, via the stress of poor diet and a hostile chemical environment, can easily upset this delicate homeostasis of his inherited biochemical being. It is up to Orthomolecular scientists to continue to search out the etiological reasons for the breakdown of nature's homeostasis. And it is very important that they do, for then instead of being incorrectly labeled and stigmatized as "psychoneurotic" or whatever, people will be properly diagnosed and treated, and thus will be given an opportunity to live a happy, healthy, and creative life of joy.

REFERENCES

1. *Low Blood Sugar: A Doctor's Guide to its Effective Control*, by J.F. Hurdle, M.D. (New York: Parker Publishers), 1970.
2. "The Significance of Selective Food and Chemical Stressors in Ecologic Hypoglycemia and Hyperglycemia," W.H. Philpott, M.D., *Journal: International Academy of Metabology, Inc.*, Volume V # I.
3. "Hypoglycemia and the New Breed of Patient," Alan Nittler, M.D., *Journal: International Academy of Metabology, Inc.*, Volume V, # I.
4. "The Significance of Selected Food and Chemical Stressors in Ecologic Hypoglycemia and Hyperglycemia," W.H. Philpott, M.D., *Journal: International Academy of Metabology, Inc.*, Volume V, # I.
5. "Effects of Vitamin Deficiency on Adrenal Cortical Function," A.F. Morgan, *Vitamin and Hormones*, 9: 162-204, 1951.

26
Domiciliary Chemical Air Pollution in the Etiology of Ecologic Mental Illness*†

THERON G. RANDOLPH

The importance of indoor or domiciliary chemical air pollution in relation to mental and related ills was presented on the program of the National Conference on Air Pollution in Washington, D.C. in 1962 [1]. That discussion will be quoted as an introductory summary of this presentation:

"Attempts to appraise the clinical significance of air pollution, as far as chemical exposures are concerned, must begin with the realization that there are two major divisions of the subject. One has to do with outdoor chemical air pollution, which you have heard discussed from various standpoints. Equally important is the subject of indoor chemical air pollution. In my experience, this indoor air contamination is such a frequent cause of chronic illness in susceptible persons that it must be evaluated and preferably controlled before one is justified in drawing deductions as to the clinical significance of chemical contamination of the outdoor atmosphere.

"Although outdoor chemical air contaminants enter homes located in contaminated areas, chemical air contamination arising within a patient's living sources of such contaminants are odors and fumes arising from leaking utility gas or the combustion products of gas, oil or coal. The gas kitchen range, gas panel heating units, and fuel-oil space heaters are the most significant, although appreciable air contamination is also derived from hot-air furnaces (irrespective of the type of fuel used), sponge rubber padding, bedding and upholstery, insecticides, paint odors, disinfectants, and various other odorous household materials. Contaminated air from the garage also often enters the house.

"These relatively constant sources of indoor chemical air pollution are rarely suspected as inciting and perpetuating causes of chronic illness. Only as patients are maneuvered in respect to these exposures may acute reactions be observed which demonstrate cause-and-effect relationships. For instance, on the

basis of observing clinical effects in moving patients in and out of their homes, and later, of maintaining the patient in his home but removing and replacing the gas kitchen range, over 800 such devices have been removed permanently from the homes of highly susceptible persons.

"A wide range of chronic illnesses result from such day-in and day-out hydrocarbon exposures. The most serious are depressions and other advanced psychotic states [2]. Lesser grade cerebral reactions manifest as mental confusion and brain fag as well as physical fatigue. Closely related manifestations are rheumatism, arthritis, myalgia, neuralgia, headache and related musculoskeletal and neurological syndromes. Any of the responses ordinarily considered as allergic, especially stuffy nose, coughing, bronchitis, bronchial asthma, are also commonly on the basis of susceptibility to airborne chemical contaminants.

"Finding and avoiding these home environmental incitants impinging on the physical and mental health of susceptible persons is opening a new experimentally orientated medical approach to many chronic illnesses."

Advanced mental illness as a manifestation of food allergy was reported preliminarily in 1950 [3]. The clinical importance of what came to be called the chemical susceptibility problem was first reported in 1952 [4]. Despite earlier suggestions that these two phenomena might be related, the full significance of domiciliary or indoor chemical air pollution was not reported as a demonstrable cause of depressions and related mental symptoms until 1955 [5]. The designation of ecologic mental illness as differentiated from psychiatrically interpreted mental illness was first applied in 1959 [6]. Observations of these relationships in extenso were reported in 1962 [2] and 1966 [7]. In the meantime, the over-all chemical susceptibility problem, of which domiciliary chemical air pollution is but one aspect, was written up in detail in 1961-1962 [8].

THE CLINICAL EFFECTS OF AIR POLLUTION

As might be expected, the first clinical manifestations associated with air pollution involved massive concentrations of

*Reprinted with permission: *The International Journal of Social Psychiatry*, Vol. XVI, No. 4, 1970.
†Sponsored by the Human Ecology Research Foundation.

ambient pollutants which were associated with a combination of predisposing geography (valleys containing heavy industry), meteorology (inversion and related absence of wind) and seasonal factors. Acute reactions largely limited to the respiratory tract and eyes predominated in the Meuse Valley, Donora and London catastrophies between 1930 and 1952.

Even in these acute air pollution episodes, it became increasingly apparent that individual susceptibility played a major role in determining the probability of reactions. Those with histories of bronchitis, bronchial asthma, emphysema and other respiratory complaints were most affected. Moreover, there was little question from a study of the epidemiology of these early episodes of the causal relationship between pollution of the ambient air and these acute localized effects.

With time and with increasingly sustained levels of air pollution, a growing concern was expressed that daily exposures to a wide range of chemicals — known to be toxic in greater concentrations — might also be contributing to chronic and more generalized effects. This possibility has been under increasingly active investigation for the past several years. But despite the accumulation of much analytical data, the twin problems of air pollution [9] and chronic illness [10] continue to multiply. Although these environmental and bodily dilemmas seem to be related from the epidemiologic and statistical standpoints, any interrelationship as far as the individual is concerned tends to remain more speculative than demonstrable.

From the ecologically oriented clinical experience of the writer, failure to demonstrate the etiological role of air pollutants seems to be largely attributable to the following: (1) Chronic illness involving ecologic relationships tends to be highly selective, inasmuch as individuality and susceptibility seem to be the cruxes of such an interrelationship. Individual susceptibility, in turn, enhances the impact of lesser exposures so that under these circumstances environmental factors become illness-inducing and illness-perpetuating. The problem is to demonstrate the existence of such relationships. (2) Since all portions of the body seem to be involved in these responses and since many portions of the environment are also suspected, any study of possible interrelationships must take into account the body as a reacting unit in response to its most intimate environment, namely, its intake of air, food and water. One cannot expect that an understanding of such an interrelationship — highly individualized to person and highly specific to parts of the environment — to yield to epidemiologic approaches and/or to analytical techniques of the type customarily employed by toxicologists and clinical investigators in studying aspects of the air pollution problem. Although biologic observations in animals may be helpful, these approaches also tend to be carried out under artificial rather than naturally occurring circumstances and to be highly analytical. Extrapolation of the results of such studies to those of human existence is fraught with hazard. (3) Whether or not a susceptible person succumbs to the hammering exposures of his potentially toxic environment and becomes chronically ill depends upon his adaptability. Efforts to demonstrate cause and effect relationships implicating the environment must be carried out in a manner which will reveal the existence of adapted, maladapted and non-adapted stages of specific reactions in the individual [11,12].

Full appreciation of the role of domiciliary chemical air pollution in mental illness awaited formulation of the concept of specific adaption in 1954, although this was not reported preliminarily until 1956 [11,12]. This concept and its practical application not only elucidated the developmental stages of the impingement of environmental exposures on susceptible persons, but it also led to the development of the technique by means of which these interrelationships are demonstrated [13,14]. This concept and related diagnostic technique — comprehensive environmental control followed by test reexposures [14] — will be described briefly before citing excerpts from illustrative case histories.

COMPREHENSIVE ENVIRONMENTAL CONTROL

One tends to remain adapted and relatively symptom-free initially when exposed constantly regularly and/or frequently to chemical air pollutants. Later, and apparently as a result of such sustained exposures, individual susceptibility increases. The impact of dosage is enhanced. Withdrawal type symptoms emerge. This gradual development beyond the ability of the afflicted person to maintain his adapted or partially adapted status by regular recourse to happenstance or arranged reexposures, is usually called the onset of the present illness. Since these increasingly troublesome withdrawal levels usually develop and manifest in the absence of any major variations in air pollutants, these are rarely suspected.

As susceptible patients were subjected to ecologically orientated techniques based on a working knowledge of the stages of specific adaptation, the following progressive levels of reaction were investigated: (1) Acute localized physical effects (rhinitis, bronchitis, asthma, eczema and gastrointestinal and other allergies). (2) Acute systemic effects (headache, fatigue, myalgia, arthralgia, neuralgia and other generalized physical syndromes). (3) Acute episodes of mental confusion, depression and more advanced cerebral and behavioral abnormalities. These alternating levels of reaction have been described elsewhere [2,15]. As chronic physical and mental syndromes were studied by means of comprehensive environmental control [14] reexposures induced diagnostically significant test reactions. It was during the course of these demonstrations that the dominant role of indoor chemical air pollution in the etiology of ecologic mental illness became apparent.

Irrespective of the stage of advancement of the process, the simultaneous avoidance of probable, potential and suspected environmental exposures reverts specifically adapted and maladapted states associated with chronic illness to maladapted stages in which reexposures induce acute test reactions. This program [14] is best accomplished by transferring a patient to an ecologic unit [16] of a hospital where maximal control of the intake and surroundings may be maintained. With fasting, avoidance of drugs and cosmetics and wearing only natural clothing while maintaining an intake of relatively less contaminated air and water, withdrawal effects are usually accentuated before they subside. Testing of previously avoided environmental exposures is carried out, incriminated exposures being avoided as detected. (1) Single commonly eaten foods, known not to have been significantly contaminated chemically [8], are tested first. (2) The cumulative ingestion of test-negative foods obtained from the commercial market, and presumably contaminated chemically in various ways, is then tested. (3) With the subject maintaining a test compatible intake of food and water and wearing compatible clothing, he returns successively to his home, work and avocations.

If a test reaction (an otherwise unexplained acute recurrence of reactive symptoms) occurs upon first returning home, either one of two courses if followed: (1) The most probable sources of domiciliary chemical air pollution are removed from the home temporarily, if this is possible. They are later returned singly, as the clinical effects of both maneuvres are observed. (2) The patient may again be removed temporarily to an environmentally controlled location and returned home a second time after certain probable sources of indoor chemical air pollution had been removed temporarily. Records of wind direction, velocity and visibility are kept throughout this home testing period as well as neighborhood activities which might increase pollution of the ambient air locally in order to aid the evaluation and differentiation of clinical effects arising from the entrance of outdoor polluted air into the home.

Other out-patient approaches in the evaluation of the chemical susceptibility problem are also helpful. In general, these are based on the same principle — namely, avoiding regular exposures temporarily and observation of the clinical response following both avoidance and reexposure. Clinical observations following a massive or rapidly absorbed exposure are also useful. A diagnostic technique of this type, the provocative hydrocarbon test employing synthetic ethanol [17] has been reported preliminarily. This and related approaches are being further investigated.

The program of comprehensive environmental control followed by test reexposures has been carried out in 3,000 patients since 1956. Approximately one-fifth of this group were studied because of their advanced mental and behavioral manifestations.

Excerpts from representative histories to illustrate the scope of the problem of domiciliary air pollution have been selected. In this selection the reader should be aware that these examples are taken out of context. The relationship of the exposure emphasized to the full range of other indoor and outdoor airborne chemical exposures as well as the other aspects of the chemical environment which commonly impinge on susceptible persons has been presented elsewhere [8]. Likewise, the levels of reaction occurring developmentally and in test responses have also been described in detail in other publications [2,15].

Fossil Fuels and Their Combustion Products

In general, air pollutants arising from gas utilities in the home constitute the greatest single source of air pollution. Since utility gas as well as the hot gaseous puffs from gas burning furnaces tend to rise, at times the worse polluted areas are those directly above such installations. Not uncommonly, a room in the attic or on the third or fourth floor may be the most offensive. Fumes arising from the storage and combustion of oil and coal are only slightly less troublesome, as has been explained elsewhere [8].

A young female artist, living in a basement apartment equipped with a gas stove, gas water heater, gas dryer and gas-fired furnace, had complained of feeling sluggish, tired and dizzy for as long as she could recall. Increasingly severe headaches, mental confusion and depression had developed more recently.

Improvement occurred in the hospital. Several acute crying spells with associated headache were induced after test feedings with single foods known not to have been significantly contami-

nated chemically, but the most severe and prolonged test reaction occurred after the first feeding of previously test-negative foods obtained from the commercial market and presumably contaminated chemically in various ways.

Although an immediate acute reaction occurred upon returning home, she moved to an enclosed porch heated electrically and remained relatively comfortable as long as she remained there. Recurrent symptoms upon returning to work necessitated changing her occupation.

Other than for seasonal hay fever, a young mother had been relatively well until the onset of her fourth pregnancy when she became increasingly tired, nauseated, achy and prone to recurrent hives and infections. Later, she developed bronchial asthma and following delivery profuse perspiration, persistent headache, myalgia, irritability and depression.

Severe headache occurred as a withdrawal reaction at the start of comprehensive environmental control. All chronic symptoms then subsided. Several reactions to common foods occurred. She became nauseated, vomited and was increasingly depressed following the first feeding of chemically contaminated foods. The gas stove had been removed while she was still in the hospital.

Although she was well upon starting for home, she became nauseated from traffic fumes and developed a severe headache on the way home. The first time that she used the gas drier, she became nauseated, shaky, headachy and depressed. Similar acute reactions occurred after exposures to hair spray and perfumes. Perineal itching followed the use of perfumed toilet paper and bathing in chlorinated water was also troublesome. She remains relatively well on her avoidance program, other than for acute reactions associated with inadvertant exposures, which controls major sources of domiciliary air pollution.

Child, age eight, who has always been subject to temper tantrums, became progressively tired and listless since moving into their new gas-fired warm air heated home containing a gas drier. He was first seen in mid-winter, having been an incorrigible behavior problem in home, school and neighborhood for the past three months. He attacked his mother, blaming her for all of his problems. He terrorized and beat up younger "playmates." The school officials said that he was not only uneducable but that his irritability, hyperactivity and fractious behavior disturbed the entire room. Psychiatric consultation and withdrawal from school had been recommended. Moreover, he had become increasingly disrespectful, hostile and sassy since the onset of the heating season. Corporal punishment had been tried and discarded.

Upon learning that an auxiliary gas-fired space heater had been installed in the wall of his bedroom the previous summer, his room was exchanged with his sister. Although his behavior improved, he still was too hyperactive and distraught to read comprehendingly. Under comprehensive environmental control, his pulse decreased from an average of 90 to 76, his behavior became normal in three days and he read incessantly — apparently for the first time with normal comprehension in months. Upon returning to school directly from the ecologic unit, his teacher was amazed at his model behavior. He developed a headache after returning home for lunch. Upon awakening the following morning, he complained of being tired and was pale with puffy eyes. By the end of the third day, he had reverted to his former tantrum-prone incorrigible self.

Although he remained well during the summertime after

removing the gas space heater and water heater, his former fractious behavior returned progressively with the onset of cold weather. By the end of November, all concerned had had enough. His father, an engineer, was convinced and finally removed the gas-fired warm air furnace, replacing it with a hot water system with combustion of fossil fuel outside the living quarters. Since this time, he has sustained an excellent scholastic and behavior record, except for recurrent reactions after exposure to massive amounts of chemically ambient air.

A middle-aged housewife and wife of an engineer complained of the "terrible Chicago weather" as the cause of her depression which worsened with the onset of cold weather each fall and persisted until warm weather in the spring. For several years she had spent winters in the South. However, her "winter depression" ceased in the hospital. Reactive depressions were induced following test feedings of given foods, but otherwise, she remained much more comfortable in the hospital than at home. Upon returning home, her headache, irritability and depression recurred. Her husband refused to remove the gas stove for a trial period on the theoretical assumption that turning off the gas at the point where it entered the house was sufficient. An acutely susceptible patient subject to sick headache and depression from gas exposures volunteered to test this house. The "tester" was well when she entered this home on the tenth day after the gas had been turned off; she lost her voice in ten minutes and within the next few minutes her eyes crossed and she lapsed into a stuporous depression. This was a convincing experience for all concerned!

Although this patient improved after complete removal of the stove and other gas appliances, she did not tolerate the "local weather" until moving into a new house constructed and furnished around this problem.

An engineer gradually came to the realization that his wife was not well in their gas-fired warm air heated home. Although she was improved in respect to her fatigue and depression after the elimination of specifically incriminated foods, maintenance therapy with house dust extract and especially following the removal of their gas kitchen range, depression in winter months remained troublesome. Suspicion of the house was strengthened by the fact that a volunteer "tester" became ill each time that she visited this home and that his son developed unexplained somnolence each time that he returned from college. Despite the installation of an extensive series of activated carbon and other filters in the heating system, his wife remained unwell and the "tester" again sickened when visiting this home — although the "tester's" reaction was less severe and more delayed.

Finally he sold this house and bought another only to find that neither of them felt well in one end of the new house; this was apparently related to a crack in the slab of that section which permitted chlordane, used in poisoning the soil for termite control at the time the house was built, to enter the living quarters. This house was also sold. He succeeded in building a new house in a semi-tropical area — an exceedingly difficult assignment — in which they both remained symptom-free except for an occasional reaction unrelated to home exposures.

A woman shopkeeper and golfer gradually lost her former muscular coordination with the development of alternating constipation and diarrhea, fatigue, headaches, irritability, mental confusion and intermittent periods of depression. All symptoms were accentuated in the mornings. With time, her depressions increased in frequency, depth and duration; they were usually initiated by a burst of energy associated with hyperactivity and ataxia and were followed by depression.

This pattern of symptoms was recapitulated after the ingestion of several common foods. After the specific food reactions came under better control, other points in her history became more apparent. Whereas formerly she had enjoyed cooking, she now detested it, noticing that she became sick shortly after entering the kitchen containing her gas stove. She not only improved following the elimination of the range, she now enjoyed cooking again and also noticed the impingement of several other lesser chemical exposures. But despite her high degree of susceptibility to inhaled chemical fumes, intolerance to chemical additives and contaminants of the diet has never been demonstrated.

A high school mathematics teacher became dull, dopey, confused and moderately depressed late each morning while at school. His classroom was located at the head of the stairs above the school cafeteria which contained many gas ranges. His symptoms improved when assigned to a room far removed from the cafeteria but did not cease until gas utilities were removed from his home.

One young mother who had complied with recommendations for removing gas utilities from her home, reported being irritable with the children and a tendency to be distraught and to cry when sitting in the living room. Despite the removal of a large plastic planter, her problem was only slightly improved. Further investigation revealed that the displaced gas water heater had been stored in the crawl space directly under her favorite davenport. With its removal to a detached garage, the emotionality in the parlor ceased.

Despite remodeling their home to comply with recommendations, another depressed patient continued to be less well in the new kitchen than elsewhere in the house. She only improved when all motors in the kitchen were quieted. This problem was handled by exteriorizing the motorized equipment of the electric refrigerator, electric freezer and electric water heater through the wall into an adjacent utility room.

A middle-aged spinster secretary living in a one-room apartment harboring a gas range improved in the course of comprehensive environmental control in the hospital only to suffer a severe "potato depression" in the course of testing major foods. Certain other foods were associated with lesser reactions. Although she was free of her long-standing depression at the time of discharge, she developed an acute depression the first night after returning home. She was advised to move from her apartment immediately. Instead, she remained, disregarded her diet instructions and came under the influence of a "friend" who persuaded her not to follow the medical advice she was receiving and to live normally." She deteriorated rapidly and committed suicide after a week.

An unemployed male in his forties living near a major source of ambient air pollution (a large paint factory) had been depressed for twenty years. When finally convinced of the correctness of the observation that he was less depressed when away from home and more depressed at home, especially when in the kitchen, the gas range and gas water heater were removed permanently. He seemed to be relatively improved. Being particularly well one day shortly following, he paid his physician an unscheduled visit to report his improvement — only to commit suicide the same evening. Apparently for the first time in months or years he became able to write the necessary messages and to organize the effort.

Solvents

Solvent exposures arising from evaporating paint, adhesives used in model building, cigarette lighters, fresh newspapers, cleaning fluids, etc. are more apt to be associated with acute than chronic reactions. However, if reexposures are sufficiently frequent, as in model building or in the use of artist's supplies, or sufficiently massive, as with extensive collections of newspapers and blueprints, chronic unexplained cerebral and behavior responses may result. Or if volatility is sustained, as from recently solvent-cleaned rugs, slowly evaporating paint and plastic surfaces, unexplained chronic reactions may also manifest.

A housewife who had been depressed for six years and who had been receiving prolonged psychiatric attention, improved following the avoidance of specifically incriminated foods and several chemical exposures. She found that she was much more comfortable when outside than when in her house, despite the elimination of several questionable furnishings. The major remaining problem was traced to the recent use of a solvent-containing adhesive employed in applying panels to the wall of a large room in the basement. Several months were required before she was comfortable in this part of the house.

A young bride, with a background of frequent colds, sore throats and occasional episodes of nausea and vomiting, became loggy, drowsy, listless and apathetic while refinishing furniture. The emotional aspects of the reaction were most troublesome in that she was alternately withdrawn and had suicidal thoughts and at other times was irritable, belligerent and ataxic.

Although she improved outside the house, persistence of residual symptoms prompted hospitalization. All symptoms subsided under controlled conditions. A few reactions to commonly eaten foods were demonstrated. The most marked test response followed the cumulative use of previously test-negative foods containing spray residues and other chemical additives and contaminants.

A housewife, subject to recurrent severe rhinitis, fatigue, headache, arthritis and moderate depression, improved greatly after avoiding specific food and chemical additives and contaminants of foods and the elimination of gas utilities from her home. Known to have been highly sensitive to house dust, her night clothing and bedding were treated with a petroleum hydrolysate recommended for controlling house dust exposures. Acute reactions consisting of severe rhinitis, sinusitis, abdominal cramps and headache with residual depression developed and persisted for several days. These symptoms occurred each time materials so treated were used and gradually subsided after their elimination.

Pesticides

Because of the frequency with which pesticides contribute to the domiciliary chemical air pollution problem and the extreme difficulty in removing such residues if a home has been so contaminated, at least persistent pesticides should never be used indoors.

A female merchandising manager complained of fatigue, aphasia, mental confusion and lapses of memory when the window of her office was open which admitted fumes from an adjacent parking lot. This problem was controlled by keeping the window closed. While on a Florida vacation she became moderately depressed while sleeping in the center of a large guest room. Two nights prior to departure, she was moved to a small room in which the head of her bed was in a corner of the room. Acute hallucinations which precluded sleep subsided immediately after leaving. It was learned in retrospect that both rooms had recently been decorated with insecticide containing paint. Her extreme intolerance to pesticides had been documented on several other occasions.

A female artist had been subject to attacks of coughing, wheezing and bouts characterized by faintness, weakness, numbness of her hands and extreme shortness of breath. She was found to be highly susceptible to several foods and especially to a wide range of chemical exposures. For a number of years after minimizing chemical exposures in her home and place of work and following a dietary program omitting several foods *per se* as well as chemical additives and contaminants of the diet, she remained well except for several acute episodes following accidental exposures. She remained particularly susceptible to perfumes and pesticides. On one occasion while sitting at her desk, she detected the odor of pesticide coming from the air conditioning ducts. Gasping, prickling sensations in her extremities, divergent vision and ataxia developed promptly and she collapsed on the way to the emergency room. Although she improved on oxygen therapy, a period of three weeks was required for complete recovery. This reaction was traced to workmen having sprayed bushes hiding the fresh air intake of the air conditioning system. Of approximately 600 others similarly exposed, she was the only one known to have sought emergency treatment. Upon another occasion she was hospitalized after eating commercially prepared broccoli, whereas broccoli known to have been grown in the absence of pesticides had been tolerated. She is also relatively intolerant to the constant levels of ambient air pollution and remains in better health since moving 100 miles away.

A middle-aged woman with a history of obstinate constipation, developed increasingly troublesome fatigue, headache, muscle and joint aching with pains in the chest, numbness of extremities, profuse perspiration and irritability and depression. There was some improvement after the elimination of the gas kitchen range, the avoidance of specifically incriminated foods and chemical additives and contaminants of food, but she again worsened after the coal-burning warm air furnace was converted to gas combustion.

Improvement occurred after moving to a new home constructed and furnished with the aim of controlling domiciliary air pollution. Severe headache, depression and related symptoms recurred immediately after a tenant in the basement apartment used an insecticide. Despite much cleaning, scrubbing and repainting, several months were required before the clinical effects attributed to the insecticide subsided.

Refrigerants and Propellants

It is sometimes difficult to distinguish the clinical effects arising from exposure to aerosolized pesticides, their solvent mixtures and the compressed gaseous propellant employed in most pressurized canisters. That the particular refrigerant and propellant that dominates the market may be a major source of illness-related domiciliary air pollution is illustrated by the following accounts.

An acutely depressed housewife, who had had several series of electroshock and insulin shock therapy, continued to be acutely depressed for the first three days of the program of comprehensive environmental control. Her almost continual crying then improved and she experienced no reactions when specific foods were tested. Acute depression recurred following the cumulative ingestion of test-negative chemically contaminated foods and also shortly after returning home. After the removal of all gas utilities from the home and following a diet and water supply omitting chemical additives and contaminants, she remained well for several weeks prior to the gradual recurrence of severe depression during a three month period. An attempt at suicide occurred during this time. On the clue that a post-prandial elevation of the pulse occurred following each meal of food which had been stored in the refrigerator, but not otherwise, the refrigerator was checked and found to contain a small gas leak. Upon questioning as to the probable duration of the leaking refrigerant, the repair technician suggested approximately three months.

An elderly woman had been subject to unexplained episodes of sudden loss of consciousness when in and about the kitchen. Although she improved as a result of the removal of the gas kitchen stove and gas water heater, the additional major cause of her unexplained falling spells was not determined until the electric refrigerator ceased to function because of the lack of its refrigerant. There were no further episodes after the removal of the defective refrigerator.

A retired secretary, complaining of gastrointestinal and genitourinary painful syndromes, denied depression. But after the induction of an acute depression starting five hours after the test feeding of wheat in which she cried for three hours, she then admitted being so depressed that she would go for days barely talking and unable to do her housework.

She lived in an all electric home except for a gas-fired hot water heating system with central air conditioning with fiberglass ducts. She became worse immediately upon coming home from the hospital. Exteriorizing the furnace in a small aluminum lined room helped. But despite avoidance of all synthetic drugs, specifically incriminated foods, chemically contaminated food and water supplies and the elimination of rubber and synthetic textiles, she did not remain well. Since acute reactions occurred each time the air conditioning system was turned on, the fiberglass duct system was replaced. She still reported an unusual odor when the system operated; this was finally traced to the slow leakage of refrigerant. Since the repairmen could not guarantee against leakage and since she remained less comfortable when the repaired system was operating than otherwise, the central system has since been discarded in favor of window units containing washable filters. Acute reactions also followed the operation of new television and radio sets until the "newness" gradually wore off after several months.

A physician and his hydrocarbon susceptible wife, prone to attacks of asthma, violently sick headaches and stuporous depressions, were visiting a technical exhibit when sprayed, without warning, with an allegedly harmless common propellant. Within a few minutes his wife became cross-eyed, ataxic, stuporous and lapsed into unconsciousness. The doctor spent the remainder of the day nursing his wife.

Rubber

Unexplained depression and related cerebral syndromes may be perpetuated chronically or precipitated acutely from air pollutants arising from the use of sponge rubber pillows, mattresses, upholstery, rug pads and typewriter pads, rubber backing of rugs and carpets and rubber-based paints. In the clinical experiences of the writer, house dust exposures induce less advanced clinical syndromes than the rubber bed which is so commonly employed in the control of dust pollution of the air.

At an early stage in the development of awareness of the chemical susceptibility problem, the writer attempted to work in a hospital unit in which sponge rubber pillows, mattresses and upholstered furniture were used exclusively as a means of dust control. Several patients failed to improve while hospitalized there. A few worsened and improved only after being transferred out. One patient, free of asthma, headaches, and depression when living in correctly engineered and furnished quarters, attempted to visit this area. She developed immediate coughing and dyspnea followed by a sick headache and an acute depression after only a few minutes exposure. Upon another occasion, the same syndrome developed as she entered the alleged "perfect home" of another patient; this reaction was traced to the inclusion of two overstuffed sponge rubber chairs in the living room.

An elderly female hydrocarbon susceptible patient, having many facets of this clinical problem, complained of insomnia, nocturnal restlessness and excessive perspiration with morning fatigue, aching and depression. This was a surprising development inasmuch as she had been relatively controlled for many previous years. It was finally learned that she was suffering from the "rubber bed syndrome," having relapsed to the use of these furnishings in a self-prescribed attempt to control her house dust allergy symptoms. These advanced constitutional manifestations subsided with substitution of cotton bedding.

An editor living in an electrically equipped home and complaining of fatigue, headache and associated mental confusion and mild depression, was no longer able to write editorials. He improved on the third day of comprehensive environmental control and reacted acutely to the test ingestion of several major foods. Although his response to the cumulative ingestion of chemically contaminated foods was questionable, he was later found intolerant to foods canned in lined tins. Recurrence of symptoms upon returning to his newly decorated home called attention to the sponge rubber upholstered furnishings and bedding. These were placed in a closed room for a week. His symptoms improved during this time and recurred promptly upon re-entering the storage room. With better control of the indoor chemical environment (removal of all sponge rubber), he acquired tolerance for several foods and regained his former mental acuity and physical vigor.

Plastics

Demonstrable home sources of air pollution also include plastic plants, flowers and toys, plastic furniture covers and plastic mattress covers, plasticized surfaces of fabrics and plastic containing textiles, plastic baggage and upholstery, plastic backing of rugs and carpets, plasticized wallpaper and plastic floors and walls (applied both with and without tar or solvent containing adhesives).

A middle-aged woman continued to have pains in her chest, to be arthritic and depressed when her food and chemical susceptibility problem had been worked out and she was maintained on a maintenance dosage of house dust therapy. The fact that her symptoms were accentuated in her home led to a house call. Six odorous plastic doors led from the central living room to various parts of the house. Her melancholia improved when the doors were removed, it recurred acutely when replaced temporarily prior to permanent removal.

A middle-aged secretary was admitted to the hospital because of generalized eczema. Although she denied depression, she admitted extreme nervousness and irritability when in reactions. Improvement occurred in the hospital and on each of several occasions when on vacations and other trips. Each time upon returning home she soon became worse.

Despite the simultaneous removal of the gas stove, plastic doors, plastic storage dishes for food and plastic and rubber furniture, symptoms continued and her pulse remained over 90. But after the additional removal of plastic tile lining the walls of both the kitchen and bathroom, her pulse dropped to the lower seventies. Upon first returning the gas range and before it became connected, she immediately felt nervous, jittery, tense and irritable. Her skin also flared acutely and her resting pulse went to 103. The range was then removed permanently. With control of the additional plastic exposures and the gas utilities she has remained relatively well.

A young housewife with a history of long standing fatigue, developed increasing post-partum depression after each of four pregnancies. She remained increasingly prone to chronic mental confusion and depression. After specific foods were identified and avoided and major sources of indoor chemical air pollution were eliminated (the warm air gas-fired furnace was replaced by hot water baseboard heating with the source of combustion of fuel located outside of the house, other gas utilities replaced, sponge rubber and most plastics removed), the chronic phase of reaction subsided. Thereafter she remained subject only to acute depressions when exposed intermittently. These included a stuporous depression characterized by prolonged crying after exposure to fumes of synthetic alcohol in physician's offices, to her husband when he used after shaving lotion, to visiting in other homes in which gas stoves were present and in talking for more than a few minutes on the telephone. The latter was helped by replacing the plastic telephone with an older less odorous bakelite model.

Textiles

Curtain and drapery materials containing plastic, synthetically derived textiles (with or without a plasticized surface), as well as chemically treated natural fabrics are major contributing factors to domiciliary air pollution. Synthetic floor coverings (with or without rubber and/or plastic backing) are particularly troublesome because of the relatively large surface involved. This problem is aggravated if installed over radiant heated floors. The treatment of fabrics for flame resistance, for mold retardation and with moth repellants also adds to the air pollution problem.

The medical problem of a young school teacher began with rhinitis but soon became associated with fatigue, headache, arthritis and depression. As she became increasingly depressed, her upper respiratory symptoms subsided. A "nervous breakdown" two years earlier had been treated successfully with electroshock

therapy. The recent recurrence of jitteriness, nervousness, insomnia and increasing depression precluded working and prompted her hospitalization.

She improved under comprehensive environmental control, reacted positively to certain foods but the most severe depression followed the initial feeding of chemically contaminated foods. She was well when she returned to her bedroom from which all cosmetics, plastics and rubber had been removed for the purpose of testing her reaction to the Acrilon carpeting which extended throughout her home. The first few hours in this room she became increasingly tense, nervous and hyperactive. She recalls being extremely confused at 3:00 a.m. At 5:00 a.m. her husband found her in a state of agitated depression and arranged for immediate hospitalization. She claimed to feel more relaxed on the way to the hospital.

She now recalled that her initial nervous breakdown occurred the first winter after obtaining the Acrilon carpeting. The carpeting was removed immediately. There was no trouble on returning the second time but she became groggy and confused each time that she attempted to wear her Nylon under garments. She also noticed a persistent headache, backache and a dazed sensation at school except when in the teacher's lounge. Inquiry revealed that the lounge was the only area not treated regularly with a deodorant. As mental confusion and depression ceased to exist, her rhinitis became more troublesome. In retrospect, she regarded the synthetic carpeting as the major health problem in her new home but she did not remain well until all gas utilities were also removed.

A middle-aged medical supply worker had had a satisfactory degree of relief as a result of the avoidance of specific foods and particulate inhalant exposures. She reported an unexplained recurrence of fatigue, aching and depression certain mornings, starting a few days after Christmas. The colder the weather, the worse the problem. Questioning finally brought out the fact that she had acquired a new Dacron bedspread for Christmas and that she had had it on her bed ever since. On warm nights, it was left over the end of the bed, but on cool nights, it was also used as a spread. Although removal of the bedspread helped, she remained subject to low grade symptoms. These did not subside until after all Dacron had been removed from her wardrobe.

A physician's wife, subject to bronchial asthma, sick headaches and stuporous depressions, purchased a new pile of bedsheets. Extreme nervousness, insomnia and delayed irritability, fatigue and mild depression developed each time that she attempted to sleep between these sheets, despite having washed them repeatedly. It was then learned that these bed linens had been plasticized. Seconds, that had escaped the final plasticizing treatment had been tolerated.

Perfumes and Hair Sprays

Hair spray (a solvent-perfume-gum mixture) and perfumes are easily the most troublesome personal exposures contributing to domiciliary air pollution and responsible for acute or chronic mental and behavioral disturbances.

An airline stewardess subject to depression was highly intolerant to hair sprays and perfumes. Upon several different occasions when working in close quarters with others or when exposed to someone spraying their hair, she would become acutely ill. Another similarly afflicted patient was riding in an airplane seat behind a woman who sprayed her hair. The hypersensitive patient developed an acute stuporous depression and required assistance in leaving the plane.

A teacher was determined to complete her tenure for retirement but was in difficulty because of chronic respiratory and gastrointestinal symptoms, and especially, fatigue, headache, myalgia and mild depression. Although she had been able to control her home exposures satisfactorily by eliminating gas utilities, sponge rubber and odorous plastics, she continued to have a major problem in connection with school exposures. The exposures to perfumes, hair sprays and hair oils (worn by her high school students) were especially effective in maintaining her daily headaches and symptoms of depression. These chronic reactions became nearly incapacitating toward the end of each week but by the start of a new week she would be relatively better.

Creosote, Tar-containing Adhesives, Lysol, Bleaches, Ammonia, Moth Balls and Miscellaneous Materials

Although creosote or carbolic acid contamination of a home is uncommon, when it does occur it presents a serious problem. Chlorine containing bleaches, ammonia and certain other odorous cleaning materials are also lesser causes of depressions and other lesser reactions occurring in susceptible persons. Moth balls and other moth repellants containing trichlorbenzene are also potentially hazardous.

A young father of several children built a "do it yourself" house, completing much of the interior after moving in. However, during the first winter he realized that something about this house was not for him, as he became progressively tired, achy and depressed when home and relatively better elsewhere. Moreover, his wife and children complained of frequent colds and were far less well in the new quarters. He had made the mistake of creosoting the sleepers (protection against termites) which were adjacent to the radiant heating elements in the ceilings of the bedrooms. Not only was there an unpleasant odor of creosote in the house which could not be dissipated, but the severity of his illness barely enabled him to complete its construction. All members of this family improved healthwise after moving.

Another young depressed female patient who improved remarkably following the elimination of the gas utilities in her home, failed to remain well after the rough wooden exterior of their home had been treated with creosote. She improved when away from this house temporarily and worsened upon returning. Maximal improvement did not occur until building and furnishing a new home in keeping with the basic principles of minimizing indoor chemical air pollution.

A young housewife with the complaints of severe chest pain, nervousness, tremulousness, sighing dyspnea, insomnia, headache, fatigue and intermittent crying spells and who had received both insulin and electroshock therapy, had not suspected her gas range or other home exposures. In more extreme reactions, she was extremely fearful of being left alone, literally clinging to her husband as he left for work. After the detection and avoidance of specifically incriminated foods and her attention had been called to this possibility, she noticed that she felt better outside the kitchen and worse during and following meal preparation. On the basis of further improvement when the stove was removed tempo-

rarily and accentuated symptoms when it was returned, it and other gas burning utilities were removed permanently. She has not only remained relatively well for the past fifteen years but during this interim has developed a gradually increasing tolerance for chemical exposures. Maximal improvement, however, did not occur until she moved from her house which was constructed with radiant hot water heating in floors over which vinyl tiles had been laid with an asphalt containing adhesive.

Depressions in another partially worked up middle-aged woman were relatively improved on vacation and accentuated at home despite avoidance of specifically incriminated foods, treatment with specific extracts and the avoidance of major sources of indoor air pollution as far as these were known. This unexplained problem occurred on a year-around basis. No apparent cause could be found until making a house call in their country house. The hunter in the family harbored seven large dogs in the basement of this home. Once a week the cement floor of the basement was washed down with a phenol-containing disinfectant in order to "decrease" the dog odor in the house. As the phenol odor disappeared with cessation of this practice, the patient's spirits improved proportionally.

A depressed middle-aged housewife reported being relatively well outdoors in the country but less well in the house. She seemed to be especially prone to a recurrence of her depression when in the kitchen and particularly in the corner of the kitchen near the stairs leading to the cellar. Although her depressions were more troublesome in the winters, they also occurred in all seasons.

Examination of the cellar revealed no obvious reason for this except for the presence of an oil-fired warm air heating system. However, on projecting shelves extending from each of the stairs to the second floor, directly above those to the basement, were stored several cases of chlorine-containing scouring powder. Although she is still not entirely well, especially when she spends much time in the house during the winter season, presumably related to the heating system, she has been relatively improved since storing this source of chlorine exposure in an outlying building.

A relatively young female theatre ticket seller became too confused, tremulous and depressed to work. However, the more she remained home, the more depressed she became. Although never well at home, she seemed to be worse after sitting in the living room.

Upon entering this home on a house call, the writer was immediately struck by the odor of moth balls. Upon sitting down on the davenport, he seemed to be "perfused with mothballness." Sticking his hand between the cushions, he came up with two moth balls. Some fifty more napthalene moth balls of various sizes were found as the three cushions were removed. They were also found in the other two overstuffed chairs.

When questioned as to why she had used so many, she seemed quite unaware that she had, simply saying that she added some from time to time when cleaning. She seemed to be equally astounded at the total number found. Needless to say, correcting this massive napthalene exposure was beneficial.

Adjacent Areas

There are subtle distinctions between the arbitrary divisions of domiciliary and ambient chemical air pollution that relate to this problem. These include air pollution arising from an adjacent garage as well as sources in the immediate vicinity of the home. Contributing to the latter are: mosquito abatement fogging and spraying; insecticide treatment of trees, lawns and gardens; herbicide treatment of lawns and gardens; decelerating fumes at street intersections and bus stops; vents of gas dryers and chimneys of adjacent dwelling; pesticides employed on adjacent golf courses, parks and playgrounds and in nearby greenhouses; fumes from adjacent tarred roofs, parking lots, alleys and roads; exhausts from gasoline-driven lawn mowers; smoke from burning previously sprayed leaves; and, incinerator smoke.

A nun complained of involuntary somnolence in chapel each morning. Knowing her tendency to snore, associates arranged to sit closely on either side, elbowing her on the slightest indication of snoring. These morning stupors were resolved by removing the parish cars from the garage beneath the chapel. Somnolence recurred as a test reaction when the cars were returned.

A school superintendent was considering retiring prematurely because of morning headache, mental confusion and depression. His problem was also solved by parking his automobile on the street. His depression and related symptoms recurred when his car was parked in the garage under his bed.

A housewife, subject to intermittent depressions, became acutely depressed each time a gasoline lawn mower was used. She was also extremely intolerant to inhalation of diesel odors and evaporating paint, developing acute recurrences of depression each of several times after such exposures.

Seasonally Accentuated Domiciliary Air Pollution

It was long assumed that winter-accentuated illness was in some way related to infection, probably attributable to greater contagiousness in closed quarters. However, increased proneness to develop infection and the wide range of respiratory manifestations in individuals reacting to house dust, animal danders and other particles to which susceptibility exists and to which exposures are also increased in wintertime has been receiving increasing attention. Whatever the precise explanation, the tendency for a relatively increased incidence of winter illness has long been recognized.

Since the advent of air conditioning, there has also been a progressive increase in summer-accentuated illness [18]. Although statistics are not available to support this clinical impression, this problem seems to focus in individuals presenting manifestations of susceptibility to chemical exposures [8]. Although mechanical filters tend to diminish the relative exposure to pollens and other noxious airborne particles, passing the same air repeatedly over the cooling coils of the air-conditioner actually increases exposure to chemical fumes arising from within the domicile. In addition, this air is frequently fouled additionally by hexachlorophene-treated filters, oil-impregnated glass wool filters, plastic duct systems or the fiberglass linings of metal ducts or adhesives employed in installing them and the volatility of motors of the system. Some persons seem to be especially susceptible to gas fueled air conditioning, although the exact source and degree of presumed gas leakage has not been identified.

A middle-aged female writer, with a long history of depression and related less advanced ecologic disturbances, had exhausted the medical and psychiatric care in her community. Upon one occasion she was referred to "another" psychiatrist, only to be told to her astonishment, that he had already seen her as a patient a year previously. For the past several years, her depression had precluded writing.

She was found to be highly susceptible to a wide range of common foods and chemical exposures. Although she has become productive again and remains reasonably well in her correctly engineered and furnished apartment and home, she becomes acutely depressed when attempting to visit gas air-conditioned homes, stores and theatre. If she is to remain consistently productive as a writer, it is necessary that such exposures be avoided during summer months.

Pine

Naturally occurring hydrocarbons, especially materials of conifir origin, have long been suspected of causing reactions in susceptible persons. Christmas tree bronchitis in children is the best known. The over-all relation of pine to other aspects of the chemical susceptibility problem [8], is based on the alleged conifir source of the coal, oil and gas deposits. The subject of reactions to naturally occurring terpenes is also receiving increasing attention [19].

A physician's wife and former cosmetics saleswoman, who had followed the usual course of developing localized reactions, systemic manifestations and increasing depression, was reported in detail previously [8]. Among various other demonstrated environmental causes, she was found to be extremely susceptible to evergreen Christmas decorations, to fumes from burning pine, to various pine-scented cleaning preparations and, for a time, her summer accentuated symptoms remained unexplained. These were later traced to the pine paneling of the interior of her summer cottage.

Upon one occasion, the airline stewardess, previously referred to, was forced to move from one apartment to a more acceptable one because of a recurrence of crying and other symptoms of depression each time that she remained in the kitchen for more than a few minutes. There was a distinct odor of pine in this kitchen, traceable to the pine lining of all kitchen cupboards. Her extreme degree of intolerance to pine-scented cleaning materials, turpentine-containing paints and other sources of pine was well known. She failed to improve until moving from this apartment.

The middle-aged wife of a judge, also subject to various lesser reactive manifestations as well as depression, was found highly intolerant to specific foods and a wide range of chemical exposures, including chemical additives and contaminants of foods. A distinctive feature of her case was the extreme degree of susceptibility to chlorinated water and several brands of treated bottled water. Her chronic symptoms did not subside in the hospital until placed on untreated water taken directly from a spring.

Her depression and related manifestations recurred upon returning home and persisted despite the elimination of all readily removable sources of domiciliary air pollution. Her problem was traced to extensive pine paneling. Maximal improvement did not occur until after moving to a new home which had been built around the knowledge of this developing field.

Tobacco Smoke

Tobacco smoke, to which individual susceptibility is a common occurrence, obviously contributes to domiciliary air pollution. Although there is no question of its localized and systemic effects [20], the contribution of tobacco smoke to the etiology of frank pyschoses has not been clearly established [20]. In the writer's opinion, its over-all effect in respect to cerebration and mental acuity is not minimal, especially in highly susceptible persons.

A woman, age 51, complained of chronic coughing, at times associated with vomiting. She was also subject to fatigue, headache, extreme nervousness, muscular incoordination and a gradually increasing level of depression. She had smoked a package of cigarettes daily for many years and stated that she had never been able to stop. With the simultaneous avoidance of tobacco and other materials in the hospital diagnostic program, she developed a violently severe headache with an associated mild depression. This withdrawal reaction subsided after three days and she remained free of headache for the first time in five years.

She experienced a sharp reaction to tomato (headache) and potato (immediate vomiting and delayed headache and depression). Both of these foods belong to the same botanical family as tobacco. Potato had long been her favorite food to which she had also been addicted. There was no obvious reaction on returning home. She did note, however, that her muscular coordination, as evidenced by her ability to play the piano and to drive her car, was greatly improved. Five days after being home, she smoked three cigarettes. Intense ringing of her ears developed immediately and she felt progressively nervous, jittery and headachy. She slept restlessly and the following morning complained of a stiff neck and depression which persisted for an additional two days.

A middle-aged business man was worried about his increasing depression which was giving him a pessimistic outlook and his impaired muscular coordination which was interfering with his golf game.

He was found sensitive to wheat and several other common foods. With the avoidance of smoking and incriminated foods, both his depression and incoordination improved. Following the avoidance of cigarettes, he noticed marked intolerance to tobacco smoke encountered in the course of business conferences. The day following such an exposure, he remained dopey and mentally lethargic. Up to two days might be required for complete recovery from the negative thinking, forgetfulness and general dullness following a massive tobacco smoke exposure.

Several years later, he drifted into an increasing level of low-grade depression; this improved following identification and avoidance of potato and major sources of chemical air pollution in the home.

Another tobacco addicted business man who had been unable to stop previously, abstained with the following characterization of his withdrawal: "The most difficult aspect of avoiding cigarettes is the fact that it nearly drives one out of his mind in that he is unable to think connectedly. The first day was the worst, but this is exactly four days without a cigarette and I am still mentally foggy and having much trouble."

Occupational Exposures

Although many occupational exposures are major contributors to indoor chemical air pollution, ordinarily these are not major factors in domiciliary chemical air pollution except as a chemically contaminated person and/or his clothing foul the home premises and as occupationally induced acute reactions initiate and accelerate the course of the chemical susceptibility problem.

The young wife of a railroad engineer became depressed each time that she washed his diesel oil-soaked clothes. Laundering these elsewhere helped. Merely wearing his work clothes home soon resulted in a similar reaction. Although taking a bath and changing to clean clothes in the roundhouse was beneficial, the few times that he short cut this decontamination process by not shampooing his hair were associated, after a night in a common bed, with morning accentuated symptoms in his wife.

She then began suspecting her brother-in-law, who lived next door and who had the habit of visiting their home Sunday mornings. Inasmuch as she was responsible for cleaning his house, upon the writers' advice, she hid his aftershaving lotion. Her Sunday afternoon depressions ceased. Disbelieving this alleged relationship, he deliberately reverted to the former practice occasionally, confirming it blindly.

A similar experience occurred in the young wife of an incense manufacturer. Despite taking all of the above precautions, he exhaled a sufficient amount of incense fumes upon returning home to be moderately troublesome in his hypersusceptible wife.

A young woman in previous excellent health, sustained a massive exposure to the fumes of burning polyurethane solution as this was spilled accidentally on a hot electric heating unit in the course of her position as a laboratory technician in an automobile manufacturing plant. She vomited after a few minutes, felt faint and lapsed into temporary unconsciousness. Despite repeated attempts to return to this position, she was unable to do so after this experience. Each time, she either developed acute headache, nausea, vomiting and, sometimes, unconsciousness or after sustained work exposures, developed chronic fatigue, headache, mental confusion and depression which precluded continuing. Moreover, the process spread rapidly to involve many related aspects of the man-made chemical environment.

She improved on the hospital comprehensive environmental control program, but failed to react either to foods *per se* or to chemical additives and contaminants of the diet or water supply. Although she remains comfortable when staying in her environmentally controlled home, she is highly tolerant of traffic fumes and many related chemical exposures which precludes visiting urban centres. She also remains unemployable.

A single young man, whose job was to disassemble fuel-pump carburetor portions of airplane engines, was the only one of a number of employees who was able to handle this position without developing a dermatitis. After several months on this job, he began hearing voices and developing paranoid behavior.

All manifestations ceased while on a vacation in the country but returned promptly each time he started to work again. By this time, however, "psychotic" manifestations did not cease as he left this employment. The continued ability of people to read his thoughts embarrassed him. In the interim he had become intolerant to various exposures in his home — especially the fumes emanating from his brother-in-law's printing press. Being unable to sleep in the house, he first tried sleeping in his car, then in a house trailer heated with bottled gas — all to no avail.

Although his symptoms improved in the hospital, he did not become entirely free of auditory hallucinations. He reacted to several common foods and, especially, to chemical additives and contaminants of the diet. He reverted promptly upon leaving the hospital and was declared unemployable as a result of several unsuccessful efforts at other jobs. After threatening his brother-in-law with physical harm, he was hospitalized in a state mental institution where he still remains as a "trustee."

DISCUSSION

It should be reemphasized that no single case report has been presented completely. They have been selected to illustrate the following specific points: the scope of the chemical environment contributing to domiciliary air pollution; the tendency for susceptibility to involve multiple environmental materials — other chemical agents as well as specific foods and other substances; inter-relationships between physical and mental syndromes; the representative range of manifestations of ecologic mental illness; and, how patients are specifically diagnosed and treated.

Many aspects of the chemical air pollution problem were not presented, especially the role of ambient air pollution in health or other aspects of indoor chemical air pollution, such as exposures associated with public places, many other occupations and avocations as well as chemical exposures associated with enclosed vehicles.

Because of the relative frequency of domiciliary chemical air pollution, it should be evaluated before assuming that a given manifestation arising from the inhalation of airborne exposures is on the basis of ambient air pollution, occupational air pollution or even personal air pollution (e.g., tobacco smoke). In general, even the possibility of domiciliary air pollution has not been considered in these contexts.

No attempt was made to correlate these finding with psychiatric observations and interpretations. Approximately one-third of the patients presented had previously been under psychiatric care. A few were referred by psychiatrists. It might be mentioned that the multiplicity of complaints of patients demonstrated to have ecologic mental illness and related physical syndromes is characteristic. Indeed, this type of history suggests the possibility of an ecologic disturbance.

Neither should one assume, in view of the relative frequency of ecologic disturbances, when cases are screened from the standpoint of ecologically oriented medical procedures, that a given manifestation is on the basis of psychogenic factors or attributable to other persons or social situations unless such relationships can be demonstrated. The position is taken that causality in mental illness is best left unassigned unless it may be demonstrated. This may be stated differently. When considering the question of cause and effect in mental illness, let us give primary consideration to apparent inter-relationships between a given individual and influences external to that person which are demonstrable and reproducible.

Although the treatment of ecologic mental illness is basically restrictive, which is sometimes not feasible for economic or for other reasons, in those instances where such a program may be applied, the results are generally good. However, this statement is based on representative cases, inasmuch as statistics supporting such a conclusion are not yet available. In view of the newness of this approach — the so-called ecologic orientation as applied to mental illness — it seems best at this time merely to report representative findings. Comparison of the over-all results with other medical approaches to the same subject will await future studies.

There is one aspect of this restrictive therapeutic approach to the treatment of chronic mental illness which should be covered by a few general statements. Both patients and their physicians may be disturbed by the extreme lobility of response, or reaction proneness, of recently diagnosed patients who are following a specifically restricted program. This initial non-adapted or hyperacute stage, in which relatively small specific exposures induce relatively severe reactions, may give the impression that the afflicted individual is less well off than when specifically exposed regularly and frequently. This is really a distinction between intermittent acute illnesses and chronic illness. The latter favors the perpetuation of chronic symptoms, their gradual increase in severity and the possibility of complications and eventual disability.

Another point has to do with prophylaxis. It should be apparent from this presentation that the home contains many potential, if not actual, hazards to health, many of which have received little general attention. If the health hazards of the constituent sources of exposure contributing to domiciliary air pollution could be recognized more widely, dangers inherent in the continued use of certain devices and accepted practices might soon become general information. This would entail a much wider application of the principles of ecologically oriented medical practices than currently. In such an event, it could be anticipated that the public demand for a greater degree of protection would make itself felt as far as public health policies and governmental regulations are concerned.

SUMMARY

Ecological mental illness is differentiated from pschiatrically interpreted mental syndromes by the ability of ecologically orientated medicine to demonstrate cause and effect relationships.

Domiciliary air pollution is more important than ambient air pollution in the etiology of ecologic mental illness.

The gas kitchen stove is the most hazardous device in the American home in contributing to domiciliary air pollution. Following closely are gas-fired fuel oil space heaters, gas dryers, gas-fired warm air furnaces and other fossil fuel burning utilities located within the home. Other major contributing exposures are pesticides; solvents and solvent-containing paints, adhesives and hair sprays; tar containing adhesives; rubber-based paints and sponge rubber bedding, upholstery and padding; plastic constructional materials, toys and furnishing; synthetic carpeting, upholstery, curtains and clothing; certain other cosmetics, pine, creosote, phenol and many others including tobacco smoke. Improper home construction permitting access of garage fumes to the house is important. More intermittent exposures occurring while visiting other homes, public places and occupational aspects are apt to be more readily recognized.

The crux of these relationships is individual susceptibility which builds up insidiously as a result of cumulative exposures, enhances the impact of domiciliary airborne substances and accounts for their selective impingement on the health and behavior of occupants of the home.

Full appreciation of domiciliary chemical air pollution awaited the development of: (1) The concept of specific adaptation which helps to explain the interrelationships between a susceptible person and this impingement of his everyday environment. (2) A full appreciation of what constitutes man's chemical environment.

Ecologic mental illness usually culminates after a long history of multiple complaints which manifest initially as lesser localized physical and/or systematic disturbances. Such chronically ill persons and/or their most immediate associates are commonly maligned by the application of speculative interpretations of causality which are not amenable to proof.

Treatment consists principally of the avoidance of incriminated exposures.

REFERENCES

1. Randolph, T.G.: *Proc. National Conference on Air Pollution.* U.S. Department of Health, Education and Welfare. Public Health Service Publication No. 1022, U.S. Government Printing Office, Washington, D.C., 1963, p. 157.

2. Randolph, T.G.: *Ecologic Mental Illness — Levels of Central Nervous System Reactions.* Proc. Third World Congress of Psychiatry, Vol. 1, Montreal, Canada, Univ. of Toronto Press, pp. 379-384, June 1961.

3. Randolph, T.G.: "Allergic factors in the etiology of certain mental symptoms." *J. Lab. & Clin. Med.,* Dec. 1950, 36, 977.

4. Randolph, T.G.: "Sensitivity to Petroleum: Including its derivatives and antecedents." *J. Lab. & Clin. Med.,* Dec. 1952, 40. 931-932.

5. Randolph, T.G.: "Depressions caused by home exposures to gas and combustion products of gas, oil and coal." *J. Lab. & Clin. Med.,* Dec. 1955, 46, 942.

6. Randolph, T.G.: "Ecologic mental illness — Psychiatry exteriorized." *J. Lab. & Clin. Med.,* Dec. 1959, 54, 936.

7. Randolph, T.G.: "Clinical ecology as it affects the psychiatric patient." *Internat. J. Social Psychiatry,* Autumn, 1966, 12, 245-254.

8. Randolph, T.G.: "Human ecology and susceptibility to the chemical environment." *Ann. Allergy,* 1961, 19, 518-540, 547-677, 779-799, 908-929; and *Human Ecology and Susceptibility to the Chemical Environment.* Springfield, Illinois; Thomas, 1962.

9. Stern, A.C. (Ed.): *Air Pollution,* New York: Academic Press, Inc., Vol. 1-3, 1968.

10. Rapaport, H.G.: "Chronic Illness." *Ann. Allergy,* 1968, 26, 230-232.

11. Randolph, T.G.: "Specific Adaptation Syndrome." *J. Lab. & Clin. Med.,* Dec. 1956, 48, 934.

12 Randolph, T.G.: *The Role of Specific Adaptation in Chronic Illness.* Submitted for publication.

13. Randolph, T.G.: "A third dimension of the medical investigation." *Clinical Physiology,* Winter, 1960, 2, 1-5.

14. Randolph, T.G.: "An ecologic orientation in medicine: Comprehensive environmental control in diagnosis and therapy." *Ann. Allergy,* 1965, 23, 7-22.

15. Randolph, T.G.: *Stimulatory and Withdrawal Phases and Levels of Chronically Occurring and Experimentally Induced Ecologic Mental Disturbances.* Program, 2nd International Congress of Social Psychiatry, August, 1969. Submitted for publication.

16. Randolph, T.G.: "The Ecologic Unit." *Hospital Management,* March 1964, 97, 45-47, and April, 1964, 46-48.

17. Randolph, T.G.: "The provocative hydrocarbon test, Preliminary report." *J. Lab. & Clin. Med.,* Dec. 1964, 64, 995.

18. Randolph, T.G.: "Man-made seasonal sickness." *J. Lab. & Clin. Med.,* 1963, 62, 1005-1006.

19. Binkley, E.L., Jr.: *Provocative Hydrocarbon Testing and Treatment, Terpenes — Naturally Occurring Hydrocarbons.* Presented on the Program, 4th Annual Meeting, Society for Clinical Ecology, Washington, D.C., April 1969.

20. Larson, P.S., Haag, H.B., and Silvette, H.: *Tobacco, Experimental and Clinical Studies.* Baltimore: The Williams & Wilkins Company, 1961.

27
The Eyes' Dual Function*
Part I

JOHN OTT

Webster's *New International Dictionary*, Second Edition, defines ophthalmology as the science which treats of the structure, functions, and disease of the eye. Traditionally, however, this seems to have been applied only to the visual aspects of the eye, possibly because until recently it was not generally recognized that the eye possessed a dual function.

Relatively recent studies suggest that the functions of the eye do go further than strictly vision and raise the question as to whether any other function should be a part of ophthalmology.

The existence of a direct connection between a photo receptor mechanism of the retina independent of vision, and the hypothalamic nuclei has been the subject of a number of discussions. The first outstanding work was that of William Rowan [1], in the early 1920's, who demonstrated that seasonal variations in the length of daylight and darkness are responsible for bird migration, as well as the mating period for some species.

In 1932, Dr. Wendell J.S. Krieg [2], professor of anatomy at Northwestern University Medical School, Chicago, described the retinal hypothalamic pathway of the albino rat. He gave an excellent review of the literature from 1872 when Meynert first described the basal optic ganglia, or supraoptic nuclei, in man.

In France the work of Benoit [3] and Assenmacher with ducks has suggested that light of different colors or wavelengths reaching the eye induces nerve impulses which affect neurosecretory cells in the hypothalamus and control gonadotropic activity. In England, Bissonnette [4] and Zuckerman [5] have done similar work with ferrets. The important point here is primarily that ferrets are mammals.

Today it is common practice in the poultry industry to increase egg production by lengthening the short daylight hours of winter with artificial lights. This response is due to the light entering the eyes and stimulating the pituitary gland.

In the May, 1964, issue of the *Journal of Vision Research*, Dr. T. Shipley [6] of the Bascom Palmer Eye Institute, University of Miami School of Medicine, Miami, Florida, stated, "Thus, not only is light itself of autonomic importance, but confirming Benoit and Assenmacher (1955) its effects are wavelength dependent. This dependency must somehow be mediated by neurochemical channels connecting the photoreceptors with the endocrine system. And these could involve photoreceptors with no visibility function."

In the March 1964 issue of *Science*, Vol. 143, there is an article entitled "Melatonin Synthesis in the Pineal Gland: Effect of Light Mediated by the Sympathetic Nervous System," by Richard J. Wurtman, Julius Axlerod, and Josef E. Fischer of the National Institute of Mental Health, Bethesda, Maryland, which states that, "Removal of both eyes resulted in a complete loss of the capacity of the pineal gland to respond to altered illumination with the accompanying changes in weight or HIOMT activity. This indicates that the action of light upon the rat pineal gland is not direct, but is mediated by retinal receptors." Such references to a photoreceptor mechanism that is wavelength-dependent and still independent of vision, but without any identification as to what or where it might be in the eye, are becoming more frequent.

More recently, Dr. Robert Y. Moore [7] of the University of Chicago and co-workers, have published a paper (February 1968) which states, "Alteration of the normal diurnal cycle of environmental lighting has effects upon gonadal function in a number of species . . . Most commonly, such effects have been attributed to a direct alteration of pituitary function mediated by central visual connections and the hypothalamo-hypophysial system. Evidence recently has been accumulated, however, indicating that the pineal also may function in mediating the neuroendocrine effects of light upon the gonads. This is of particular interest because of its relevance to the wellknown, but poorly understood, relation between the pineal and gonadal function in both rat and man."

Since 1927 I have been taking time-lapse pictures that have resulted in a number of interesting observations on plant and animal growth that seem to tie in directly to variations in the wavelength distribution, periodicity, and intensity of light. The effects of artificial lights used for photographic purposes and also supplemental growing lights necessitated because of restricted daylight conditions, gave evidence of influencing physiological growth responses in both plants and animals. such growth responses [8] included development of all staminate or pistallate buds on a pumpkin vine, the influence on sex ratio of guppies, mice, and other animals, especially chinchillas, born of parents kept under different types of light. Even a significant difference in the time required for spontaneous tumor development in the C_3H strain of mice is particularly susceptible to spontaneous tumor development.

Microscopic time-lapse pictures of the streaming of chloroplasts [8], small particles within the cells of Elodea Grass,

*Reprinted with permission: *The Eye, Ear, Nose and Throat Monthly*, Volume 53, July, 1974.

showed all the chloroplasts streaming actively to the full extremities of the cells under direct sunlight unfiltered through ordinary window glass. When sunlight was filtered through ordinary window glass, blocking most of the ultraviolet that normally penetrates the earth's atmosphere, most of the chloroplasts continued streaming, but some moved to the center of each cell and remained motionless.

When different colored filters, permitting only specific bands of wavelengths to pass, were placed in the light source, certain chloroplasts would continue streaming in each instance to the full extremities of the cell. Some would move to the center, some to one end of the cell remaining practically motionless, and others would establish different patterns of motion, forming short circles from one end of the cell to the center, instead of the normal continuous flow to the full extremities of the cells. Removing the colored filters and supplementing the incandescent microscope light with a low intensity long wave length ultraviolet artificial light to duplicate natural sunlight, as nearly as possible, would make virtually all the chloroplasts become active again and resume their normal streaming pattern.

Variations in the distribution of the wavelengths from that of natural sunlight, brought variations in the pattern of streaming of the chloroplasts within the cells of Elodea Grass.

Toward the end of each 12-hour light period the activity of the chloroplasts would slow down noticeably. After dark the chloroplasts would virtually become inactive and, regardless of how much the intensity of the artificial light source was increased, would require their normal dark period before resuming their streaming patterns in response to light energy.

Streaming of the chloroplasts goes on in connection with the process of photosynthesis, which is a conversion of light energy into chemical energy which the cell then uses in various ways. Therefore, it seems reasonable to assume that if the characteristics of the source of energy responsible for this conversion to chemical energy are altered, the end result will likewise be altered. In other words, through the process of photosynthesis the chemistry of the cells and the plants they are a part of will be influenced by the characteristics of the light energy under which they are growing.

The intensities of ultraviolet used were within the range only of those capable of influencing the pattern of the streaming of the chloroplasts within the cells influencing the process of photosynthesis or growth responses over a period of extended time; they were not of sufficient intensity to cause noticeable browning or physical injury to the leaf.

Viruses are sometimes described as abnormal chemicals or chemical compounds within the cell. It is suggested that there may be a relationship between the abnormal cell chemistry associated with viruses responding through the process of photosynthesis to an incomplete or unbalanced light spectrum, and that a direct relationship may exist between viruses and light energy that should be further investigated.

Time-lapse cinemicrographic studies [9], utilizing the tissue culture method of growing pigment epithelial cells of the retina of a rabbit's eye in vitro, also revealed variations in the responses of the pigment granules when subjected to alterations in the intensity, periodicity, and wavelengths of light. These cells are located right where the rods and cones terminate and are thought to have no visibility function.

This project was originally undertaken as a drug toxicity study to observe the effects of various tranquilizer drugs on the pigment epithelial cells of a rabbit's eye, as abnormal side effects from a number of tranquilizers had been reported in the pigment epithelial cells in humans. From the beginning of the experiment it became apparent that there were far greater abnormal responses in these cells, depending on the color of the filter placed in the light source of the phase contrast microscope, than from the drugs that were being tested. This would seem to indicate the need for serious consideration of what similar abnormal effects might result from placing various colored filters in the form of sunglasses, or tinted contact lenses, in the light source entering the human eye.

When the slides were freshly prepared, all the pigment granules appeared to move actively throughout the entire cell. After 12-hour daily exposure for ten days to an incandescent light, an estimated 90 percent of the pigment granules became sluggish in their action and remained virtually motionless at one end of the cell. By adding a very low intensity of black light or near ultraviolet to the ordinary incandescent light source, all the pigment granules would become active again amd move in their normal pattern within the cell. No method of measuring the intensity of the ultraviolet was available, but was arrived at by trial and error in connection with the previously mentioned experiment which showed similar results with the chloroplasts in the cells of Elodea Grass.

Increasing the intensity of the ultraviolet from the artificial light source resulted in an abnormal action and death of the pigment epithelial cells within a period of two hours.

The daily and seasonal range of intensities and periodicity of different wavelengths of light to which various types of cells are normally exposed is indeed critical. Prolonged exposure to high intensities of narrow bands of wavelengths, especially in both the short and long (black light) wavelengths of ultraviolet, produces abnormal growth responses and frequently ultimate death of the cells. An ultraviolet light source by itself cannot be considered as representative of natural sunlight.

Microscopic time-lapse pictures of many different animal cells [10] in the tissue culture also show variations in growth patterns when different colored filters are placed in the photographic light source. A blue filter that transmits only the shorter wavelengths produced an undulating or boiling motion, not noticeable at normal speed, but only apparent when the action is speeded up many times through time-lapse photography. This abnormal activity closely resembles cells being attacked by viruses. When a red filter was used in the light source, restricting all but the longer wavelengths at the other end of the visible spectrum, the final death of the cell resulted from a rupturing of the cell membrane. In each instance a water cooling condenser was used to remove all heat from the light source that otherwise might vary considerably with red or blue filters alone.

Mitosis would not occur when the cells had been exposed to either blue or red light for approximately three hours or more, but only under a white light containing a more complete wavelength spectrum. Fresh media is also important for mitosis, but adding fresh media to the slide chambers at constant incubator temperature would not encourage mitosis. When the feeding of the cells with fresh media was done at room temperature and the tissue culture slides then placed in the incubator, greatly accelerated mitosis would take place in approximately 16 hours. Toward the end of the normal daytime period, the activity of the pigment granules would noticeably slow down. Similar to the actions of the chloroplasts, the pigment granules also required a dark period uninterrupted by light before again resuming their normal responses to light energy.

It is suggested that the responses of the chloroplasts and pigment granules may be "tuned" to the natural light spectrum under which all life on this earth has evolved. With respect to the ultraviolet range of wavelengths the matter of intensity seems to be particularly critical. The normal intensity of the near ultraviolet, that is the ultraviolet wavelengths above 290 millimicrons at which point the earth's atmosphere filters out the shorter wavelengths of far ultraviolet, may be an essential part of the natural sunlight spectrum.

It is suggested that the chemistry of the plants might be affected by the various responses of the chloroplasts to both the periodicity of light and darkness, intensity, and distribution of wavelengths influencing the process of photosynthesis. It is further suggested that the similar responses of the pigment granules in the pigment epithelial cells might be the photoreceptor mechanism that stimulates the retinal-hypothalamic-endocrine system in animals and influences the hormonal balance or body chemistry. Thus, it would appear that the basic principal of photosynthesis in plants, as a growth regulating factor, might carry over and be equally as important as a growth regulating factor in animal life through control of the chemical or hormonal activity.

In placing a filter of any particular color in a white light source, only the wavelengths of light representing that particular color are permitted to pass through. On first thought it might seem that any abnormal growth responses might be caused by the wavelengths of the color involved. However, these wavelengths that do pass through the filter are part of the total spectrum of the original source of white light, and the filter cannot add any additional energy. Therefore, it would appear that any altered growth responses must be due to the absence of the wavelengths blocked by the filter, and that the lack of these wavelengths would cause a biochemical or hormonal deficiency in both plant and animal cells.

This might be referred to as causing a condition of malillumination similar to malnutrition which results primarily from what is lacking from a well-balanced diet. When certain wavelengths of light energy are missing in artificial light sources, or blocked from entering the eyes by eyeglasses and especially sunglasses of different colors or tinted contact lenses, then the various pigment granules in the epithelial cells that respond to these particular wavelengths that are missing will not be activated as also is the case with the chloroplasts in the cells of a leaf. Therefore, in the cells of a leaf a full or complete process of photosynthesis is not taking place nor is the endocrine system in animals being fully stimulated through the photoreceptor mechanism in the eye in which the pigment granules are now indicated as having an important role.

In 1969 an interesting experiment was conducted by Philip Salvatori, F.I.A.O. Mr. Salvatori is chairman of the board of directors of Obrig Laboratories, one of the largest manufactures of contact lenses. He is also one of the trustees of the Environmental Health and Light Research Institute, of which I am chairman and executive director. The experiment consisted of fitting a patient with an ultraviolet transmitting contact lens for one eye and a non-ultraviolet transmitting lense over the other eye.

Indoors under artificial light containing no ultraviolet, the size of both pupils appeared the same, but outdoors, under natural sunlight, there was a marked difference. The pupil covered with the ultraviolet transmitting lense was considerably smaller. This would seem to indicate that the photoreceptor mechanism that controls the opening and closing of the iris responds to ultraviolet wavelengths as well as visible light. When the ultraviolet wavelengths are blocked from entering the eye, the pupil remains larger than it would otherwise normally be, and the visible part of the spectrum would then seem brighter. This could explain why some people feel a greater need for dark glasses.

In recognition and application of the eyes' dual function there are now several light related products available. These include the clear and the neutral grey ultraviolet transmitting spectacle lenses* and also full spectrum cathode shielded fluorescent tubes† both of which carry the symbol of approval of Environmental Health and Light Institute of Sarasota, Florida.

The respiratory system in animals is much more complicated and sophisticated than the way plants actually breathe through the pores in their leaves. The digestive system in animals is similarly more advanced than the way plants absorb nutrients through their roots, but these more complicated systems in animals can be related back to the more simpler forms of plant life.

However, photosynthesis, which is probably the most important life process in plants and is sometimes described as a conversion of light energy into chemical energy, has not been recognized as jumping the gap to animal life in any way. It has been recognized that animals are dependent on photosynthesis but only indirectly as the result of eating the plants. However, if light energy entering the eyes ultimately influences the endocrine system and hormonal balance, then this would seem to indicate that, through evolution and in a much more sophisticated way, possibly the basic principals in photosynthesis of coverting light energy into chemical energy do carry over to animal life. In addition to the known effects of light on the skin, light also entering the eyes may be extremely important in affecting man's general health, both physical and mental.

In view of the indications of the growing importance for increased communications between different disciplines in both medicine and science, it becomes more obvious how closely the eye is tied into the endocrine system and what an influence it has on total body functions. Thus a strong need for broadening the areas of interest in the field of ophthalmology is indicated.

REFERENCES

1. Rowan, William: Relation of Light to Bird Migration and Developmental Changes. Nature, 155, pages 494-495, 1925.
2. Kreig, Wendell J.S.: The Hypothalamus of the Albino Rat, Journal of Comparative Neurology, Vol. 55, No. 1, May 1932.
3. Benoit, J. and Assenmacher, I.: The Control of Visible Radiations of the Gonadotropic Activity of the Duck Hypo-

* Armorlite Lens Co., Inc., 727 South Main Street, Burbank, CA 91505.
† Specto Lite Company, 1621 Blue Jay Drive, Holiday, FL. 33589. Complete full spectrum light fixture: Solar Lighting Corporation, 1520 West Fulton Street, Chicago, Ill. 60607.

physis. Recent Progress in Hormone Research, Vol. 15, pages 143-164. New York, Academic Press, 1955.

4. Bissonnette, T.H.: Light and Sexual Cycles in Starlings and Ferrets. Quarterly Review Biology, 8 pages 201-208, 1933.

5. Zuckerman, Sir Solly: Light and Living Matter. Trotter-Patterson Memorial Lecture, in Transactions of Illuminating Engineering, Vol. 24, No. 3, London, 1959.

6. Shipley, T.: Rod-cone Duplexity and the Autonomic Action of Light. Vision Research, Vol. 4, pages 155-177, May 1964.

7. Moore, R.Y., Heller, A., Bhatnager, R.K., Wurtman, R.J. and Axelrod, J.: Central Control of the Pineal Gland: Visual Pathways, Archives Neurology, Vol. 18, pages 208-218, February, 1968.

8. Ott, J.N.: Effects of Unnatural Light. New Scientist (London) Vol. 25, No. 429, pages 294-296, February 4, 1965.

9. Ott, J.N.: Some Observations of the Effect of Light on the Pigment Epithelial Cells of the Retina of a Rabbit's Eye. Recent Progress in Photobiology. E.J. Bowne (ed). Oxford, Blackwell, 1965.

10. Ott, J.N.: Some Responses of Plants and Animals to Variations in Wavelengths of Light Energy, Annals of the New York Academy of Sciences, Vol. 117, Art. 1, pages 624-636, September 10, 1964.

Part II
(The Eyes' Dual Function)

That part of the total electromagnetic spectrum within the range of human vision, commonly referred to as light, has become a subject of considerable interest in research dealing with plants, laboratory animals, and people [1]. However, standard research procedures have mostly dealt with light and responses to it only in connection with what the human eye sees plus ultraviolet. Beyond this it is generally considered darkness with the connotation that no further radiant energy exists that could produce a pathobiological or photosynthetic response. Some similar responses that have been observed to take place in so-called "darkness" have been called chemosynthetic because of the theoretical absence of any light energy in accordance with this quite obviously erroneous definition.

Light within the range of human vision represents only a very narrow part of the total electromagnetic spectrum, and there are many shorter and longer wave lengths of similar characteristics that are capable of penetrating most types of building materials as readily as visible light penetrates ordinary window glass. Though similar in nature to visible light, these wave lengths are frequently referred to as general background radiation.

Certain photobiological responses in seed germination and flower development have been shown to react to quite narrow bands of wave lengths within the visible spectrum. However, other responses such as circadian rhythms, where the petals and leaves of some species of plants open and close each day and night, are attributed to a so-called biological clock system that works somehow independently of light and darkness within the definition of light being only what the human eye can see. For example, the sensitive plant (mimosa Pudica) folds its leaves together tightly and all the petioles or little leaf branches on the main stem hang in a more downward position as soon as the sun sets; they remain in this nighttime position during the dark period until sunrise when they again resume their normal daytime position. This action is thought to be controlled by a so-called biological clock because it will continue an established rhythm even though the apparent light-dark cycle is altered. If the sensitive plant is placed in a dark closet during the daytime, its leaves remain open and the leaf stems in their upward position until the sun sets. Only after sunset will they assume their normal nighttime positions. Then the leaves and the stems "wake up" and resume their daytime positions as the sun rises the following morning even though they remained in the dark closet.

But some of these wave lengths of general background radiation beyond the range of human vision that penetrate most building materials are very much present in the so-called "dark" closet. Possibly something like cosmic rays, which readily penetrate ordinary lead shielding that stops most x-rays, might be controlling the day-night responses of the sensitive plant.

The only practical shielding against cosmic rays is a massive amount of earth. Accordingly, an experiment [2] was set up in which six sensitive plants were taken to the bottom of a coal mine, at noon time, 650 feet below the surface of the earth. The leaves and leaf branches of all six plants immediately assumed their nighttime positions, not waiting for the sun to set. Furthermore, the area where the plants were placed was lighted with regular incandescent bulbs. This suggests that the day-night responses of the leaves and leaf branches of the sensitive plant react to some form of radiation capable of penetrating through the building material surrounding the "dark" closet at the surface of the earth, but not to the bottom of the coal mine, 650 feet down. This also suggests that these particular responses are not influenced by the wave lengths of light energy produced by an ordinary incandescent light bulb.

Another experiment confirmed what might be expected; that the degree of loss of response to the general background radiation was proportionate to the amount of shielding material involved.

The buds of the hoya vine and some other night blooming (nocturnal) plants will only open during the nighttime, whether or not they are placed in a dark closet at the surface of the earth during the daytime. This further suggests the opening action of these buds is not due to the absence of visible light, but possibly to the presence of some form of nighttime radiation.

Some species of nocturnal laboratory animals have been noted to be more active during the nighttime when located in a one story frame building compared to the basement area of a tall solid masonry structure [3]. It therefore becomes apparent that some biological responses in both plants and animals react to certain areas of the so-called general nighttime background radiation in a positive way rather than to merely the absence of the visible light during the dark nighttime period.

What is possibly of greater significance is the indication of biological responses in both plants and animals to such minor variations of extremely low levels of radiation. Here again it is quite customary to think of general background radiation as only natural radiation from not only the sun, but other stars and outer space. In our modern civilization today there are increasing amounts of man-made radiations that are present in far greater intensities than the natural background radiation. A very serious question now exists as to whether or not this artificial radiation is causing any biological responses in plants, laboratory animals, or people.

The November 6, 1964, issue of *Time* carried a very interesting and provocative article entitled "Those Tired Children." It told of a report presented by two Air Force physicians at a meeting of the American Academy of Pediatrics in New York City. No explanation for the symptoms of 30 children being studied could be found after doing all the usual tests for infectious and childhood illnesses. Both the food and water supplies were checked. The symptoms included nervousness, continuous fatigue, headaches, loss of sleep, and vomiting. Only after further checking was it discovered that this group of children was all watching television three to six hours a day during the week and six to ten hours on Saturdays and Sundays.

The doctors prescribed a total abstinence from TV. In 12 cases the parents enforced the rule and the childrens' symptoms vanished in two to three weeks. In 18 cases the parents cut the TV time to about two hours a day and the children's symptoms did not go away for five or six weeks. But in 11 cases the parents later relaxed the rules and the children were back again spending their usual time in front of the picture tube. Their symptoms returned as before.

The report concluded that watching TV, in itself, is not necessarily bad, but that some children become addicted to it and fall into a vicious cycle of viewing for long hours. Thus they become too tired to do anything more strenuous than to continue watching the TV set. Other reports have suggested over-psychological stimulation in children from the program content of too many western thrillers and murder mysteries. Little or no consideration seems to have been given to the question of possible radiation problems. However, epileptic seizures in some children have been reported as being caused by flicker from TV sets in the visible light range, and some further questions have been raised regarding possible effect of sonic energy.

It will be remembered that the x-ray type shoe-fitting machines, commonly used in many shoe stores, were found to be giving off excessive x-rays and were banned from use.

In order to determine if there might be any basic physiological responses in plants or laboratory animals to some sort of radiation or other form of energy being emitted from TV sets, an experiment [4] was set up in our laboratory at Environmental Health and Light Institute using a large screen color TV. One-half of the picture tube was covered with one-sixteenth inch solid lead, which is customarily used to shield x-rays, and the other half was covered with ordinary heavy black photographic paper that would stop all visible light but allow other areas of radiation to penetrate. Six pots, each containing three bean seeds, were placed directly in front of the portion of the TV tube covered with the black photographic paper; six pots were placed outdoors at a distance of 50 feet from the green house where the TV set was located. At the end of three weeks all the young bean plants, in the six pots outdoors and the six pots behind the lead shielding, showed approximately six inches of normal appearing growth. All the bean plants in the six pots shielded only with the black photographic paper showed an excessive vine type growth

ranging up to 13 1/2 inches. Furthermore, the leaves were all approximately 2 1/2 to 3 times the size of the outdoor plants, or those protected with the lead shielding. The bean plants in front of both the black paper and the lead shielding, that were placed at the highest point so that the bottom of the pot was approximately in line with the top of the TV set, showed considerable root growth emerging from the top surface of the soil. The bean plants in front of both the black paper and the lead shield, directly in front of the center horizontal line of the picture tube or near the bottom of the TV set, and those at a distance of 50 feet showed no such upward directional growth of the roots causing them to emerge from the top surface of the soil in the pots.

Such hard to explain results prompted setting up an additional similar experiment [5] using white laboratory rats. Two rats, approximately three months old, were placed in each of two cages directly in front of the color television tube, and the set was turned on for six hours each weekday and ten hours on Saturday and Sunday. One cage was placed in front of the half of the tube covered with black photographic paper, and the other cage in front of the lead shielding which was increased to one-eighth inch thickness. The sound was turned off, but it should be pointed out that turning off the audible sound does not rule out the possibility of sonic energy in the range of fifteen kilocycles that can in some instances be produced by the action of the picture scanning device.

The rats, protected only with the black paper, showed stimulated abnormal activities from three to ten days and then became progressively lethargic. At 30 days they were extremely lethargic and it was necessary to push them to make them move about the cage. This experiment was repeated three times and the same results were obtained.

When the color television set was placed in the greenhouse area of our laboratory the location was 15 feet from our animal breeding room with two ordinary building partitions in between. We observed that immediately following the placing of the color television set in the greenhouse our animal breeding program, which had been going on very successfully for over two years, was completely disrupted. Whereas litters of the rats had previously averaged eight or twelve or more young, this immediately dropped off to one or two. Many of these did not survive. After removal of the TV set approximately six months time was required before the breeding program was back to normal.

Susan Korbel [6] and William D. Thompson, at Baylor University, conducted a study in 1965 in which 20 male albino rats were used in determining behavioral effects of ultra high frequency radiation. Experimental animals were exposed to low intensity, and low frequency UHF radio waves for 47 consecutive days. Radiated rats were more active than nonradiated rats during the early part of the experiment, but they became less active as the days of radiation increased. The UHF group was more emotional than the non-UHF group and showed a gradual increase in the latency of recovery from electro-shock convulsion. Results suggest that some time is required for UHF to have a consistent effect on behavior, and the effects on behavior may be non-thermal and related to neurophysiological substrates.

In 1965, Allan H. Frey [7] at the Institute for Research, State College, Pennsylvania, also reported that electromagnetic energy is an important factor in the biophysical analysis of the properties and function of living systems, and it is now being used as a research tool, both by study of its emission by living organisms and also by applying it to the organism. He used new techniques to detect neural activity, brain impedance shifts and behavior, and the influence of UHF energy on behavior. He concluded that though these areas are in the embryonic stage of development, most are potentially of great significance in the understanding of the nervous system and behavior.

During the 1972-73 school year the Environmental Health and Light Research Institute of Sarasota, Florida, undertook a study of the effects of lighting on behavioral problems of first grade students.

In a pilot project conducted in four windowless elementary classrooms [8], children showed such dramatic reactions to an improved lighting environment that the Sarasota County School Board authorized an expanded comprehensive study which is currently under way.

Under their normal classroom lighting, some first graders in the study demonstrated nervous fatigue, irritability, lapses of attention and hyperactive behavior. After installing full spectrum lighting, with lead foil shields over the cathode ends of the fluorescent tubes to stop suspected soft x-ray, and an aluminum screen grid over the entire fixture to stop known RF radiation, which is characteristic of all fluorescent tubes, a marked improvement appeared in the youngsters.

Without any use of drugs, the first graders settled down and paid more attention to their teachers. Nervousness diminished and teachers reported that overall classroom performance improved. The children were unaware of the special cameras mounted near the ceiling that snapped sequences of time-lapse pictures during the class day. With the standard type of unshielded lights still in operation, students could be observed fidgeting to an extreme degree, leaping from their seats, flailing their arms and paying little attention to their teachers. After the full spectrum shielded lighting was installed, the same children were filmed two and three months later. Behavior was entirely different. Youngsters appeared calmer and far more interested in their work. One little boy, who stood out in the first films because of his constant motion and who was inattentive to everything, had changed to a quieter child, able to sit still and concentrate on routine. According to his teacher, he was capable of doing independent study and had even learned to read during the short period of time.

This may indicate that hyperactivity is a radiation stress condition. The improvement occurred when that part of the visible spectrum, which is lacking in standard artificial light sources, was supplied and excessive radiation was eliminated.

The fact that no drugs were used is of particular significance since warnings are now being heard about the widespread use of amphetamines and other psychoactive drugs on children thought to be hyperactive. As child psychiatrist Mark Stewart of the University of Iowa points out (*Time* Magazine, Feb. 26, 1973), the danger is that "by the time a child on drugs reaches puberty, he does not know what his undrugged personality is."

Estimates of the number of children in this country now taking drugs range as high as one million; a situation which prompted the Committee on Drugs of the American Academy of Pediatrics to propose regulations to the U.S. Food and Drug Administration to prevent abuses. Psychoactive drugs have been shown helpful in treating hyperkinesis, a restlessness that some experts believe derives from minimal brain damage or chemical imbalances. What will become of the hyperactive boy in the pictures and the many other children like him? If he gets relief through drugs from stress caused by malillumination and radiation, will that lead to later addiction to drugs or alcohol? Dr. Irving Geller [9], chairman of the Department of Experimental Pharmacology at Southwest Foundation for Research and Education in San Antonio, has found that abnormal conditions of light and darkness can affect the pineal gland, one of the master glands of the endocrine system.

Experimenting with rats, Dr. Geller discovered that rats under stress preferred water to alcohol until left in continuous darkness over weekends. Then they went on alcoholic binges. Nobel prize winner Dr. Julius Axelrod [10] earlier found that the pineal gland produces more of the enzyme melatonin during dark periods. Injections of melatonin to rats on a regular light-dark cycle turned these rats into alcoholics.

We have found that many biological responses are to narrow bands of wave lengths within the total light spectrum. If these are missing in an artificial light source, the biological receptor responds as in total darkness. That alcoholism may be related to the pineal gland is also under study by Kenneth Blum, a pharmacologist at the University of Texas Medical School. (See *Science News*, April 28, 1973). Under near total darkness rats with pineals drank more alcohol than water while rats without pineals drank more water than alcohol. When the animals were returned to equal periods of light and dark, rats with pineals retained their liking for alcohol. Applied to humans, Dr. Blum says "it is possible that alcoholics may have highly active pineals."

The hyperactive reaction to radiation from unshielded fluorescent tubes may have a correlation to the hyperactivity symptoms and severe learning disorders triggered by artificial food flavors and colorings. (See *Newsweek*, July 9, 1973.) Dr. Ben F. Feingold of the Kaiser-Permanente Medical Center, found that a diet eliminating all foods containing artificial flavors and colors brought about a dramatic improvement in 15 of 25 hyperactive school children studied. Any infraction of the diet led within a matter of hours to a return of the hyperkinetic behavior.

This points out the possibility of an interaction between wavelength absorption bands of these synthetic color pigments and the energy peaks caused by mercury vapor lines in fluorescent tubes. This could explain the reaction or "allergy" to fluorescent lighting. (Increased sunburn reactions have been found to occur in individuals taking particular drugs, who are not so "sunreactive" when not on medication.)

This reaction could be eliminated two ways: by eliminating the absorbing material consumed when the child eats artificial coloring, or by eliminating the energy peaks in fluorescent tubes.

At the American Association for the Advancement of Science meeting in Chicago, December 26-31, 1970, Lewis W. Mayron, Ph.D., presented a paper entitled "Environmental Pollution: Its Biological Effects and Impact on the Bioanalytical Laboratory," in which he explored the biological effects of radiation from television sets and fluorescent lighting tubes.

In discussing the published results of our experiments with the bean plants and white rats placed in front of a television set, Dr. Mayron comments as follows:

"Thus it appears that the radiation emitted from the TV set has a physiological effect both on plants and animals and it is likely that this effect, or these effects, are chemically mediated. If 'Those Tired

Children' are any indication of a trend, the bioanalytical laboratory may be called upon to chemically determine low-grade radiation toxicity.

"Although there is as yet no indication of the body chemicals involved in the physiological effects of TV radiation, there is some indication of a chemical effect of the radiation of Ultra High Frequency (UHF) radio fields. Gordon (*Science* 133: 444, 1961) has found that UHF fields result in the accumulation of acetylcholine along nerve fibers. Korbel and Thompson (*Psychological Reports* 17: 595-602, 1965) reported on the behavioral effects of stimulation by UHF radio fields, which just happens to correlate with the behavior of the rats in front of the color TV screen and which also correlates with behavioral effects due to the accumulation of acetylcholine. Acetylcholine in small concentrations lead to a decrease in activity (Crossman and Mitchell, *Nature* 175: 121-122, 1955; Koshtoiants and Kokina, *Psychological Abstracts* 32: 3584, 1957; Russell, *Bulletin British Psych. Society* 23: 6, 1954 [abstract]). Nikogosyan found significant reductions in blood cholinesterase activity in rabbits after a program of UHF exposure (in Letavet and Gordon, Eds., *Biological Action of Ultra-high Frequencies*, OTS 62-19175, Moscow; Academy of Medical Sciences USSR, 1960). Thus, perhaps cholinesterase activities ought to be determined on man and laboratory animals exposed to TV radiation. An interesting addendum to this story on TV radiation is a series of experiments performed by Dr. Ott, using bean seeds and seedlings and fluorescent light tubes."

Dr. Mayron then relates the procedures and results of the bean seed experiments with the fluorescent tubes and further comments: "The implications of this are enormous when one considers the magnitude of the use of fluorescent lighting in stores, offices, factories, schools and homes."

The fluorescent cathode, as a source of soft x-ray, has been recognized by such scientists as Dr. K.G. Emeleus, professor of physics at Queens' University, Belfast, in his book "The Conduction of Electricity Through Gases."

Soft x-rays from the cathodes of fluorescent tubes were first suspected as a result of timelapse pictures made by John Ott Pictures, Inc. of flowers for the Barbara Streisand film "On a Clear Day You Can See Forever." Flowers nurtured under high power fluorescent lights didn't grow as well near the end of the tubes. Additional tests on bean sprouts showed abnormal growth when near the ends of fluorescent tubes. TV x-ray measuring equipment detected slight measurements of x-rays at the ends of the tubes which would penetrate aluminum foil, but not lead foil.

In our experiments we found the trace amount of suspected x-radiation from the ends of fluorescent tubes was not consistent and that as a rule it varied significantly between one end and the other end of the same tube. Some tubes seem to give off more radiation than others and generally speaking, the older the tube, the more noticeable were the abnormal growth responses in the bean plants. This is a similar situation to the problem of x-ray emission from TV tubes which also varied considerably from one tube to another as far as the amount of x-ray emissions.

REFERENCES

1. Ott, J.N.: "Effect of Wavelengths of Light on Physiological Functions of Plants and Animals," Illuminating Engineering, Vol. LX, No. 4, Section 1, April 1965, pp. 254-261.
2. Ott, J.N.: Paper presented to Eleventh International Botanical Congress, September 1, 1969, "Influence of Ionizing Radiation of Directional Growth of Roots and Biological Clock Rhythms in Plants."
3. Lloyd, C.: Worchester Foundation, conversation and correspondence, 1965.
4. Ott, J.N.: Paper presented to the Society of Motion Picture and Television Engineers, October 3, 1966, "Time-Lapse Cinematography."
5. Ott, J.N.: "Responses of Psychological and Physiological Functions to Environmental Radiation Stress," Journal of Learning Disabilities, Part II, Vol. 1, No. 6, June, 1968.
6. Korbel, Susan and Thompson, William D.: "Behavioral Effects of Stimulation by UHF Radio Fields." Psychological Reports, 1965, 17, 595-602.
7. Frey, Allan H.: "Behavioral Biophysics," Psychological Bulletin, Vol. 63, No. 5, May 1965.
8. Mayron, L.W., Nations, R., Mayron, E.L., Ott, J.N.: Paper to be presented to The American Society for Photobiology, July, 1974, "Initial Studies on the Effects of Full-Spectrum Lighting and Radiation Shielding on Classroom Behavior and Scholastic Achievement."
9. Geller, Irving: "Ethanol Preference in the Rat as a Function of Photoperiod," Science, Vol. 1973, pp. 456-459, 1972.
10. Wurtman, Richard J. and Axelrod, Julius: "The Pineal Gland" Scientific American, July, 1956, pp. 50-58.

28
A Legal Triumph for Orthomolecular Medicine*

DWIGHT K. KALITA

Preface

For the past fifteen years, I have been badgered and at odds with my colleagues, hospitals, Blue Shield and many insurance carriers, concerning hypoglycemia. My real bout came with the local peer review committee. Here are a group of physicians that don't know anything about hypoglycemia (except what little information you get out of "Cecil Loeb's Medical Textbook") making an attempt to govern my practice.

This patient came to me with the complaint of passing out on a stressful job. He had visited the usual company doctor, several internists, and finally a psychiatrist, and they all came up with the diagnosis of "psychoses." The insurance company would not accept the diagnosis of hypoglycemia, although the patient, in a short time was able to return to work. He found a good attorney and we went before a jury. We won the case. We have very little problem with hypoglycemia acceptance now. The following article by Dr. Dwight Kalita tells the story.

J.M. Baron, D.O.
June 2, 1975

INTRODUCTION

In order to maintain the integrity of the position that treatment of mental disease is best accomplished by supplying an optimum, nutritional, molecular environment for the mind, and more specifically, by supporting the optimum concentration of substances normally present in human chemistry, some orthomolecular psychiatrists have found it necessary to go to court. But, of course, the discovery of oneself in the battleground of the legal arena is nothing new for those who have vigorously challenged the status quo of the scientific community.

THE LEGAL CHALLENGE: BACKGROUND

Such a legal challenge was recently made by Dr. John M. Baron, Cleveland, Ohio. He went to court in defense of Mr. Conley Dockery. The story began around January 18, 1972,

when Mr. Dockery visited Harold Barker, M.D., who represented the Metropolitan Life Insurance Company. Mr. Dockery had recently lost his job; he complained of severe dizziness, headaches, insomnia, indigestion and extreme weakness, all of which plagued his vocational effectiveness. And in order for Mr. Dockery to collect unemployment insurance, his symptoms had to be proven as being organic in origin. Dr. Barker saw the patient five subsequent times after the initial meeting. "I could not find anything organically wrong with this gentleman except his obesity of 215 lbs.," testified Dr. Barker while appearing before the Honorable A.D. Arnson at Shaker Heights Municipal Court, Shaker Heights, Ohio (9:00 A.M., 9/5/74). "There is no organic disease;" he continued, "the patient is psychoneurotic ... His symptoms are related to something referrable to the nervous system." Dr. Barker was then asked whether he had run a five-hour glucose tolerance test. He replied, "I did not feel that a five-hour glucose tolerance test would help ... Hypoglycemia clinical syndrome is not a serious syndrome. If the individual will eat more than three times a day or take any form of sugar, that will alleviate attacks." The lawyer then continued his questioning: "What about a person doing something – like driving – and the attack comes on? Can he get to this candy, or whatever you want him to eat, fast enough to control the condition?" "Here," Dr. Barker replied, "you smoke a cigarette in traffic ... Hypoglycemia is relatively mild all the time. It is never very serious unless it is associated with certain organic diseases. We do not feel that clinical hypoglycemia syndrome is sufficient to make anyone disabled for work. Its symptoms are usually weakness, thirst, and they may or may not have dizziness, and this is probably relieved by eating or taking sugar, like hard candy."

THE PROBLEM: HYPOGLYCEMIA

It so happened, and luckily so, that during the time of his troubles our "dizzy" patient stumbled one day directly into Dr. John Baron's office. Dr. Baron, who specializes in "nutrition, preventative medicine, and Orthomolecular Psychiatry," has been practicing nutritionally oriented medicine since 1939. He is certified by the American College of Applied Nutrition and the American College of Bariatric Physicians, and is a member of the

*Reprinted with permission: *Journal of Preventive Medicine*, Volume 2, # 2.

Cleveland Academy of Osteopathic Medicine and the American College of Neuropsychiatry. Upon seeing the patient for the first time, he immediately gave him a five-hour glucose tolerance test. "He complained," testified Dr. Baron, "of severe dizziness, headaches, insomnia, indigestion and poor appetite; he also craved sweets." Since Dr. Baron has tested and treated over 1000 similar cases, he easily recognized Mr. Dockery's symptoms as being those of a clinical hypoglycemia syndrome. Hypoglycemia, according to Dr. Baron, is an abnormality of carbohydrate metabolism. As a result of a patient's inability to tolerate processed carbohydrates, sugar, white flour, etc., his blood sugar level drops below normal, and the commonly expressed symptoms of anxiety, weakness, depression, insomnia, irritability, dizziness, therefore quickly ensue. A special diet of "high protein, low carbohydrates," along with "megavitamins, and injections of adrenal cortex extract, which relieves the adrenal glands from 2-6 hours so it can recuperate," was recommended by Dr. Baron to his patient.

THE LEGAL CHALLENGE: IN COURT

In court, Dr. Baron was asked, "Based on your experience in dealing with hypoglycemia, can you state whether or not many people who have hypoglycemia have been diagnosed as being psychoneurotic prior to having their hypoglycemia condition diagnosed?" Dr. Baron's answer was emphatic: "Definitely! But Orthomolecular Psychiatry is a new field that has been developed to look at the view of psychiatric problems (i.e., psychoneurosis, psychosis, etc.) from a biochemical aspect." The lawyer pursued his point: "Could Mr. Dockery have remained at work by carrying hard candy on him and eating it whenever he became weak and dizzy?" "No," responded Dr. Baron, "because candy would develop just the adverse reaction we are seeking to eliminate. The pancreas, reacting to the processed carbohydrate, sugar, etc., would seek to enter the bloodstream; its insulin would continue to keep pouring because it had been reacted. The insulin increases and the sugar starts to drop. Therefore, candy is only a temporary measure as far as hypoglycemia is concerned. Two to three hours after this type of ingestion of food, the hypoglycemia would become worse."

THE IMPLICATIONS

There is really nothing new with, or surprising about, a doctor like Dr. Barker, failing to see hypoglycemia as a serious organic disease. Nor is there anything new — although it is startling — about a medical doctor prescribing candy for a hypoglycemia patient. But I begin to wonder about our supposedly learned scientific community when some members therein actually suggest, under oath, smoking a cigarette to alleviate a drop in blood sugar. Suppose, for example, that a jet airplane pilot with severe case of hypoglycemia was cruising at 40,000 feet, and 85 people were on board. The flight is between New York and California. Also imagine that a Dr. Jones, as a member of our scientific community, is one of those passengers, and that he is summoned as an M.D., after take-off, to the cockpit because the pilot is feeling dizzy and weak. "Here," Dr. Jones would probably say, "smoke this cigarette and take this

sweet candy." By the time the plane approached the Rocky Mountains, our poor pilot's blood sugar level would be dropping even more quickly, and for that matter, so might the plane. Ouch! that idea hurts. Failing to see that our hypoglycemia pilot might also be cerebrally allergic to tobacco, Dr. Jones would wonder why, after a short time, the plane was suddenly so unstable. Up goes the allergic reactions; down goes the sugar level, and down goes the jet airplane!

But Mr. Dockery, and thousands of people just like him, are fortunate to have orthomolecular physicians like Dr. Baron. It is men like him, who have the integrity of their convictions and the internal fortitude to fight the general medical population's appalling ignorance of this now "epidemic-like" (Ross) organic disease.

A HAPPY ENDING

By the way, Dr. Baron did come out the victor during his day in court. Mr. Dockery was awarded his unemployment insurance by the Metropolitan Life Insurance Company. Mr. Dockery was not psychoneurotic, and one hundred hours on the couch of a psychoanalyst would not have alleviated his problem, for it was strictly organic. Due to many factors — environmental, allergic, genetic, etc., — his ability to utilize processed carbohydrates was impaired during his lifetime. If his treatment had been along the lines of symptomatic relief (i.e., shock, psychoanalysis, drug therapy), Mr. Dockery would have been doomed to a miserable life. But it was not. Root causes behind the manifested symptoms were discovered. As a result, treatment was etiological.

CONCLUDING OBSERVATIONS

All good scientists are aware that for every effect, there must be a cause(s). But too often, and tragically so for some people, some doctors center their attention only on the effect. They try to repress it, tranquilize it, ignore it, punish it, shock it, or just plain talk it down, and in this maddening process they create mental, emotional and spiritual vegetables who are shunned by society and often locked up in the back wards of our now overcrowded mental institutions. And what is far more serious, these institutions create a hostile environment for already overly sensitive, malfunctioning body chemistries. They feed schizophrenics high carbohydrate dinners because it is "inexpensive"; to compound the problem, they permit potential allergens such as tobacco, sugar, wheat, corn, etc., to literally abound for consumption; cerebral allergies are not even tested; a glucose tolerance test is rarely seen as diagnostically important; a hair analysis test is frowned upon and the diet is enough to destroy any healthy biochemical mechanism given enough time. Amino acids, vitamins and minerals, substances which are normally present at the cellular level, are, of course, ignored. And on and on and on!

I believe our problem all goes back to a basic philosophy of life. Do we seek to "have dominion over nature?" That is, do we seek to manipulate desired ends by synthetic intervention into the processes of nature, or do we seek to be harmonious with nature, discover her mysterious and majestic laws, and then live our lives, and this includes our medical lives, in tune with our discoveries? I think the latter is the correct path. Today, a few brave scientists are emerging who know that our human biochemical mechanism is an extremely complex, delicately balanced dynamism of millions upon millions of chemical reactions. They also know that man, via the stress of poor diet and a hostile chemical environment, can easily upset this delicate homeostasis of his inherited biochemical being. It is up to us, as orthomolecular scientists, to continue to search out the etiological reasons for the breakdown of nature's homeostasis. For if we can, men like Mr. Dockery, instead of being incorrectly labeled and stigmatized as "psychoneurotic," will be properly diagnosed and treated, and thus will be given an opportunity to live a happy, healthy and creative life.

Robert Frost once wrote, "Two roads diverged on a country road, and I took the one less traveled by. And it has made all the difference." Orthomolecular scientists have taken the scientific road "less traveled by" but the empirical success they have seen in their own patients, I'm sure you will all agree, "has made all the difference."

29
Orthomolecular Therapy
Review of the Literature*

KAY HALL

An increasing number of research studies point to a biochemical etiology of mental illness in which transient factors, like history, and experience, play much the same role as in other physical disorders. This paper will review such research.

DEFICIENCY DISEASES

Mental illness, associated with physical disease, results from a low concentration in the brain of any one of the following vitamins: thiamine (B_1), niacin (B_3), pyridoxine (B_6), cyanocobalamin (B_{12}), pantothenic acid, folic acid, and ascorbic acid (C). Mental function and behavior may also be affected by changes in the concentration in the brain of other substances that are normally present, such as the amino acids and various minerals (Pauling, 1968; Cott, 1970).

Vitamins

Vitamin B_1 (thiamine). Thiamine deficiency causes loss of appetite, generated by cell malnutrition in the hypothalamus (Williams, 1971). Other symptoms include depression, irritability, confusion, loss of memory, inability to concentrate, fear of impending doom, and sensitivity to noise. These symptoms, related to mild mental disease, disappear when thiamine is administered (Williams, 1971; Bruno, 1973).

Vitamin B_3 (niacin). The earliest manifestations of pellagra, created by a severe deficiency of niacin, are anxiety, depression, fatigue, and vague somatic complaints (Joliffe, 1939; Joliffe et al., 1940; Frostig and Spies, 1940; Hoffer, 1973a). Frostig and Spies (1940) examined 60 patients with subclinical and mild pellagra, with an initial syndrome of hyperesthesia, hyperactivity, depression, apprehension, fatigue, headache, and insomnia. This pattern readily fits into the standard classification of anxiety neuroses (Hoffer, 1973a).

As the disease progresses, patients often complain of failing vision, hypersensitivity to light, illusions, vertigo, visual and auditory hallucinations, hyperacute sense of smell, dulled sense of taste, and persistent salty taste. These perceptual changes are, of

course, very similar to those produced by schizophrenia and by the hallucinogens (Hoffer and Osmond, 1966).

Acute cases of pellagra quickly respond to 0.5 to 1.0 g of niacin per day, but chronic cases respond very slowly (Aring and Spies, 1939; Aring et al., 1939; Gillman and Gillman, 1951; Hoffer, 1973b).

Vitamin B_6 (pyridoxine). Of the 12 known disorders involving genetic vitamin dependency, pyridoxine is involved in five (Rosenberg, 1970). This vitamin is a precursor to 50 enzymes, necessary for the metabolism of all amino acids and required for the maintenance of a stable immunologic system (Axelrod and Trakatellis, 1964; Davis et al., 1970; Ellis, 1973; Philpott, 1974).

Vitamin B_{12} (cyanocobalamine). A higher incidence of low B_{12} concentrations has been found in mental patients than in the population as a whole. Deficiencies of vitamin B_{12} can cause pernicious anemia, with mental symptoms ranging from poor concentration to stuporous depression, severe agitation, and hallucinations. Administration of vitamin B_{12} sometimes corrects the mental symptoms only slowly and, occasionally, incompletely (Hart, 1971).

Pantothenic acid. Both animals and humans withstand stress better after receiving large doses of pantothenic acid (Williams, 1971). Volunteers fed a diet deficient in pantothenic acid became easily upset, irritable, quarrelsome, sullen, depressed, tense, dizzy, and numb (Wormsley and Darragh, 1955; Eiduson et al., 1964). The wide variance observed in reactions of the subjects suggests that requirements for pantothenic acid vary greatly (Williams, 1971).

Folic acid. Several surveys revealed low folic acid levels in the blood of 40 to 80 percent of elderly psychiatric patients. A significant number of subjects were benefited by folic acid administration (Williams, 1971). However, deficiency reappeared unless sufficient vitamin C was supplied to convert folic acid into a usable form (Scheid, 1952; Greenberg, 1957; Herbert, 1963).

Vitamin C (ascorbic acid). Ascorbic acid is present in all tissues of higher animals during development and occurs in greater concentrations in the tissues of higher metabolic activity (Martin, 1961). Research indicates that almost any physical or mental stress significantly lowers vitamin C levels in plasma (Urbach et al., 1952; Maas et al., 1961; Baker, 1967). Deficiencies of the vitamin can cause listlessness, decreased epinephrine response, and increased susceptibility to vascular stress (Dayton and Weiner, 1961).

*Reprinted with permission: Orthomolecular Psychiatry, Vol. 4, No. 4, 1975, 297-313.

The amount of ascorbic acid, 20 mg a day, necessary to prevent scurvy is well established for man. How much beyond this minimum is necessary for optimal functioning is still controversial. The unstressed normal rat synthesizes ascorbic acid at the rate of 70 mg/kg of body weight per day, and the stressed rat increases this to 215 mg/kg per day (Conney et al., 1961). This is equivalent to the production of 4.9 to 15.0 g of ascorbic acid per day calculated to the 70 kg weight of an adult human (Herjanic, 1973).

Minerals

Potassium. In a single week, healthy volunteers fed a refined diet developed muscle weakness, extreme fatigue, indifference, and lack of feeling. All symptoms quickly disappeared following administration of 10 g potassium chloride (Black, 1952; Wormsley and Darragh, 1955).

Magnesium. Persons deficient in magnesium are nervous, irritable, quarrelsome, and apathetic (Shils, 1964). In one reported case, magnesium deficiency accompanied severe paranoid psychosis, which was remitted when magnesium was administered (Williams, 1971). Magnesium plus salt and water has been successfully used to treat delirium tremens (Goodhart, 1957).

Zinc. Normally found in all human tissues, zinc is essential for the synthesis of protein and the action of more than 30 enzymes (Wohl and Goodhart, 1968; Hurley, 1969; Rodale, 1973b). It helps the body use up lactic acid developed during exercise (Mayer, 1972). Zinc deficiency affects taste, smell, and appetite and may cause lethargy and apathy (Rodale, 1973c, 1974).

The high-phosphorus diet consumed by many Americans may produce zinc deficiency and thus interfere with the nucleus formation of each cell in the body (Wohl and Goodhart, 1968). Animals lacking sufficient zinc during early brain formation made more errors during experimental tests than normal controls (Rodale, 1973a). Deficiencies of zinc and the amino acid taurine have been linked to epileptic seizures (Barbeau in Rodale, 1974).

Chromium. Biochemically, chromium is an active compound that forms many complexes with protein, stimulates several enzyme systems, and may stabilize certain nucleic acid structures. It is present in exceptionally high concentrations in brain tissue, particularly in the caudate nuclei (Mayer, 1971).

Chromium is essential for the body to utilize sugar properly. Diabetes may be caused, in part, by a deficiency of this trace metal. Hypoglycemia has been corrected by daily administration of 250 mcg of chromium (Mayer, 1971, 1972; Schroeder, 1973).

Manganese. This trace metal activates numerous enzymes and aids in fat utilization. A high-phosphorus diet reduces the absorption of manganese (Pfeiffer, 1973).

Animals deficient in manganese show retarded growth, hyperactivity, abnormal bone structure, joint deformities, poor equilibrium, and uncoordinated movements. In some animals, choline and inositol supplements prevent the deficiency symptoms (Josephson, 1961).

Amino Acids

The dry material in the brain is over one-third protein; thus, brain function depends upon the amino acids. Stress so increases the demand for protein that it becomes difficult for the body to produce sufficient amounts of the nonessential amino acids (Tui, 1953).

A protein deficiency or an imbalance of amino acids can cause mental depression, apathy, peevishness, irritability, and a desire to be left alone (Knox, 1960; Williams, 1971).

In animals fed diets lacking any of the essential amino acids, production of uric acid increases (Bicknell and Prescott, 1953). Uric acid levels in children appear to be associated with self-mutilating behavior (Cott, 1971).

DEPENDENCY DISEASES

Vitamin deficiencies are acquired and respond to usual physiological doses. In contrast, vitamin dependencies reflect genetic disturbance, leading to specific biochemical abnormalities affecting only one reaction catalyzed by a vitamin. Such dependencies respond only to large, pharmacologic doses (Hoffer, 1973b).

SCHIZOPHRENIA

Genetic Transmission

Huxley (1964) suggested that schizophrenia is caused by a dominant gene with an incomplete penetrance of about 25 percent, determined in some cases by other genes and by the environment. Pauling (1973) suggested that the other genes may be those that regulate the metabolism of vital substances and that cause the development of brain cell membranes with a decreased permeability for the passage of essential nutrilites from the blood.

Karlsson (1966) proposed a two-independent-gene theory. The dominant gene predisposes toward thought disorder and occurs in one out of 15 people, and the recessive gene occurs homozygous in one out of six people. Hoffer (1973b) suggested that the dominant gene controls the formation of adrenolutin and is related to perceptual changes plus thought disorders and that the recessive gene controls conversion of tryptophan to nicotinamide adenine dinucleotide (NAD) by some unknown mechanism.

According to Karlsson (1966), his theory accounts for the known distribution of schizophrenia in the population. A breakdown is as follows: (1) 75 percent SSPp or SSPP; normal production of adrenolutin and adequate NAD, (2) 15 percent SSpp; normal production of adrenolutin with a dependency of niacin, creating a vulnerability to alcohol and to drug-induced psychosis, thus accounting for the success of niacin in treatment of alcoholics (Hawkins, 1968; Smith in Cheraskin and Ringsdorf, 1971; Hoffer, 1973b), (3) 5 percent SsPP or SsPp; excessive adrenolutin with normal NAD, creating susceptibility to schizophrenia induced by a decreased consumption of niacin, (4) 1 percent Sspp; too much adrenolutin and too little NAD, creating schizophrenia, (5) 0.1 percent SsPp or ssPp; double dose of adrenolutin in the presence of normal NAD and niacin, possibly representing autism, thus accounting for the nonresponse of autistic children to niacin (Rimland, 1968) and suggesting treatment which decreases production of adrenochrome using gluthathione, vitamin

C, and other reducing agents, or penicillamine and other substances which divert adrenochrome into the inert indole leuco-adrenochrome rather than into the hallucinogen adrenolutin (Hoffer, 1973b), (6) 0.01 percent sspp; lethal condition of inadequate NAD plus double-dose adrenolutin. These are, of course, hypotheses, useful principally in directing further research.

Biochemical Defects

Research indicates that schizophrenia is not a single disease resulting from a single biochemical disorder, but more probably a constellation resulting from many biochemical disorders (Cott, 1970).

Methylation. One of the most likely biochemical defects is an overactive methylation process. Methylation of any biogenic amine results in a compound with greater lipid solubility and greater brain stimulant effect (Pfeiffer et al., 1973), creating over-arousal. Goldstein and Beck (1965) and Kornetsky and Mirsky (1966) agree that overstimulation is inherent in schizophrenia.

Nicotinamide adenine dinucleotide (NAD). In schizophrenia, there appears to be an endogenous failure to deliver enough NAD to vital areas of the brain (Hoffer, 1973b). Nicotinic acid but not nicotinamide elevates blood NAD levels in animals and in humans (Altschule, 1964; Burton et al., 1962).

Tryptophan. Tryptophan, niacin, and pyridoxine are essential precursors of NAD. The body is unable to quickly metabolize tryptophan, the most toxic of the essential amino acids (Gullino et al., 1956). When amine oxidase, one of the enzymes which helps destroy tryptophan, is blocked, tryptophan becomes more toxic. Overloading with tryptophan is harmful, because it increases the psychologically powerful indoles (Hoffer, 1973b). Olson et al. (1960) found that 10 g of L-tryptophan caused perceptual and mood changes in 16 normal subjects but not in chronic alcoholics.

Indoles. When indole derivatives polymerize *in vitro* to melanins, hydrogen peroxide is generated. The brain is deficient in enzymes to destroy hydrogen peroxide (Cohen and Hochstein, 1963), and thus cell membranes and other lipid-containing cellular components may be damaged (Altschule and Hegedus, 1973).

Adrenolutin. Adrenochrome may be produced from adrenaline and non-adrenaline substances made in the body from tyrosine and possibly serotonin (Altschule and Hegedus, 1973). In schizophrenia, adrenochrome is converted to toxic adrenolutin. In non-schizophrenia, adrenochrome is converted into non-toxic leucoadrenochrome. This change is facilitated by the presence of sufficient amounts of vitamin C and the amino acids, gluthathione and cysteine (Cott, 1972; Hawkins, 1973).

Adrenochrome is a potent inhibitor of glutamic acid decarboxylase (Osmond and Hoffer, 1966), which assists synaptic transmission. Thus, inhibition of glutamic acid decarboxylase disrupts transmission of neural impulses, producing abnormal neurophysiological activity (Krippner, 1972).

Ceruloplasmin, a protein present in normal blood, can combine with and remove adrenolutin. The blood of some schizophrenics has more ceruloplasmin than others, and Heath (1966) found that these were more often the ones who recovered.

Taraxein. The brain of schizophrenics may be sensitized to substances like adrenolutin by the toxic protein taraxein. Taraxein, which Heath (1966) isolated in ceruloplasmin from the blood of schizophrenics, made monkeys psychotic and produced EEG tracings like those found in chronic schizophrenics. Human subjects, injected with taraxein, showed behavior similar to that seen in schizophrenic patients.

Gultamic acid. Glutamic acid removes intracellular ammonia and other toxic wastes in the brain. The metabolite of glutamic acid, glutamine, is involved in the maintenance of cerebral tissues. Glutamic acid is metabolized, in part, into the amine gamma amino butyric acid (GABA), which is believed to coordinate and regulate electrical activity at postsynaptic junctions and to aid the depolarized nerve to recover and fire once more. Thus, GABA inhibits neural fatigue and, conversely, enables the neural fibers to be receptive to continuous stimulation. This may underlie the increased attention, persistence, and ability to perform simple repetitive tasks reported to follow administration of glutamic acid (Vogel et al., 1966).

Vitamins B_3 and B_6. A deficiency of vitamin B_6 interferes with the metabolism of amino acids, proteins, and biogenic amines. L-dopa may induce pyridoxine deficiency (Golden et al., 1970). Some psychotic symptoms caused by L-dopa administration to psychiatric patients are blocked by administration of nicotinic acid (Yaryura-Tobias, 1973). The action of nicotinic acid is potentiated by pyridoxine, possibly by opening up the kynurenine cycle of tryptophan metabolism and thereby decreasing the formation of indoles (Ananth et al., in Hawkins, 1973).

Alpha-2-Globulin. Studies in molecular biology indicate that the function of the molecule depends on its geometry, symmetry, and other three-dimensional attributes. All forms of chronic schizophrenia may be associated with an abnormal molecular conformation of the alpha-2-globulin. Increased metabolic activity in 60 percent of the subjects in a study by Gottlieb et al. (1971) was associated with preponderance of the alpha-helix form of this protein, while in normal controls the beta-conformation predominated. Such increased activity altered intracellular levels of tryptophan and affected catecholamine ratios. In the 40 percent of the patients lacking the alpha-helix and the beta-conformation forms of the alpha-2-globulin, the molecule had a unique shape, which could be artificially reproduced in the laboratory only by exposure to a "leaked" intracellular protein destroying all alpha-helix forms (Lucas et al., 1971; Hawkins, 1973).

Catecholamine. A survey of psychiatric patients indicated that urinary catecholamine levels tended to increase in acute but not in chronic schizophrenics. It appeared that excretion of catecholamines may be modified by emotional and physical factors, but that overall metabolism of catecholamines is normal in schizophrenics (Ridges, 1973).

Kryptopyrrole (mauve factor). The EEGs of kryptopyrrole excretors were more frequently abnormal or borderline abnormal, showing low alpha content, high beta content, and sometimes delta activity, but no paroxysmal response to photic stimulation. Large excesses of beta waves have been associated with kryptopyrrole (Irvine, 1973).

Infections

Papez (1952, 1954), in studies of brain cultures, reported the consistent presence of a pleomorphic organism in the brains of schizophrenics. Philpott (1974) found bacterial infections in the urine of a majority of 30 schizophrenics. Ten of these showed progenitor cryptocides, a pleomorphic organism.

Orthomolecular Treatment

Symptomatology. The early stages of schizophrenia are marked by perceptual distortions resulting in altered subjective experiences of the self and the world. The illness may remain mild and never progress beyond this stage, aptly termed "metabolic dysperception" (Kowalson, 1973).

Posthypnotic suggestions to normal subjects indicated some of the profound effects which altered perceptions have on the human mind (Aaronson, 1967). Induced alterations of time and space resulted in elation or dysphoria, catatonia or hypomania. Suggesting that the world appeared two-dimensional resulted in depression and flattening of affect. Suggestions of altered perception of depth, size, constancy, and time rates produced paranoid reactions, schizoid behavior, and proprioceptive changes with alterations of posture, speech, and gait (Fogel and Hoffer, 1962; Aaronson, 1967).

The perceptual distortions in schizophrenia appear to occur independently of their subjective meaning to the patient. The disease process seems independent of the patient's personality and psychological type, although the patient's stability and psychological strengths determine to some degree at which point in the illness he becomes incapacitated (Hawkins, 1973).

Diagnosis. Perceptual disorders and the degree of schizophrenia can be measured by the Hoffer-Osmond Diagnostic Test (HOD) and the Experiential World Inventory (EWI). The HOD consists of 145 true-false statements, read and answered by the patient, which are designed to measure visual, auditory, olfactory, touch, taste, and time dysperceptions, as well as thought and mood disturbances (Hoffer and Osmond, 1961a, 1961b, 1966; Kelm, 1967). The EWI consists of 400 true-false statements measuring perceptual, affective, and ideational components and determining the relative contribution of perceptual and nonperceptual phenomena to each category of disturbance (El-Meligi and Osmond, 1973).

Prognosis. In general, the higher the HOD or EWI score, the greater the likelihood of response to orthomolecular therapy. The grown-up childhood schizophrenic, with the low score, postural stigmata of proprioceptive deficit, and primarily visual perceptual distortions, in particular the loss of depth, is the least likely to benefit. This type of patient appears to belong to a different biochemical category of the subtypes of the schizophrenias (Hawkins, 1973).

Treatment with vitamins. Appreciable drops in HOD or EWI scores and/or obvious clinical improvement have been seen following regular, daily treatment with combinations of the following: 20 mg to 1 g B_1, 20 mg B_2, 1 to 4 g B_3, 75 to 200 mg B_6, 15 mg pantothenic acid, 3 to 4 g C, 600 to 1,200 I.U.E. (Hoffer, 1962; Le Claire, 1972; Adams, 1973; Hawkins, 1968, 1973; Robie, 1973).

Interference with absorption of medications taken orally is, in some cases, a significant factor in those patients who respond poorly to treatment or who do not respond at all. Improvement can be speeded up by parenteral injections of the megavitamin (Cott, 1967, 1971).

A 48-week double-blind controlled study demonstrated the significant therapeutic effect of pyridoxine alone, nicotinic acid alone, and the two together. The effect of nicotinic acid was found to be potentiated by pyridoxine (Ananth et al., in Hawkins, 1973).

However, another double-blind study failed to demonstrate any therapeutic effect of the oral administration of nicotinamide (3 grams daily for one year) in the treatment of a consecutive series of 265 schizophrenic patients (McGrath et al., 1972).

Side effects observed in treating over 5,000 patients with megavitamins have been minimal and minor. Vitamins B_6, C, and E produced no side effects, although vitamin C may reputedly cause diarrhea. Niacinamide in a dosage of 4 g a day can produce nausea, particularly in adolescent girls. Niacin produces occasional nausea and an initial flush due to the release of histamine from the mast cells. The main contraindications to niacin are peptic ulcer, hypertension, diabetes, and gout (Hawkins, 1973).

Treatment with trace minerals. Many elements, needed by the body in trace amounts for specific enzyme action (Pfeiffer et al., 1973), compete with each other in biological systems, so an excess of one can block other minerals from an active enzyme site (Nicolson et al., 1966). Trace element levels in the body may be determined by testing such tissues as hair, nails, skin, and leukocytes (Pfeiffer et al., 1973).

Brain autopsies of schizophrenics revealed less zinc than brains of other patients. Offspring born of zinc-deficient rats and mice have learning deficits. Rats on a zinc-free diet have a 38 percent drop in serum zinc levels within 24 hours, indicating a lack of easily mobilized zinc reserves in body tissues. Zinc is necessary for RNA synthesis and for adrenal corticoid action involving protein synthesis (Pfeiffer et al., 1973).

Manganese, like reserpine, increases the activity of acetylcholine acetylase. In 1929, English (in Pfeiffer et al., 1973) treated 181 schizophrenic patients with intravenous injections of manganese chloride and found that half showed improvement.

Copper is high in the blood serum of some schizophrenics (Angel et al., 1957; Horwitt et al., 1957). Hypercupremia can aggravate depression and other symptoms in the schizophrenic. In one study, approximately 20 percent of 240 schizophrenic outpatients had elevated copper levels, 11 percent had low serum zinc levels, 12 percent had high iron levels, and 8 percent had low iron levels (Pfeiffer et al., 1973).

High serum copper levels, tremor of the hands, ataxia, and intermittent schizophrenic symptoms with wide mood swings may indicate mercury poisoning. In a group of 200 outpatient schizophrenics, four suffered from mercury poisoning. This may mean that 2 or more percent of mental patients are suffering from mercury poisoning (Pfeiffer et al., 1973).

Histamine levels. Pfeiffer et al. (1973) found that 50 percent of a group of schizophrenic patients had low blood histamine (H-) with a rise as they improved, while 20 percent had high blood histamine (H+) with a decrease as they improved. The H- group was characterized by a low incidence of allergies, a low basophil count, freedom from head colds, and slowness in achieving ejaculation or orgasm. Their main psychiatric symptoms were thought disorder, paranoia, and sometimes hallucinations. These patients generally responded to the usual antischizophrenic therapies and sometimes responded dramatically to folic acid therapy plus vitamin B_{12}. Dilantin, a folate antagonist, made them worse. H+ schizophrenics were characterized by a normal or high incidence of allergies and a basophil count above 0.6 percent. These patients were obsessed with suicidal depression and did not respond to the usual antischizophrenic therapies. They did respond to zinc and manganese and to histamine-releasing methadone.

Pfeiffer et al. (1973) suggested the following daily vitamin and mineral supplements for an adult histapenic (H-): 3 g vitamin C, 200 I.U. vitamin E, 3 g vitamin B_3, 200 mg vitamin B_6, 2 mg folic acid, 100 mg rutin, a multivitamin without minerals plus 1 mg B_{12} by injection each week; for an adult histadelic (H+): 2 g vitamin C, 200 I.U. vitamin E, 1 g calcium lactate, 200 mg niacin.

Oxidation levels. Watson and Currier (1960) and Watson (1965, 1972), studying over 200 mentally ill persons exhibiting a wide range of psychological disorders, established two basic types of subjects and two basic classes of vitamins and minerals for treatment. Blood studies showed significant differences between the group means of plasma pH, plasma bicarbonate, dissolved carbon dioxide plus carbonic acid, while the blood sugar difference was not quite significant at the 0.05 level.

Biochemical differences between groups disappeared and every subject showed psychological improvement when treated daily with the following supplements:

Type 1: 30 mg vitamin B_1, 30 mg vitamin B_2, 30 mg vitamin B_6, 75 mg niacin, 75 mg para-aminobenzoic acid, 900 mg vitamin C, 7,500 I.U. vitamin D, 900 mg potassium citrate, 300 mg magnesium chloride, 0.6 mg copper gluconate, 30 mg manganese oxide, 200 mg ferrous sulfate.

Type 2: 50,000 I.U. vitamin A, 200 I.U. vitamin E, 20 mcg vitamin B_{12}, 400 mg niacinamide, 100 mg calcium pantothenate, 100 mg choline, 180 mg inositol, 100 mg vitamin C, 100 mg bioflavonoids, 660 mg calcium, 500 mg phosphorus, 0.45 mg iodine, 20 mg zinc sulfate.

Type 1 subjects were, on the whole, made more ill by administration of Type 2 vitamins, and the contrary was true of Type 2 subjects.

A consideration of the metabolic roles of the vitamins suggested two major types of disturbances in intermediary metabolism, (1) slow oxidation of carbohydrates and glucogenic amino acids, resulting in a slow but preferential utilization of fats and ketogenic amino acids (Type 1 subjects), and (2) fast oxidation of carbohydrates and glucogenic amino acids, together with a slower but still more rapid than normal oxidation of fats and ketogenic amino acids (Type 2 subjects). Intense psychological stress resulted in decreases in the oxidation rates of Type 1 slow oxidizers and increases in the oxidation rates of Type 2 fast oxidizers (Watson, 1965, 1972).

Other studies of metabolism in schizophrenia (Kety et al., 1948; Gordon et al., 1955) have not found oxidation variations. However, representative samples were not tested, according to Watson (1972). In Watson's terms, 20 of Kety's 22 subjects were fast oxidizers, and 21 of Gordon's 24 subjects were slow oxidizers.

Fasting. Fasting has been successfully used to treat seriously disabled schizophrenics who have not responded to other means of treatment (Nickolayev in Cott, 1969; Lilliston, 1972; Meiers, 1973). Acidosis provoked by fasting and its compensation reflect a mobilization of detoxifying defense mechanisms, which may neutralize toxins associated with the schizophrenic process. As the acidosis decreases, the blood sugar level rises. The pH and other blood parameters remain constant after acidosis decreases.

Fasting mobilizes the proteins in the body, which are higher in schizophrenics than in nonschizophrenics. After fasting, the protein level becomes normal, but tends to rise to the prefast level after three to six months, even when patients eat a meat-free diet. Therefore, recurrent short fasts are necessary to maintain

nonschizophrenic protein levels (Nickolayev in Cott, 1969).

The presence of neurological allergies may also explain the benefits derived from fasts. Abstention from food and drink permits the withdrawal of allergens from the patient's internal environment, creating improved mental and physical functioning. Over 90 percent of the schizophrenics studied by Philpott (1973) displayed neurological reactions to common foods.

Gluten. Hoffer (1973b) believes the gluten in wheat and other grains may decrease absorption of niacin. A high association has been found between gluten enteropathy (celiac disease) and schizophrenia (Dohan, 1969).

Dohan et al. (1969) found a significant relationship between wheat consumption and hospitalization of schizophrenics. In Norway, Finland, Sweden, and Canada, consumption of wheat decreased by 30 percent from 1936 to 1939 and likewise the mean annual hospital admissions decreased by about 30 percent. In Canada, in 1943, wheat consumption rose and hospital admissions again increased.

In a controlled study by Dohan et al. (1969), a milk-and-cereal-free diet (CF) or a somewhat high-cereal diet (HC) were fed all men admitted to a locked psychiatric ward. Of the 47 CF relapsed schizophrenics, 62 percent were released from the ward to full privileges before the end of the median day, compared to 36 percent of the HC patients. The CF schizophrenics were discharged from the hospital significantly sooner than the HC group. When wheat gluten was secretly added to the CF diet, the difference in release rates disappeared. Such dietary changes had no effect on nonschizophrenics.

CHILDHOOD SCHIZOPHRENIA AND AUTISM

Although numbering only three or four per 10,000 among their age group, children afflicted with childhood schizophrenia and autism are victims of one of the most disabling illnesses known (Rimland, 1964). The most common means of treatment, based on psychoanalysis and related forms of psychotherapy, have been evaluated in numerous controlled studies and have invariably been shown to be of no discernible benefit. (For review, see Lewis, 1965.) Drugs have also been widely used in the treatment of such children, but few believe the drugs currently available provide more than stopgap assistance.

Several psychiatrists have experienced encouraging results using megavitamins. Green (1969) has successfully used several grams each of niacinamide and ascorbic acid daily, along with a highprotein, low-fat diet. Bonisch (in Rimland, 1973) reported that 12 of 16 autistic children became more interested and accessible when treated with vitamin B_6. Heeley and Roberts (in Cott, 1972) reported that 11 of a group of 19 psychotic children exhibited an abnormality of trytophan metabolism, which responded to supplemental vitamin B_6.

Cott (1972) successfully treated 500 children between 1966 and 1972 with 1 to 3 g niacinamide, 200 to 400 mg vitamin B_6, 400 to 600 mg calcium pantothenate, and 1 to 3 g vitamin C. Frequently folic acid, vitamin B_1, vitamin B_2, vitamin E, and glutamic acid were added. Cott's records indicated that those beginning treatment early in life, between ages three and seven, responded better than those further advanced in age. Children 11 years and older had the dimmest prognosis.

Rimland (1968, 1973) treated 190 schizophrenic children in

a controlled study, with daily administrations of two multiple vitamins plus 200 mg pantothenic acid, 1 to 3 g vitamin C, 1 to 3 g niacinamide, and 150 to 450 mg vitamin B_6. Vitamin B_6 brought the most obvious and dramatic changes. It not only seemed to stimulate speech but also to create a pressure to talk, a finding supported by Bonisch (in Rimland, 1973). Vitamin C seemed to increase alertness, social awareness, and sociability, a finding supported by Milner (1963) and VanderKamp (1966). Niacinamide seemed to quell bizarre behavior in some children but in others to produce irritability and hyperactivity. The children benefited by pantothenic acid seemed to become more alert, calmer, and more accessible, but the behavior of some children seemed to worsen with the addition of this vitamin (Rimland, 1968, 1973).

For a child to receive a "definite improvement" score, he not only had to improve during the three months of treatment but also to regress during the no-treatment period. Many children regressed within a matter of days, others took a month, and still others took longer. This suggested that the child who deteriorated very rapidly may have had a deficiency process quickly remedied or partially remedied by the added vitamins. In the slowly responding children, the process might instead have been one of gradual accretion of some toxic product of metabolism (Rimland, 1968, 1973).

Fifty-nine percent of the 37 austistic children showed definite improvement, as compared with 63 percent of the remainder of the sample. Among the children in the study showing the greatest improvement were six autistic children taking Dilantin along with the vitamins. Children taking Mellaril also showed unusually good improvement on the vitamins but unlike Dilantin, Mellaril showed no special interaction with autism. No other drugs seemed beneficial (Rimland, 1968, 1973).

LEARNING DISABILITIES

Genetic Transmission

Multiple occurrences in siblings and a history of familial psychiatric disorders point toward genetic transmission of learning disabilities (Wender, 1973). A high percentage of adults developing schizophrenia exhibited hyperactivity and/or learning disabilities as children (Cott, 1972). A study of 112 dyslexic children revealed that 90 percent had parents and/or siblings with similar problems, compared to 10 percent among the first-degree relatives of the control group (Hallgreen in Wender, 1973). Fifty percent of a small sample of fostered-away full sibs were hyperkinetic, whereas only 15 percent of the half sibs were so diagnosed (Safer in Wender, 1973).

Etiology

Almost any insult to the nervous system at a critical point of maturation may result in poor development of motor control, perception, language, or impulse inhibition. However, research points to a biochemical rather than an anatomical defect in children with learning disabilities (Wender, 1973).

Allergic insults in early infancy may impair some of the subtle interactions of the brain. Kittler (1970) reported that feed-ing difficulty, with repeated formula changes, is almost always part of the neonatal history of children with learning disabilities.

Characteristics

Clinically, children with learning disabilities appear to be hyperaroused, with high motor activity, sleep difficulties, poor attention span, and poor figure-ground discrimination. In many respects, they appear similar to children in early schizophrenic and manic excitement (Wender, 1973).

Children with learning disabilities and/or hyperkinesis were reported by Cott (1972) to eat a heavily salted diet high in cereals, carbohydrates, sweets, and sugary processed foods. Hypoglycemia occurred frequently. The glucose-tolerance test generally revealed either a flat curve, in which glucose levels showed little or no response to the ingestion of glucose, or a sawtooth profile. The flat curve is produced by an overproduction of insulin and the sawtooth curve by an erratic production of insulin (Shaw in Cott, 1972).

Lead and copper levels tend to be high in the hair of learning disabled children (Cott, 1972), while zinc, potassium, sodium, and manganese tend to be low (von Hilsheimer, 1971). This picture has frequently been reported for schizophrenics (Pfeiffer et al., 1973) and for allergic patients (Philpott, 1973, 1974).

Treatment

In a parental evaluation of the reactions of children with learning disabilities to various treatments, Mellaril, the drug with the best results, helped 15.8 percent. In a later study, parents indicated that 45 percent of the children taking high dosages of vitamins were definitely helped (Rimland in Lilliston, 1972).

Other encouraging results have been reported using combinations of 1 to 3 g niacinamide or niacin, 1 to 3 g ascorbic acid, 50 to 60 mg calcium pantothenate, 50 to 400 mg vitamin B_6, 300 to 600 I.U. vitamin E, 250 to 500 mg calcium, 8 to 15 mg lecithin granules, plus a high-protein, low-carbohydrate diet accompanied by digestive enzymes (Hoffer, 1973b; Cott, 1972; Fredericks, 1972; Powers, 1973; Vogel, 1973; Green, 1969, 1974). Some children react unfavorably to vitamin B_6, probably because it interacts with magnesium in such a way that it is removed from the body. Addition of 100 to 500 mg magnesium promptly corrects the deficiency (Martin, 1974).

Many children with learning disabilities respond to a rotation diet and allergy treatment, including 2 to 4 g ascorbic acid given immediately after exposure to a known allergen (Green, 1974). A well-established function of niacin in flushing histamine seems to have a long-term positive effect as an allergy treatment (von Hilsheimer, 1971).

As a pilot study, 20 children with abnormal electroencephalograms (EEGs) and a history suggestive of allergy were placed on a rotation diet free of foods to which they were sensitive. After six weeks, nine EEGs reverted to normal. Two more showed marked improvement. Scores on the Wechsler Intelligence Scale for Children (WISC) showed improvement following the dietary restrictions for those children initially scoring in the normal range. Those children with initial lower scores (50 to 80 I.Q.) showed no consistent change (Kittler, 1970).

MENTAL RETARDATION

Injections of vitamin B_{12} markedly enhanced learning in rats (Enesco et al. in Krippner, 1972). An absence of vitamins B_3 and B_{12} has been identified as a possible cause of brain dysfunction and/or mental retardation in animals (Brozek, 1961a, 1961b; Brin, 1967).

Nearly half the retarded children in a London study had higher lead levels than the maximum found in the control group of normal children. It does not necessarily follow that lead caused the children's mental retardation, but it is a possibility that lead at levels too low to cause obvious poisoning might result in mental retardation (Moncrieff, 1964). Animal studies revealed that any level of lead affects the functioning of the enzyme ALA dehydratase, in both the blood and the brain (Millar et al., 1970).

A study by Careddu et al. (1963) indicated that mental retardates excreted slightly less N-methylnicotinamide than normal subjects, although mongoloids excreted over twice as much N-methyl-6-pyridone-5-carboxamide. When given 2mg/kg of nicotinic acid intramuscularly, excretion of the 6-pyridone derivative increased slightly in mongoloids and in normal subjects and more than doubled in retardates.

Carter (1970) recommends treating various types of mental retardation with the following vitamins: cystathioninuria, vitamin B_6; homocystinuria, choline and vitamin B_6; hydroxy-kynureninuria, niacin; infantile spasms, vitamin B_6; methyl-malonic aciduria, low-protein diet and vitamin B_{12}; hyper-B-alaninemia, vitamin B_6; Lowe's syndrome, vitamin D, sodium and calcium; Fanconi's syndrome, vitamin D, sodium, and potassium bicarbonate; hepato-lenticular degeneration, low-copper diet. Potent concentrates of wheat germ oil have also been successfully used with retardates (Fredericks, 1972).

Perry et al. (1970) found that a deficiency of plasma glutamine was more characteristic of the degree of mental retardation in phenylketonuria than an excess of phenylalanine. Several investigators reported improvement in personality and an increase in intelligence of 5 to 20 I.Q. points for patients with mild to moderate deficiencies after administration of 10 to 20 mg daily of glutamic acid (Zimmerman and Ross, 1944) or glutamine (Vogel et al., 1966).

Turkel (1972) developed a formula of 50 different substances, including enzymes, hormones, vitamins, and minerals, which he successfully used to clear the mongoloid's blood and tissues of their excess metabolites. Retardation, he believes, is caused by accumulation of these metabolites, by-products of enzymes produced by genes contained in the extra chromosome in each cell. These aggregates cause water retention and calcification and prevent assimilation of nutrients and elimination of wastes.

In Russia, promising results in treating retardates have been obtained from vitamin B_{15}, pangamic acid, which aids in respiration of brain tissue (Blumina in Cott, 1972). Adequate tissue respiration is required for proper brain function. Warburg (in Himwich, 1951) reported that vitamins B_3 and C are important in respiration of all body tissues.

Fredericks (1974) reported that current, as yet unpublished, research indicates the megadoses of vitamin B_6, manganese, and zinc may prove to be the bridge to normal function for some of the retarded.

ALCOHOLISM

Alcohol's primary metabolite, acetaldehyde, competitively inhibits nicotinamide-adenosine-dinucleotide-linked aldehyde dehydrogenase (NADase), which interferes with the metabolism of dopamine, producing aberrant metabolites. Prolonged consumption of alcohol enhances the activities of the enzyme-reduced NAD phosphate oxidase (Davis and Walsh, 1970; Lieber and DeCarli, 1970). Alcoholics have been found to have a lower level of leukocyte ascorbic acid than control groups (Goldberg in Hawkins, 1973).

In 1972, an estimated 20,000 to 25,000 alcoholics were taking megavitamins. Cure rates ranged from 50 to 80 percent for alcoholics and alcoholic-schizophrenics, with improvement generally appearing between the third and sixth months (Hawkins, 1968, 1973). Using vitamins B_3, B_6, and C, Hoffer and Osmond (in Cheraskin and Ringsdorf, 1971) obtained a cure rate of 75 percent, as compared with a cure rate of 30 percent of alcoholics not treated with megavitamins.

In curing alcoholism and in relieving the intoxicated crises in alcoholics (Smith in Hawkins, 1973) and in LSD psychosis (von Hilsheimer, 1971; von Hilsheimer et al., 1967), niacin appears to be more effective than niacinamide. This may relate to the ability of niacin to release histamine from the mast cells, pointing to allergies, probably of grains (Cordas, 1975).

DRUG ADDICTION

Heroin addiction causes a considerable increase in the body's acid and also depletes the body's potassium and calcium. Blackman et al. (1973) used sodium bicarbonate to neutralize the acid, potassium bicarbonate to replace the lost potassium, and calcium carbonate to replace the lost calcium.

In a controlled study of 19 heroin addicts, Blackman et al. (1973) administered to each a salts mixture with a weight ratio of 6 $NaHCO_3$ to 3 $KHCO_3$ to 1 $CaCO_3$. A dose of one-tenth gram of the mixture per kilogram of body weight was administered with an eight-ounce glass of water every half hour for a two-hour period. Following a two-hour break, the salts were again administered with water for two hours at half-hour intervals. When symptoms occurred, an additional dose of the salts was administered.

All volunteers said the salts either eliminated withdrawal symptoms or considerably alleviated those symptoms that appeared. In 16 of the 19 cases, the volunteers reported no severe withdrawal symptoms; minor symptoms did occur, but only of short duration. In the other three cases, most symptoms were relieved within 30 minutes by additional doses of salts, and no symptoms lasted more than four hours (Blackman et al., 1973).

NEUROSES

A biochemical basis apparently exists for at least some anxiety neuroses. This is underlined by a strong familial tendency toward anxiety neuroses. Inherited biochemical individuality may be a factor. Excessive metabolic lactate production or excessive adrenaline secretion may be the metabolic fault. Perhaps anxiety neurotics need far more calcium than others. The antifatigue characteristics of ascorbic acid may point to a greater need for this vitamin (Williams, 1971). Many neurotic patients are greatly helped by the hypoglycemic diet, particularly when the presenting symptoms are depression, anxiety, phobia, fatigue, irritability, or hypochrondia (Hawkins, 1973).

Mild or heavy exercise produced significantly higher levels of lactate in anxiety neurotics than in control groups (Wendel and Beebe, 1973). Anxiety attacks were precipitated in susceptible neurotics by the infusion of lactate into the blood. But when calcium ions were infused with the lactate, the subjects did not experience anxiety symptoms (Williams, 1971).

ALLERGIES

Although most allergy patients have multiple organ-specific reactions, some have central nervous system (CNS) reactions as the primary organ-specific target. In such cases, sensitivities to specific foods, chemicals, or inhalants may be responsible for emotional reactions, not unlike the symptomatology commonly labeled "neurotic" or "psychotic" (Campbell, 1970). Confusion, mental blocking, dullness, lethargy, tenseness, irritability, dissociation, and perceptual distortions are some of the more common CNS allergic responses (Rinkel et al., 1951; Randolph, 1962; Philpott, 1974).

Acetylcholine is thought to be a major factor in CNS allergic reactions and is one of the synaptic junction transmitters in tension states. Both carbon dioxide and sodium bicarbonate destroy acetylcholine (Speer, 1970). Alkaline therapy with sodium and potassium bicarbonate (2:1 ratio) also effectively treats the acidification characteristically occurring during an allergy reaction (Randolph, 1962; Philpott, 1974).

Maladaptive reactions to foods and chemicals can generally be relieved by the administration of appropriate nutrients. This reinforces the thesis that enzyme deficiencies are involved in these reactions and that these nutrients are priming essential enzyme production (Philpott, 1974).

The most important nutrients for treatment are vitamins B_3, B_6, and C, calcium, magnesium, and manganese. Of lesser importance are vitamins A, B_1, B_2, D, and E, pantothenate, and other essential minerals. However, doses of appropriate nutrients reduce but do not completely prevent maladaptive reactions. Nutritional treatment works best when combined with initial avoidance of incriminating substances and a four-day dietary rotation by food families (Philpott, 1974).

HYPOGLYCEMIA

Research indicates that some individuals are unable to tolerate the American diet with its heavy emphasis on sugar, coffee, cola, and alcohol. In response to such dietary stress, some persons develop hypoglycemia (Yudkin, 1963), with such symptoms as fatigue, apathy, tension, irritability, confusion, anxiety, listlessness, trembling, sweating, and headaches (Portis, 1950; Mason, 1958). In schizophrenics, the marked drop in blood sugar, indicative of hypoglycemia, may precipitate suicidal depression, rage, or catatonia (Buckley, 1969).

Research studies indicate that hypoglycemia occurs in 30 to 70 percent of psychiatric patients (Cott, 1967; Hawkins, 1973; Meiers, 1973) and in 90 percent of alcoholics and alcoholic-schizophrenics (Hoffer and Osmond, 1962; Meiers, 1973, Hawkins, 1973).

Hypoglycemia may be caused or aggravated by shortages of zinc and chromium, vital to insulin and pancreatic action but often dissipated by excess starch (Pfeiffer et al., 1973). Recent animal studies showed that a high-carbohydrate diet or an increase in blood insulin altered tryptophan and serotonin levels in the brain (Fernstrom and Wurtman, 1971).

Most hypoglycemics respond favorably to frequent feedings of a low-carbohydrate, high-protein diet lacking caffeine, alcohol, and cigarettes (Fredericks, 1972; Hawkins, 1973; Meiers, 1973).

PSYCHOTHERAPY

During the acute phases of a mental illness, when the patient's HOD score is elevated, the most effective psychotherapy is probably an educational approach, which benefits both the patient and his family. This may be followed by supportive practical advice as the patient recovers and goes through the successive stages of recovery, including changes which may lead the patient erroneously to conclude he is getting worse (Hawkins, 1973).

After the patient's HOD score has returned to normal, specific conflicts may be handled either by supportive, individual therapy or by group therapy. At this stage, recurrence of symptoms accompanied by elevated HOD scores indicates that the cause is biochemical and should be treated by a change in the medical regimen. Symptoms unaccompanied by a rise in the HOD score, on the other hand, probably stem from interpersonal or psychological conflicts and, therefore, may be treated psychotherapeutically (Hawkins, 1973).

SUMMARY

Slight changes in molecular concentrations of common substances may affect the brain in such a way as to bring on major changes in behavior, mood, and perception. These phenomena can be commonly observed, easily demonstrated, experimentally induced, and therapeutically utilized.

REFERENCES

Aaronson, B.S.: Hypnosis, responsibility and the boundaries of self. American Journal of Clinical Hypnosis. 9:229:46, 1967.

Adams, R., and Murray, F.: *Megavitamin Therapy*. New York: Larchmont Books, 1973.

Atlschul, R.: Niacin in vascular disorders and hyperlipemia. Springfield, Ill.: Charles C Thomas, 1964.

Altschule, M.D., and Hegedus, Z.L.: The Adrenochrome Hypothesis of Schizophrenia. 1972. The Role of Rheomelanin Formation in Some Toxic Effects of Catecholamine Derivatives. In: Hawkins, D., and Pauling, L. (Eds.): Orthomolecular Psychiatry, Treatment of Schizophrenia. San Francisco: W.H. Freeman and Co., 1973.

Angel, C., Leach, B.E., Martens, S., Cohen, M., and Heath, R.G.: Serum Oxidation Levels. Archives of Neurological Psychiatry 78:500, 1957.

Aring, C.D., Evans, J.P., and Spies, T.D.: Some Clinical Neurologic Aspects of Vitamin B Deficiencies. Journal of the American Medical Association 113:2105, 1939.

Aring, C.D., and Spies, T.D.: A Critical Review: Vitamin B Deficiency and Nervous Disease. Journal of Neurological Psychiatry 2:335, 1939.

Axelrod, A.E., and Trakatellis, A.C.: Relationship of Pyridoxine to Immunological Phenomena. Vitamins and Hormones 22:59, 1964.

Baker, E.M.: Ascorbic Acid Metabolism in Man. American Journal of Clinical Nutrition 19:583, 1967.

Bicknell, F., and Prescott, F.: The Vitamin in Medicine. Milwaukee: Lee Foundation, 1953.

Black, D.A.K.: Experimental Potassium Depletion in Man.Lancet 1:244, 1952.

Blackman, D., Blackman, S., Thomason, A., and Thomason, N.: The Blackman-Thomason Salts Technique for Treating Opiate Addiction. Berkeley (unpublished manuscript), 1973.

Brin, M.: Newer Methods of Nutritional Biochemistry. New York: Academic Press, 1967.

Brozek, J.: Nutritional research in the Soviet Union: I. Some general aspects. Nutrition Reviews 19:129-32, 1961a.

Brozek, J.: Nutritional research in the Soviet Union: II. Some specific aspects. Nutrition Reviews 19:161-4, 1961b.

Bruno, M.: There's Psychotherapy in the B Vitamins. Prevention 25(4): 75, 1973.

Buckley, R.E.: Hypothalamic Tuning, Hypoglycemia Episodes and Schizophrenic Responses. Schizophrenia 1:1, 1969.

Burton, R.M., Salvador, R., Smith, K., and Howard, R.E.: The effect of chlorpromazine, nicotinamide and nicotinic acid on pyridine nucleotide levels of human blood. Annals of the New York Academy of Science 96:195, 1962.

Campbell, M.B.: Allergy and Behavior: Neurologic and Psychic Syndromes. In: Speer, F. (Ed.): Allergy of the Nervous System, Springfield, Ill.: Charles C. Thomas, 1970.

Careddu, P., Tenconi, L.T., and Sacchetti, G.: Transmethylation in Mongols. Lancet 1:828, 1963.

Carter, C.H.: Handbook of Mental Retardation Syndromes. Springfield, Ill.: Charles C. Thomas, 1970.

Cheraskin, E., and Ringsdorf, W.M.: New Hope for Incurable Diseases. New York: Exposition Press, 1971.

Cohen, G., and Hochstein, P.: Enzymatic mechanisms of drug sensitivity in brain. Diseases of the Nervous System 24:44, 1963.

Conney, A.H., Bray, G.A., Evans, C., and Burns, J.J.: Metabolic interactions between L-ascorbic acid and drugs. Annals of the New York Academy of Science 92:115, 1961.

Cordas, S.: Personal Correspondence. Eulis, Texas, 1975.

Cott, A.: Treating Schizophrenic Children. Schizophrenia 1:3, 1967.

Cott, A.: Continued Fasting Treatment of Schizophrenics in the U.S.S.R., J. Schizophrenia 1:44, 1969.

Cott, A.: Orthomolecular Treatment: a Biochemical Approach to Treatment to Schizophrenia. New York: Huxley Institute for Biosocial Research, 1970.

Cott, A.: Megavitamins: the Orthomolecular Approach to Behavioral Disorders and Learning Disabilities. J. Schizophrenia 3:1, 1971.

Cott, A.: Megavitamins: the Orthomolecular Approach to Behavioral Disorders and Learning Disabilities. Academic Therapy 7:245, 1972.

Davis, S.D., Nelson, T., and Shepard, T.H.: Teratogenecity of Vitamin B_6 deficiency: Omphalocele, skeletal and neural defects, and splenic hypoplasia. Science 196:1329, 1970.

Davis, V.E., and Walsh, M.J.: Alcohol, amines and alkaloids: a possible biochemical basis for alcohol addiction. Science 167:3920, 1970.

Dayton, P.G., and Weiner, N.: Ascorbic acid and blood coagulation. Annals of New York Academy of Science 92:302, 1961.

Dohan, F.C.: Is celiac disease a clue to the pathogenesis of schizophrenia? Mental Hygiene 53:4, 1969.

Dohan, F.C., Grasberger, J.C., Lowell, F.M., Johnston, H.T., and Abbegast, A.W.: Relapsed schizophrenics: More rapid improvement on a milk and cereal free diet. British Journal of Psychiatry 115:522, 1969.

Eiduson, G., Geller, E., Yuwiler, A., and Eiduson, B.T.: Biochemistry and Behavior. Princeton: Van Nostrand, 1964.

Ellis, J.M.: Vitamin B_6: the Doctor's Report. New York: Harper Row, 1973.

El Meligi, A.M., and Osmond, H.: The Experiential World inventory in Clinical Psychiatry and Psychopharmacology. In: Hawkins, D., and Pauling, L. (Eds.): Orthomolecular Psychiatry, Treatment of Schizophrenia. San Francisco: W.H. Freeman and Co., 1973.

Ferstrom, J.D., and Wurtman, R.J.: Brain Serotonin Content: Increase Following Ingestion of Carbohydrate Diet. Science 174:1028, 1971.

Fogel, S., and Hoffer, A.: The use of hypnosis to interpret and to reproduce an LSD-25 experience. Journal of Clinical and Experimental Psychopathology 23:44, 1962.

Fredericks, C.: Eating Right for You. New York: Grosset and Dunlap, 1972.

Fredericks, C.: Hotline to Health. Prevention 26 (10):59, 1974.

Frostig, J.P., and Spies, T.D.: The initial syndrome of pellagra and associated deficiency diseases. American Journal of Medical Science 199:268, 1940.

Gillman, J., and Gillman, T.: Perspectives in Human Malnutrition. New York: Grune and Stratton, 1951.

Golden, R.L., Mortati, R.S., and Schroeter, G.A.: Correspondence. Journal of the American Medical Association 213:628, 1970.

Goldstein, L., and Beck, R.A.: Amplitude analyses of the electroencephalogram. International Reviews of Neurobiology 8:125, 1965.

Goodhart, R.S.: The role of nutritional factors in the cause, prevention and cure of alcoholism and associated infirmities. American Journal of Clinical Nutrition 5:612, 1957.

Gordon, G.S., Estess, F.M., Adams, J.E., Bowman, K.M., and Simon, A.: Cerebral oxygen uptake in chronic schizophrenic reactions. Archives of Neurological Psychiatry 73:544, 1955.

Gottlieb, J.S., Frohman, C.E., and Harmison, C.R.: Schizophrenia: New Concepts. Southern Medical Journal 64:743, 1971.

Green, R.G.: Correspondence. Canadian Medical Association Journal 100:586, 1969.

Green, R.G.: Correspondence. Canadian Medical Association Journal 110:617, 1974.

Greenberg, S.M.: Iron absorption and metabolism. Journal of Nutrition 63:19, 1957.

Gullino, P., Winitz, M., Birnbaum, S.M., Cornfield, J., Otey, M.C., and Grunstein, J.P.: Studies on the metabolism of amino acids and related compounds in vitro. Archives of Biochemistry 64:319, 1956.

Hart, R.J.: Psychosis in vitamin B₁₂ deficiency. Archives of Internal Medicine 128:596, 1971.

Hawkins, D.R.: Treatment of Schizophrenia. J. of Schizophrenia 2:3, 1968.

Hawkins, D.R.: IV. A Practical Clinical Model. In Hawkins, D., and Pauling, L. (Eds.); Orthomolecular Psychiatry, Treatment of Schizophrenia. San Francisco: W.H. Freeman and Co., 1973.

Heath, R.G.: Schizophrenia: Biochemical and Physiologic Aberrations. International Journal of Neuropsychiatry 2:597, 1966.

Herbert, V.: A palatable diet for producing experimental folate deficiency in man. American Journal of Clinical Nutrition 12:17, 1963.

Herjanic, M.: Ascorbic Acid and Schizophrenia. In: Hawkins, D., and Pauling, L. (Eds.): Orthomolecular Psychiatry, Treatment of Schizophrenia. San Francisco: W. H. Freeman and Co., 1973.

Himwich, H.E.: Brain Metabolism and Cerebral Disorders. Baltimore: Williams and Williams, 1951.

Hoffer, A.: Niacin Therapy in Psychiatry. Springfield, Ill.: Charles C. Thomas, 1962.

Hoffer, A.: Correspondence. Canadian Medical Association Journal 107:112, 1972.

Hoffer, A.: Correspondence. Canadian Medical Association Journal 109:574, 1973a.

Hoffer, A.: Mechanism of Action of Nicotinic Acid and Nicotinamide in the Treatment of Schizophrenia. In: Hawkins, D., and Pauling, L. (Eds.): Orthomolecular Psychiatry, Treatment of Schizophrenia. San Francisco: W.H. Freeman and Co., 1973b.

Hoffer, A., and Osmond, H.: Double-Blind Clinical Trials. Journal of Neuropsychiatry 2:221, 1961a.

Hoffer, A., and Osmond, H.: In reply. Journal of Neuropsychiatry 3:262, 1961b.

Hoffer, A., and Osmond, H.: The Chemical Basis of Clinical Psychiatry, Springfield, Ill.: Charles C. Thomas, 1962.

Hoffer, A., and Osmond, H.: Some Psychological Consequences of Perceptual Disorders in Schizophrenia. International Journal of Neuropsychiatry 2:1, 1966.

Horwitt, M.K., Meyer, B.J., Meyer, A.C., Harvey, C.C., and Haffron, D.: Serum copper and oxidase activity in schizophrenic patterns. Archives of Neurology and Psychiatry 78:275, 1957.

Hurley, L.S.: Zinc deficiency in the developing rat. American Journal of Clinical Nutrition 22:1332, 1969.

Huxley, J.: Evolution: the modern synthesis. Heredity 9:1, 1964.

Irvine, D.G.: Kryptopyrrole in Molecular Psychiatry. In: Hawkins, D., and Pauling, L. (Eds.), Orthomolecular Psychiatry, Treatment of Schizophrenia. San Francisco: W.H. Freeman and Co., 1973.

Joliffe, N.: Effects of vitamin deficiency on mental and emotional processes. Research of Nervous and Mental Disease 19:144, 1939.

Joliffe, N., Bowman, K.M., Roseblum, L.A., and Fein, H.D.: Nicotinic acid deficiency encephalopathy. Journal of the American Medical Association 114:307, 1940.

Josephson, E.: Thymus, manganese and myasthenia gravis. New York: Chedney, 1961.

Karlsson, J.L.: The Biological Basis of Schizophrenia. Springfield, Ill.: Charles C. Thomas, 1966.

Kelm, H.: An Evaluation of the Hoffer-Osmond Diagnostic Test. J. Schizophrenia, 1:90, 1967.

Kety, S.S., Woodford, R.B., Harmel, M.H., Freyhan, F.A., Appel, K.E., and Schmidt, C.F.: Cerebral blood flow and metabolism in schizophrenia. American Journal of Psychiatry 104:765, 1948.

Kittler, F.J.: The effect of allergy on children with minimal brain damage. In: Speer, F. (Ed.): Allergy of the Nervous System. Springfield, Ill.: Charles C. Thomas, 1970.

Knox, W.E.: An evaluation of the treatment of phenylketonuria with diets low in phenylalanine. Pediatrics 26:1, 1960.

Kornetsky, C., and Mirsky, A.: On certain pharamacological and physiological differences between schizophrenics and normal persons. Psychopharmacology 8:309, 1966.

Kowalson, B.: Metabolic Dysperception: the Role of the Family Physician in its Diagnosis and Management. In: Hawkins, D., and Pauling, L. (Eds.): Orthomolecular Psychiatry, Treatment of Schizophrenia. San Francisco: W.H. Freeman and Co., 1973.

Krippner, S.: Illicit drug usage: Hazards for learning disabled students. Orthomolecular Psychiatry 1:1, 1972.

LeClair, E.R.: A Report on the Use of Orthomolecular Therapy in a California State Hospital. Orthomolecular Psychiatry 1:2 and 3, 1972.

Lewis, W.W.: Continuity and intervention in emotional disturbance: a review. Exceptional Children 31:467, 1965.

Lieber, C.S., and DeCarli, L.M.: Reduced Nicotinamide Adenine Dinucleotide Phosphate Oxidase: Activity Enhanced by Ethanol Consumption: Science 170:3953, 1970.

Lilliston, L.: The Megavitamin Controversy. Los Angeles Times, November 26, 1972.

Lucas, A.R., Warner, K., and Gottlieb, J.S.: Biological studies in childhood schizophrenia: Serotonin uptake by platelets. Biological Psychiatry 3:123, 1971.

Maas, J.W., Gleser, G.C., and Gottschalk, L.A.: Schizophrenia, anxiety, and biochemical factors. Archives of General Psychiatry 4:109, 1961.

Martin, G.R.: Studies on the tissue distribution of ascorbic acid. Annals of the New York Academy of Science 92:141, 1961.

Martin, P.: Mentally ill children respond to nutrition. Prevention 26(2): 95, 1974.

Mason, A.S.: Endocrine and metabolic disorders. British Journal of Clinical Practice 12:732, 1958.

Mayer, J.: Chromium in medicine. Postgraduate Medicine 49:235, 1971.

Mayer, J.: Human Nutrition. Springfield, Ill.: Charles C. Thomas, 1972.

McGrath, S.D., O'Brien, P.F., Power, P.J., and Shea, J.R.: Megavitamin treatment of schizophrenia. Schizophrenia Bulletin 5:74, 1972.

Meiers, R.L.: Relative Hypoglycemia in Schizophrenia. In: Hawkins, D., and Pauling, L. (Eds.): Orthmolecular Psychiatry, Treatment of Schizophrenia. San Francisco: W.H. Freeman and Co., 1973.

Millar, J.A., Goldberg, A., and Hernberg, S.: Lead and delta-aminolevulinic acid dehydratase levels in mentally retarded children and in lead-poisoned suckling rats. Lancet 2:695, 1970.

Milner, G.: Ascorbic acid in chronic schizophrenic patients: a controlled test. British Journal of Psychiatry 109:294, 1963.

Moncrieff, A.A.: Lead poisoning in children. Archives of Diseases in Children 39:1, 1964.

Nicolson, G.A., Greiner, A.D., McFarlane, W.J.G., and Baker, R.A.: Effects of penicillamine on schizophrenic patients. Lancet 2:344, 1966.

Olson, R.E., Gursey, D., and Vester, J.W.: Evidence for a defect in tryptophan metabolism in chronic alcoholism. New England Journal of Medicine 263:1169, 1960.

Osmond, H., and Hoffer, A.: A Comprehensive Theory of Schizophrenia. International Journal of Neuropsychiatry 2:303, 1966.

Papez, J.W.: Form of living organisms in psychotic patients. Journal of Nervous and Mental Disease 116:375, 1952.

Papez, J.W.: The hypophysis cerebric in psychosis. Journal of Nervous and Mental Disease 119:326, 1954.

Pauling, L.: Orthomolecular Psychiatry: Varying the concentrations of substances normally present in the human body may control mental disease. Science 160:265, 1968.

Pauling, L.: Orthomolecular Psychiatry. In Hawkins, D., and Pauling, L. (Eds.): Orthomolecular Psychiatry, Treatment of Schizophrenia. San Francisco: W.H. Freeman and Co., 1973.

Perry, T.L., Hansen, S., Tischler, B., Bonting, R., and Diamond, S.: Glutamine depletion in phenylketonuria. New England Journal of Medicine 282:761, 1970.

Pfeiffer, C.C., Iliev, V., and Goldstein, L.: Blood Histamine, Basophil Counts, and Trace Elements in the Schizophrenias. In Hawkins, D., and Pauling, L. (Eds.): Orthomolecular Psychiatry, Treatment of Schizophrenia. San Francisco: W.H. Freeman and Co., 1973.

Philpott, W.H.: Ecologic and supernutrition methods of determining values of orthomolecular psychiatry treatment (unpublished), November, 1973.

Philpott, W.H.: Methods of relief of acute and chronic symptoms of deficiency-allergy-addiction maladaptive reactions to foods and chemicals. Paper presented at the meeting of Seventh Advanced Seminar in Clinical Ecology, Fort Lauderdale, Florida, January 9, 1974.

Portis, S.A.: Emotions and hyperinsulinism. Journal of the American Medical Association 142:1291, 1950.

Powers, H.W.S.: Dietary measures to improve behavior and achievement. Academic Therapy 9:3, 1973.

Randolph, T.G.: Human ecology and susceptibility to the chemical environment. Springfield, Ill.: Charles C. Thomas, 1962.

Ridges, A.P.: The methylation hypothesis in relation to "pink spot" and other investigations. In: Hawkins, D., and Pauling, L. (Eds.): Orthomolecular Psychiatry, Treatment of Schizophrenia. San Francisco: W.H. Freeman and Co., 1973.

Rimland, B.: Infantile Autism: the Syndrome and Its Implications for a Neural Theory of Behavior. New York: Appleton-Century-Crofts, 1964.

Rimland, B.: High-Dosage Levels of Certain Vitamins in the Treatment of Children with Severe Mental Disorders. San Diego: Institute for Child Behavior Research, 1968.

Rimland, B.: High-Dosage Levels of Certain Vitamins in the Treatment of Children with Severe Mental Disorders. In: Hawkins, D., and Pauling, L. (Eds.): Orthomolecular Psychiatry, Treatment of Schizophrenia. San Francisco: W.H. Freeman and Co., 1973.

Rinkel, H.J., Randolph, T.G., and Zeller, M.: Food Allergy. Springfield, Ill.: Charles C. Thomas, 1951.

Robie, T.R.: A Review of Ten Years' Experience Utilizing Niacin in Treating Schizophrenia with an Evaluation of Metabolic Dysperception as a Clarifying Diagnostic term. In: Hawkins, D., and Pauling, L. (Eds.): Orthomolecular Psychiatry, Treatment of Schizophrenia. San Francisco: W.H. Freeman and Co., 1973.

Rodale, R.: The Zinc Story. Prevention 25(7):21, 1973a.

Rodale, R.: Putting More Zinc into Your Life. Prevention 25(8):21, 1973c.

Rodale, R.: You Can Solve Your Zinc Problem. Prevention 25(9): 21, 1973c.

Rodale, R.: Creeping Vegetarianism Creates Zinc Hunger. Prevention 26(7):21, 1974.

Rosenberg, L.E.: Vitamin-Dependent Genetic Disease. Hospital Practice p. 59, 1970.

Scheid, A.S.: Comparison of methods for determination of vitamin B_{12} potency. Journal of Nutrition 47:601, 1952.

Schroeder, H.A.: The Trace Elements and Man. Old Greenwich, Conn.: Devin-Adair, 1973.

Shils, M.E.: Experimental human magnesium depletion. American Journal of Clinical Nutrition 15:133, 1964.

Speer, F. (Ed.): Allergy of the Nervous System. Springfield, Ill.: Charles C. Thomas, 1970.

Tui, CO.: The fundamentals of clinical proteinology. J. Clinical Nutrition 1:232, 1953.

Turkel, H.: New Hope for the Mentally Retarded. New York: Vantage, 1972.

Urbach, C., Hickman, K., and Harris, P.L.: Effect of individual vitamins A, C, and E and carotene administered at high levels on their concentration in the blood. Experimental Surgery 10:7, 1952.

Vanderkamp, A.: A biochemical abnormality in schizophrenia involving ascorbic acid. International Journal of Neuropsychiatry 2:204, 1966.

Vogel, M.J.: Correspondence. Canadian Medical Association Journal 108:959, 1973.

Vogel, M.J., Broverman, D.M., Diaguns, J.G., and Klaiber, E.L.: The role of glutamic acid in cognitive behaviors. Psychological Bulletin 65, 378, 1966.

Von Hilsheimer, G.: A Point of View for Teachers and Parents of Special Children Regarding Vitamins and Orthomolecular Medicine. Address presented to Texas Association for Children with Learning Disabilities, Dallas, 1971.

Von Hilsheimer, G., Klotz, S.D., McFall, G., Lerner, H., Van West, A., and Quirk, D.: The Use of Megavitamin Therapy in Regulating Severe Behavior Disorders, Drug Abuse and Frank Psychoses. J. Schizophrenia 3:1, 1967.

Watson, G., and Currier, W.D.: Intensive vitamin therapy in mental illness. Journal of Psychology 49:67, 1960.

Watson, G.: Differences in intermediary metabolism in mental illness. Psychological Reports 17:563, 1965.

Watson, G.: Nutrition and Your Mind: the Psychochemical Response. New York: Harper and Row, 1972.

Wendel, O.W., and Beebe, W.E.: Preliminary Observations of Altered Carbohydrate Metabolism in Psychiatric Patients. In: Hawkins, D., and Pauling, L. (Eds.): Orthomolecular Psychiatry, Treatment of Schizophrenia. San Francisco: W.H. Freeman and Co., 1973.

Wender, P.: Some speculations concerning a possible biochemical basis of minimal brain dysfunction. Annals of the New York Academy of Science 205:21, 1973.

Williams, R.: Nutrition against Disease. New York: Pitman, 1971.

Wohl, M.G., and Goodhart, R.S.: Modern Nutrition in Health and Disease. Philadelphia: Lea and Febiger, 1968.

Wormsley, G.H., and Darragh, J.H.: Potassium and sodium restrictions in the normal human. Journal of Clinical Investigation 34:456, 1955.

Yaryura-Tobias, J.A.: Levodope and Mental Illness. In: Hawkins, D., and Pauling, L. (Eds.): Orthomolecular Psychiatry, Treatment of Schizophrenia. San Francisco: W.H. Freeman and Co., 1973.

Yudkin, J.: Myocardial infarction and other diseases of civilization. Lancet 1:1335, 1963.

Zimmerman, F.T., and Ross, S.: Effect of glutamic acid and other amino acids on maze learning in the white rat. Archives of Neurological Psychiatry 51:446, 1944.

Index

30
Appendix
Proteolytic Enzyme and Amino Acid Therapy
in Degenerative Disease

Two articles by William H. Philpott, M.D. (1. *The Significance of Reduced Proteolytic Enzymes in the Diabetes Mellitus Disease Process and in the Schizophrenia Syndrome Variable*; 2. *Ecologic Stimulus Evoked Pancreatic Insufficiency in Chronic Degenerative Disease in General and Cardiovascular Disease in Particular*) were condensed and edited by Dwight K. Kalita, Ph.D. for this one single presentation. Although all points of discussion in the two articles could not be presented, the Editor emphasized Dr. Philpott's ideas concerning proteolytic enzyme and amino acid therapy in degenerative disease.

CURRENT STATUS OF CLINICAL ECOLOGY

Successions of medical practitioners since the 1920's have been recording individualized idiosyncratic maladaptive reactions to foods and chemicals observed as emerging during controlled systematic test exposures. These reactions are especially acute after a four to six day period of avoidance of incriminated substances. These reactions have been varyingly characterized as allergic, hypersensitivity, non-reaginic allergies, maladaptive reactions, idiosyncratic reactions, enzymatic deficiency reactions, and acute metabolic acidosis reactions. Substances evoking these reactions are far beyond the anticipated allergic reactions to protein substances, and include all food categories and chemicals especially those frequently contacted. The types of reactions evoked are as varied as the many tissues and organ systems of the human body; therefore, mental as well as physical symptoms are included.

Due to the numerous substances evoking reactions, some of which are obviously beyond the evidence of the immunologic mechanisms, there has developed in medicine a clinical ecology practice which honors the fact of reactivity whether immunologic or non-immunologic in its origin. Clinical ecology has developed significant methods of diagnosis and treatment of a wide assortment of physical and mental reactions (diseases).

By and large clinical ecology has viewed these maladaptive reactions in terms of the significance of individualized reactions. Recent monitoring of shifts in chemistry comparing the non-reactive state with the reactive state reveals the reactions to be the building blocks of degenerative diseases. Thus an acute arthralgia reaction when evoked numerous times which damages tissue becomes arthritis, acute muscle pains become chronic myocitis; acute mental reactions when chronic become named as mental diseases; acute hyperglycemia when it progresses to a chronic state is named as diabetes mellitus. Monitoring of before and after reactions in the areas of blood sugar shifts, pH shifts, porphyric reactions, thyroid reaction, liver function, triglycerides, and cholesterol gives convincing evidence that these acute discrete maladaptive reactions are indeed chronic degenerative diseases in miniature.

THE PANCREAS AS A PRIMARY SHOCK ORGAN TO ECOLOGIC FOOD AND CHEMICAL FACTORS

The pancreas is the first endocrine-exocrine organ to be influenced by the ecologic contact with ingested foods and chemicals. We can well understand the predisposition of the pancreas as a primary shock organ to ingested foods and chemicals. The pancreas has the monumental task of making useful metabolic products from the ingested foods and chemicals and also buffering against reactions to foods and chemicals. An overstimulated pancreas follows the same general law that other overstimulated tissues and organ systems follow, and that is that overstimulation eventually leads to inhibition of function. Besides the mechanism of inhibition of function by overstimulation, the pancreas has a mechanism of self injury by the mechanism of activation of proteolytic enzymes while still in the pancreas producing pancreatitis. Pancreatitis states may be severe or mild, but often they are mild attacks which are easily dismissed as mild gastritis attacks.

It is well documented that addiction to alcohol leads to pancreatic insufficiency. What has been little appreciated is that all addictions lead to pancreatic insufficiency of varying degrees. B.M. Frier, et al., made a most pertinent observation about diabetes mellitus observing it to be a state of generalized pancreatic insufficiency. This generalized pancreatic insufficiency occurs in all types of diabetes mellitus whether juvenile, adult onset, or of known pancreatitis origin. Most affected in this pancreatic insufficiency is the bicarbonate production followed by enzyme production and least of all, insulin production.

To understand the significance of pancreatic insufficiency, we need to examine the physiology of pancreatic function especially its exocrine function. Gastric digestion occurs in an acid media (pH of 1.8 to 3 and functions best at a pH of 1.8 to 2) while the small intestine functions in an alkaline medium pH of 6.8 and higher and most optimum at a pH of 8 to 9). The pancreas produces bicarbonate and the fluids coming from the pancreas normally have a pH of 8. Proteolytic enzymes from the pancreas function in a neutral to alkali media, and at optimum value at a pH of 8 to 9. These enzymes are destroyed in an acid media. Optimum function of proteolytic enzymes require the presence of the lipid digestive enzyme lipase. Proteolytic enzymes (trypsin, chymotrypsin, carboxypeptidase) digest proteins to amino acids which are then used as building blocks for enzymes, hormones, and tissues. An important systemic function of proteolytic enzymes is a regulatory mechanism for inflammatory reactions from any source and as well as regulatory mechanism over kinins which are tissue hormones. Inflammation has two sources: 1. Histamine-mediated inflammation (immunologic). 2. Kinin-mediated inflammation (non-immunologic). Proteolytic enzymes have a regulatory and inflammation resolving control over both types of inflammations, but is of special importance in kinin-mediated reactions since proteolytic enzymes are capable of blocking the rise in kinins thus preventing the kinin-mediated inflammatory reactions from occurring. This fact becomes of special import when we realize there is test information justifying the conclusion that two-thirds of the maladaptive reactions to ecologic substances are kinin-mediated inflammatory reactions and only one-third histamine-mediated inflammatory reactions. The common denominator between histamine and kinin inflammatory reactions such as edema and an acid state makes these reactions clinically indistinguishable. However, kinin inflammatory reactions are more prone to be painful than histamine inflammatory reactions since kinins evoke pain when in contact with nerve endings.

The consequences of insufficient pancreatic bicarbonate are: 1. Acute metabolic acidosis post meal since the pancreatic bicarbonate has not neutralized the acid from the stomach as it empties into the duodenum. 2. Inactivation of and/or destruction of proteolytic enzymes from the pancreas (trypsin, chymotrypsin, carboxypeptidase) and intestine (prolinase, amino peptidase, cathepsin, A, B, and C).

The consequences of insufficient pancreatic proteolytic enzymes are: 1. Poor digestion of proteins to amino acids. 2. Unusable inflammatory evoking protein molecules absorbed through the intestinal mucosa and circulating in the blood reaching tissue in undigested form, evoking both immunologic (histamine) as well as non-immunologic (kinin) inflammatory reactions. 3. Low systemic proteolytic enzymes (a) allowing inflammatory reactions from any source to go unresolved and (b) a rise in tissue kinins evoking inflammatory reactions in response to specific substances, (c) the evoking of severe inflammatory reactions injuring lysosome membranes which start a chain of inflammation, a cell degeneration, and carcinogenic potential.

The consequences of amino acid deficiency are: 1. Inability to make enzymes, hormones, tissues, and antibodies against infection in adequate quality or quantity. 2. Excessive demands for vitamins and minerals, especially B_6 and its helpers, zinc and magnesium, thus setting up a chain of deficiencies. 3. Infectious invasion due to unhealthy tissues and low immunologic defense which set in motion another chain of inflammation, tissue destruction, and bacterial and viral toxins poisoning vital metabolic processes as well as some of the infectious microbes having known carcinogenicity such as Progenitor Cryptocides.

The significance of this information comes into sharp focus when we appreciate that clinical ecology has demonstrated adaptive addiction to be common and that biochemical monitoring of these maladaptive reactions to foods and chemicals reveals the presence of pancreatic insufficiency of varying degrees ranging from mild to severe and from reversible to non-reversible.

PROTEOLYTIC ENZYME THERAPY IN DEGENERATIVE DISEASE

Proteolytic enzymes digest proteins into amino acids. Without adequate proteolytic enzymes, amino acid deficiency results. The guiding principal of treatment is to be sure to use an adequate amount for the maximum inhibition of inflammation.

The schedule can vary from three to six doses in twenty-four hours and it is likely best to have at least one dose during the night although some will do well with three daytime doses.

1. *With meals* (x3)
   Thirty minutes before meals — Two tablets of pancreas compound with duodenum.
2. *At the beginning of the meal.*
   If the gastric acid has been demonstrated to be low, then give glutamic acid HCL and/or betaine HCL or a digestive enzyme tablet containing these plus pepsin and pancreatic concentrate.
3. *End of meal.*
   Two tablets of pancreas compound with duodenum.
4. *Thirty minutes after end of meal.*
   One tablet pancreas compound with duodenum.
   One tablet bromelain with papain.
   Ten to twenty grains of sodium bicarbonate or one-fourth to one-half tsp. of sodium bicarbonate and potassium bicarbonate (two-thirds to one-third).
5. *At bedtime.*
   Five tablets of pancreas compound with duodenum.
   Two bromelain tablets with papain.
6. *At 2 A.M.*
   Five tablets of pancreas compound with duodenum.
   Two tablets of bromelain with papain.

Maintain this program for two to four months and then reduce according to patient's needs.

The sodium bicarbonate is necessary to produce the alkali necessary for activation of the pancreatic enzymes. This is given thirty minutes after the meal so as not to interfere with the acid gastric phase of digestion. The alkali should be given earlier than one half hour if there is an epigastric discomfort with eating. The determination of the amount of alkali needed for each person can be roughly judged by taking readings of saliva pH using Phydrion paper before the meal, thirty minutes after the meal, and one hour after the meal. The normal saliva pH is 6.4 to 6.8. If the saliva is below 6.4 before the meal, this is an indication that the patient is producing too much gastric HCL and certainly should not have any supplemented acid with the meal. If the pH is around 6.8 or especially if higher than this, it is presumptive evidence of a need to supplement acid with the meal. If the saliva pH at thirty minutes post meal is below 6.4, it is a definite indication for a need of alkali supplementation. Even if the pH is in the 6.8 range, the alkali should be given since the desired pH of the small intestine during ingestion is 8 to 9. If the saliva pH one hour post meal is 6.8 to 7 and above then this systemic alkalosis is presumptive evidence that the local small intestine pH may be around 8 to 9. Bear in mind that the goal is to have the local intestinal alkali high enough to provide an alkaline media for the function of the proteolytic digestive process as well as providing absorption of proteolytic enzymes and also systemic post-meal activation of the systemic proteolytic enzyme pool so as to prevent kinin-mediated inflammatory reactions occurring in response to the absorbed foods.

CASE HISTORIES

Catatonia Schizophrenia — Woman Age 26

I. *Cheddar Cheese Test Before and After Proteolytic Enzymes.*
Initial Reaction: Markedly sweating hands followed by tension which progressed to rigid catatonia.

Cheddar Cheese Test After Proteolytic Enzymes.
(1) 1,670 mg. concentrated pancreatic enzymes in enteric coated tablets. Glutamic Acid HCL, and Pepsin also in the non-enteric coated part of the tablet. Blood sugar 75 mg.%.
(2) Thirty minutes after step one blood sugar was 80 mg.%.
(3) Fifty minutes after step one, 1,670 mg. concentrated pancreatic enzymes enteric coated was given.
(4) Fifty-five minutes after step one she ate one pound of cheddar cheese.
(5) Thirty minutes after the test meal, one-fourth tsp. sodium bicarbonate plus potassium bicarbonate (two-thirds to one-third) given. Blood sugar was 80 mg.%.
(6) One hour after test meal blood sugar was 90 mg.%.
Results of test: No tension or catatonia. She was mentally clear. The only symptom was minor sweating of hands.

II. *Test for Irish Potato and Dairy Butter Before and After Proteolytic Enzymes.*
Test for Butter Without Enzymes.
Nausea and vomiting. Blood sugar 110 mg.%.

Test for Irish Potato Without Enzymes.
Hands cold, tense, and nervous. Feels hot and breathing labored.

Test for Dairy Butter Plus Irish Potato After Proteolytic Enzymes.
(1) Blood sugar was 80 mg.% and symptom free. 1,670 mg. pancreatic enzymes enteric coated tablets plus Glutamic Acid HCL, Betaine HCL, and Pepsin administered.
(2) Thirty minutes after step one blood sugar was 80 mg.% and she was symptom free. Test meal of Irish potato and dairy butter given.
(3) Thirty minutes after the test meal, one-fourth tsp. alkali salts was given. Blood sugar was 80 mg.%.
(4) One hour after the test meal blood sugar was 100 mg.%.
Results of Test: The only symptom was slight nausea.

III. *Test Meal of Peanuts Before and After Proteolytic Enzymes.*
The initial reaction to a test meal of peanuts was irritability, depression, crying, and dissociation.

A test meal after proteolytic enzymes was on the order of 1,670 mg. pancreatic concentrate forty minutes before the meal, and another 1,670 mg. at the time of the test meal. The blood sugar remained stable.
Results of Test: The only symptom was slight sweating of the hands.

IV. *Test Meals of Beef Before and After Proteolytic Enzymes.*
The initial test meal without proteolytic enzymes produced tension, a desire not to talk, a wish to be alone, and feeling like screaming.

The test meal using proteolytic enzymes was on the order of 1,670 mg. pancreatic concentrate plus Glutamic Acid HCL, Betaine HCL, and Pepsin before the meal followed by one-fourth tsp. alkali salts thirty minutes after the meal.
Results of Test: No symptoms developed.

V. *Repeat of the peanut test on the second day using powdered pork source pancreatic concentrate of 1,225 mg. thirty minutes before and 1,225 mg. with the meal.*
She became catatonic one hour after the meal. She promptly recovered when given the following intravenously: B_6, 1,000mg.; Vitamin C, 12.5 grams, B_5, 1,250mg.; B-Complex, 5cc.; Calphosan, 10cc.; Magnesium Chloride, 2 grams; Heparin, 20,000 units. On several other occasions she had recovered promptly from catatonic states after test meals by the use of the vitamins and minerals only without the Heparin. Heparin was given for the theoretical reason of raising the systemic proteolytic enzyme pool. Heparin alone has been administered with success in relieving symptoms in a number of patients. Some trials have been failures presumably because of using a pork source of pancreatic enzymes in pork sensitive patients or even more likely the inability to raise the proteolytic capacity of the blood in the brief thirty minutes to one hour before the test exposure. Also we should never assume that proteolytic enzyme therapy will be more than a partial answer.

Inhibition of Cytoxic Reaction by Proteolytic Enzymes Plus Amino Acids:

I. Schizophrenic — Age 30: (1) ten tablets pancreas compound (325 mg.) with duodenum. Ten tablets Bromelain (100 mg.) plus papain (10 mg.). Fifteen grams free amino acids as predigested protein. (2) One half hour after Step 1: Five pancreas compound tablets with amino acids. Five tablets Bromelain plus papain. (3) Cytotoxic test one half hour after Step 2.

Before and After Proteolytic Enzymes and Amino Acids:
CYTOTOXIC TEST:

BEFORE	AFTER
+++ Cigarette Tobacco	+ Cigarette Tobacco #1
++ Burley Tobacco	+ Cigarette Tobacco #2
	+ Burley Tobacco #1
	+ Burley Tobacco #2

For five days before the test, the patient had been given selective foods she seldom used for the purpose of an avoidance of commonly used foods. There was no smoking during these five days.

II. Manic depressive — Age 51: (1) Ten tablets pancreas compound (325 mg.) with duodenum. Ten tablets Bromelain (100 mg.) with papain (20 mg.). Fifteen grams free amino acids as predigested protein. (2) One half hour after Step 1: Five pancreas compound with duodenum. Five tablets Bromelain with papain. (3) Cytotoxic test one half hour after Step 2.

Before and After Proteolytic Enzymes and Amino Acids:
CYTOTOXIC TEST:

BEFORE		AFTER	
++	Rice	0	Rice
I ++	Eggs	+	Eggs
++	Potatoes	+	Potatoes
++	Cheddar Cheese	+	Cheddar Cheese
+++	Navy Beans	++	Navy Beans
+++	Peanuts	++	Peanuts

Sublingual Petrochemical Hydrocarbon Test Before and After Proteolytic Enzymes Plus Amino Acids:

Schizophrenic — Age 23: Sublingual auto exhaust test before exposure to proteolytic enzymes and amino acids. Symptoms: Marked negativism, loss of insight, loss of motivation, reduced ability to concentrate, reduced comprehension, and painful tension in back and neck.

Sublingual test for auto exhaust after proteolytic enzymes. (1) Five pancreas compound (325 mg.) plus duodenum. Five Bromelain (200 mg.) plus papain duodenum. (2) Thirty minutes after Step 1: Five pancreas compound plus duodenum. Five Bromelain plus papain. (3) Thirty minutes after Step 2 Sublingual test for auto exhaust was given.

Symptoms: Talkative, spaced out feeling, poor concentration, difficulty reading, poor comprehension of what is read, tension, tapping of feet, and headache.

Sublingual test for auto exhaust with proteolytic enzymes plus amino acids: (1) Five pancreas compound with duodenum. Five Bromelain with papain. Fifteen grams free amino acids as predigested protein. (2) Thirty minutes after Step 1: Five tablets pancreas compound with duodenum. Five tablets Bromelain with papain. Fifteen grams free amino acids as predigested protein. Twenty grains sodium bicarbonate. (3) Thirty minutes after Step 2 auto exhaust given as sublingual test.

Symptoms: A question of increased visual light sensitivity when he went out into the sunlight. Minor brief nasal stuffiness at the beginning of the test. No mental symptoms occurred and no other physical symptoms occurred.

CONCLUSIONS

It was necessary to add free amino acids to proteolytic enzymes in order to obtain test evidence of symptom relief to petrochemical hydrocarbons. Deficient proteolytic enzymes lead to deficient essential amino acids. Amino acids need to be routinely supplemented in pancreatic insufficiency. At the beginning of therapy, amino acid supplementation is of equal importance to supplementing proteolytic enzymes. Free amino acids can be supplied as capsules, tablets, or predigested protein as liquid free amino acids. Approximately fifteen grams four times a day of free amino acids should be supplied for a minimum of one month and then reduced according to the individual needs.

After one week of proteolytic enzyme therapy plus amino acids this patient had complete relief from reactions to all petrochemical hydrocarbon exposures. Whereas, before even while on mega-vitamins and a diet of avoidance of incriminated foods on a four day rotation diet he was severely reacting to contact with auto exhaust, perfume, gas stove, and so forth. Before enzyme therapy began, he violated his diet by eating a meal of Mexican foods, and suffered numerous and severe symptoms. One week after enzyme therapy plus amino acids he purposely as a test ate again a meal of Mexican food with the result of no symptoms occurring.

These tests give evidence that proteolytic enzymes plus amino acids can be used to reduce or eliminate cerebral allergic reactions in severe degenerative disease. More definitive studies need to be made after longer term therapy with proteolytic enzymes and amino acids.

Chronic Schizoaffective Reaction — Woman Age 27

I.   Test for Raisins Before and After Proteolytic Enzymes

Test for Raisins Without Proteolytic Enzymes.
One hour after test meal for raisins, the blood sugar was 400 mg.%. Symptoms were marked tension, trembling, irritability, and unprovoked anger at mother.

Test Meal With Proteolytic Enzymes.
(1) Symptom free. Blood sugar 100 mg.%. 1,670 mg. pancreatin enzyme concentrate enteric coated tablets plus the Glutamic Acid HCL, Betaine HCL, and Pepsin.
(2) Thirty minutes after Step 1 blood sugar was 100 mg.%. Symptom free. 1,670 mg. pancreatin enzyme concentrate and other items as given in Step 1. Meal of raisins given.
(3) Thirty minutes after test meal blood sugar was 160 mg.%. Symptom free. One fourth tsp. sodium bicarbonate given.
(4) One hour after test meal blood sugar was 120 mg.%. Symptom free.
Results of Test: No symptoms developed. Blood sugar remained normal.

II.   Pineapple Test Before and After Proteolytic Enzymes

Pineapple Test Without Proteolytic Enzymes.
Blood sugar was 260 mg.% forty-five minutes after test meal. No subjective or objective symptoms observed.

Pineapple Test With Proteolytic Enzymes.
(1) Symptom free. Blood sugar 80 mg.%. 1,225 mg. concentrated pancreatic enzyme powdered pork source.
(2) Thirty minutes after Step 1 blood sugar was 80 mg.%. Symptom free. Test meal of pineapple given. 1,225 mg. pancreatin enzymes given.
(3) Thirty minutes after the test meal the blood sugar was 80

mg.%. Symptom free. One fourth tsp. sodium bicarbonate given.
(4) One hour after test meal blood sugar was 130 mg.%. Symptom free.
Results of Test: Hyperglycemia was present on test without proteolytic enzymes. Blood sugar remained normal on test after proteolytic enzymes.

III. Apple Test Before and After Proteolytic Enzymes.

Apple Test Without Proteolytic Enzymes.
Blood sugar was 200 mg.% at one hour after the test meal. There were symptoms of nervousness, marked tension, trembling, and anger in response to the test meal.

Apple Test With Proteolytic Enzymes.
(1) Blood sugar was 80 mg.%. Symptom free. 1,670 mg. pancreatic enzyme concentrate enteric coated tablet plus Glutamic Acid HCL, Betaine HCL, and Pepsin.
(2) Thirty minutes after Step 1 the patient was symptom free.

Apple test meal given.
(3) Forty-five minutes after the test meal, blood sugar was 80 mg.%. Symptom free. One fourth tsp. sodium bicarbonate given.
Results of Test: Test meal of apple without proteolytic enzymes produced hyperglycemia and marked symptoms. Test meal of apple with proteolytic enzymes produced no symptoms and blood sugar remained normal.

POST INFLUENZA PANCREATIC SUPPRESSION

Following influenza, a woman complained of dizziness, marked weakness, and a response of abdominal bloating to every food she ate. 1,335 mg. of concentrate of pancreatic enzymes plus Glutamic Acid HCL, Betaine HCL, and Pepsin accompanied each meal followed by one-fourth tsp. sodium bicarbonate thirty minutes after each meal. By the third day there was no dizziness, her strength had returned, and no foods evoked abdominal bloating.

It has been known for some time that infections may set the stage for maladaptive reactions to foods and chemicals. Some of these reactions including involving the pancreas and the small intestine are of great importance and justify the diagnosis of diabetic visceral neuropathy (Harvey et al., 1972) occurring in both the chemical as well as clinical stages of diabetes mellitus.

DISCUSSION

My study based on biochemical monitoring of glucose before and during induction test exposures to foods and chemicals reveals the evidence that schizophrenia and many other emotional reactions as well as many other chronic degenerative diseases are variants of the diabetes mellitus stage in which a hyperinsulinism evoked hypoglycemia is frequent. This occurs during the addictive adaptation stage. When the addiction adaptation is reversed by a four to six day period of avoidance then there usually emerges a hyperglycemia at about one hour after the test exposure thus revealing the evidence of a chemical diabetes mellitus phase of the disease process. Brambilla et al. (1976) observed schizophrenics to be in the chemical diabetes mellitus state. Weiss and Kaufman (1971) observed the relatives of emotional patients to have a high incidence of disordered carbohydrate metabolism and postulated a relationship between a carbohydrate disorder and emotional disorder.

Low enzymatic production by the pancreas would have serious consequences such as reduced digestion of starch, reduced digestion of fats, reduced splitting of proteins to amino acids, and reduced systemic levels of proteolytic enzymes. Inability to split proteins would produce (1) a deficiency of essential amino acids needed in many metabolic functions. The reduced essential amino acids would produce a selective nutritional deficiency and thus encourage inflammatory reactions to numerous substances. In a small sample of schizophrenic subjects, I found four essential amino acids missing on their hair test. One reason these could be missing is that adequate proteolytic enzymes are not available to split them from proteins. (2) Undigested, and therefore unusable proteins passing through the intestinal mucose and producing kinin evoked inflammatory reactions.

While there are a few who have low gastric hydrochloric acid and need hydrochloric acid supplementation for the gastric phase of digestion, there are large numbers needing bicarbonate supplementation for small intestine digestion. In fact anyone reacting maladaptively to foods needs bicarbonate supplementation for small intestine activation of proteolytic enzymes as well as bicarbonate activation of systemic proteolytic enzymes thus preventing maladaptive inflammatory reactions to foods and chemicals at the cellular level as well as providing for rapid resolution of inflammatory reactions whether kinin or histamine evoked. The value of systemic application of bicarbonate in relieving maladaptive reactions to foods and chemicals has been documented (Randolph, 1976).

A mild to severe degree of epigastric distress is frequent as a response to test meal foods. One patient with a history of wine addiction with associated episodes of pancreatitis had an acute pancreatitis attack lasting three days in response to a test meal of grape juice (Mandell and Philpott, 1972). It seems evident from clinical experience that mild acute pancreatitis is frequently evoked as a maladaptive response to foods, chemicals, toxins, and infections. Once the pancreatic function is reduced, there is a rapid spread of maladaptive reactions to foods, chemicals, inhalants, and infections due to the inherent metabolic defects that low pancreatic function produces.

Even though acute pancreatitis may temporarily provoke an over production of the pancreatic secretions, the damage done by the episodic pancreatitis is in the direction of reduced function of the pancreas (Guyton, 1971), and it finally becomes so curtailed that supplementation of its enzymes, bicarbonate, and hormones may be necessary. The evidence is that bicarbonate is the most inhibited followed by enzymes, and least affected is insulin production (Guyton, 1971; Frier, 1976). Bicarbonate and enzymes are inhibited at all stages of the disease process except acute pancreatitis while insulin production fluctuates between excess production to inhibition of production during the chemical diabetes stage and only in the clinical diabetes stage is it always in the direction of inhibition of insulin and even in the clinical stage most adult onset diabetics are capable of the recovery of the insulin production if all substances to which they are reacting are discovered, avoided, and/or spaced so that rea - tions do not occur. Furthermore, supplementing the proteolytic enzymes has been observed to aid in normalizing the hormonal production of the pancreas. The presence of pancreozyme could help explain insulin regulation when supplementing with pan- creatic concentrate (Harvey, 1972). There is a known inhibitor (Guyton, 1971) of proteolytic enzymes in the pancreas which maintain these enzymes in an inactive form while in the pancreas. Pancreatitis is thought to be due to a blocking of this enzyme inhibiting factor in which the active proteolytic enzymes damage the pancreas. One could logically postulate that there are reactions to foods, chemicals, bacterial toxins, and so forth which block the proteolytic enzyme inhibitor with results of damage to pancreatic tissue. The damaged pancreatic tissue reduces pan- creatic function further each time a reaction occurs. The only way to stop the progression of damage is to isolate through induction testing these substances evoking pancreatitis. The sup- plementation of the enzymes alone would not stop the pro- gression of the damage and disease progression even though it would materially lessen non-pancreatic reactions. Thus a satisfac- tory treatment regimen requires a discovery of the maladaptive reacting substances as well as supplementation of all pancreatic enzymes, bicarbonate, and in the most severe cases, insulin as well. Only in the most severely damaged cases will insulin supplementation be required since insulin production has a better recovery capacity than enzyme and bicarbonate production. The islets of Langerhans are the least damaged area of the pancreas from attacks of pancreatitis (Guyton, 1971).

FORMULA OF MALADAPTIVE CHAIN REACTION

I. Adaptive addiction caused by:
(1) Frequency of contact making enzymatic over demands.
(2) Any other stress factor such as infection, heat, cold, fatigue, and emotion.
(3) Genetic disposition.

II. Leading to disordered pancreatic function producing:
(1) Disordered carbohydrate metabolism.
(2) Hyperinsulinism and resultant hypoglycemia during addictive adaptation and evidence of chemical diabetes mellitus evidenced by hyperglycemia during induction testing after a period of avoidance.
(3) Clinical diabetes mellitus if and when and for what- ever reason the adaptive addiction cannot be meta- bolically maintained.
(4) Disordered lipid metabolism due to reduced lipase. A high fat content in circulating blood has been shown to evoke inflammatory reactions (kinin mediated).
(5) Disordered carbohydrate metabolism due to reduced amylase.
(6) Low proteolytic enzymes producing:
a. Impaired digestion of protein with the con- sequences of not providing essential amino acids for metabolic function as well as unusable and inflam-

matory evoking proteins reaching varied tissues by the circulating blood.
b. Low systemic proteolytic enzymes encourage kinin mediated inflammation reactions to occur as well as reducing the efficiency of resolving inflam- matory reactions once they occur whether these be histamine or kinin mediated.

FORMULA FOR CORRECTION OF MALADAPTIVE REACTIONS TO FOODS, CHEMICALS, AND INFECTIONS

(1) Correct Addictive Adaptation by:
a. Avoidance of symptom incriminated substances.
b. Spacing contacts below reaction level.
(2) Pancreatic substitution therapy of bicarbonate, lipase, amylase, and most important of all proteolytic enzymes. Keep the proteolytic enzymes systemically high enough to block kinin production.
(3) Adequate over all general nutrition of proteins, carbohy- drates, fats, and so forth.
(4) Daily vigorous exercise.
(5) Remove any demonstrated infections by appropriate medical measures. Provide autogenous and stock vaccines to produce optimum defense against opportunist microbes.
(6) Pancreatic insufficiency sets the stage for amino acid deficiency which in turn through excessive demands sets the stage for vitamin and mineral deficiencies. The intestinal absorption of amino acids and the metabolic use of amino acids make demands for B_6 which in turn demands associa- ted nutrients especially B_2, zinc, and magnesium. Nutritional deficiencies can result out of these excessive demands even in the face of theoretical adequate diet. The observation is also pertinent that few people have even a theoretical adequate diet.

A proposed optimum supernutrition program is on this order:
Vitamin C — 2-4 grams three times a day. Powder is the best tolerated. Calcium ascorbate has the highest tolerance.
B_6 — 100-500 mg. three times a day.
B_5 —100-500 mg. three times a day. (Note: B_5 is Panto- thenic Acid)
B_2 — 100-500 mg. three times a day.
B_1 — 100-500 mg. three times a day.
B_3 — 500-1,000 mg. three times a day as either niacin or niacinamide.
PABA — 100-500 mg. three times a day.
L-Glutamine — 100-500 mg. three times a day.
Vitamin E — 200-800 units three times a day.
Vitamin A — 10,000-20,000 units three times a day.
Folic Acid — 400-800 mcg. three times a day.
Magnesium as a chelate — 75-150 mg. three times a day.
Manganese as a chelate — 10-20 mg. three times a day.
Zinc as a chelate — 10-20 mg. three times a day.

Maintain these high doses for one to two months and then consider reduction. An initial hair test which also should be repeated in six months to one year should serve as a guide to supplementation of calcium, magnesium, potassium, manganese, zinc, and chromium as well as the possibility of a toxic level of lead, mercury, cadmium, or arsenic.

The supplementation of essential amino acids is of prime importance. A survey for essential amino acids classically reveals several to be missing in chronically ill patients. Amino acids can be provided in capsules, tablets, or liquid predigested collagen. The following is recommended: Liquid predigested protein as free amino acids, 15 grams (2 tbsp.) four times a day for one month, reduced to 7½ grams four times a day for one month, and then 7½ grams twice a day for maintainance.

CONCLUSIONS

To further clarify the metabolic situation, the following terms and states have been observed as applicable to varying stages of the diabetes mellitus disease process leading to chronic physical and chronic mental diseases.

(1) Disordered carbohydrate disorder of hypoglycemia and hyperglycemia.
(2) Addiction adaptation to foods and chemicals.
(3) Intestinal malabsorption syndrome.
(4) Digestive disorder.
(5) Deficient proteolytic enzymes both at the pancreatic-intestinal level as well as the systemic-cellular level.
(6) Episodic pancreatitis as a maladaptive reaction to foods, chemicals, and infections (usually undiagnosed due to its mild degree and brief duration).
(7) Acute nutritional deficiency with essential amino acid deficiency as a prominent feature due to a proteolytic enzyme inability to adequately split amino acids from proteins.
(8) Episodic small intestine acidosis due to decreased pancreatic bicarbonate production.
(9) Episodic systemic acidosis due to decreased pancreatic bicarbonate as well as from incomplete metabolism of carbohydrates, lipids, and proteins.
(10) Secondary infectious invasion.

To understand these varied states in terms of a disease process provides a valuable framework for treatment of that disease process whether its presenting symptomatology be mental or physical. Treating rationally the basic underlying disease process makes it much easier to achieve success in also treating the specific maladaptive tissues named as the specific mental or physical degenerative disease.

It would seem unwise to use only proteolytic enzymes applied to schizophrenia or other chronic degenerative diseases in the hopeful expectation of a miraculous cure. The dynamic functions of the human organism must be kept in mind such as nutrition, metabolic errors, infections, physical stresses, and emotional stresses. To achieve a dynamic homeostasis equilibrium all isolatable factors should be treated appropriately and simultaneously. It seems apparent that proteolytic enzyme supplementation, in some cases better characterized as substitution, will play an important role in the treatment of many chronic degenerative diseases including the major mental reactions such as schizophrenia, manic-depressive reactions, psychotic depression, autism, and so forth.

Although this presentation has centered around the illness schizophrenia, it should be understood that schizophrenia is one of the chronic degenerative diseases and has common denominators with several other chronic degenerative diseases. The problem of low proteolytic enzymes is an important common denominator in several chronic degenerative diseases. The most obvious disease to which these observations apply is diabetes mellitus, and especially clinical adult onset type.

REFERENCES

Bell, Iris R.: The Kinin Peptide Hormone Theory of Adaptation and Maladaptation in Psychobiological Illness. Unpublished Manuscript. Doctorial Thesis. Stanford University, Stanford, California, 1974.

Brambilla, F., Guerrini, R.; Riggi, F.; Rovere, C.; Zanoboni, A.; and Zanoboni-Muciaccia, W.: Glucose-Insulin Metabolism in Chronic Schizophrenia. *Dis. Nerv. Sys.*, Vol. 37, No. 2, February, 1976.

Bullock, T.M., M.D., and Carroll, F.M., M.D.: Personal Consultation, 1977.

Davis, Bernard D., M.D., et al.: *Microbiology*. Second Edition. Harper & Row Publishers, Inc., New York, New York, 1973. P. 1464.

Dickey, Lawrence D., M.D.: *Clinical Ecology*. Thomas, Springfield, 1976.

Dohan, F.C., M.D., and Grasberger, J.C.: Relapsed Schizophrenics: Earlier Discharge from the Hospital After Cereal-Free, Milk-Free Diet. *Am. J. Psychiatry,* 130:6. June, 1973. Pp. 685-688.

Dohan, F.C., M.D.: Schizophrenia: Possible Relationship to Cereal Grains and Celiac Disease. In *Schizophrenia – Current Concepts and Research.* Edited by Siva Sankar DV. Hicksville, New York, PJD Publications, 1969, Pp. 539-551.

Frier, B.M.: Exocrine Pancreatic Function in Juvenile-Onset Diabetes Mellitus. *Gut.* 17:685-691m, 1976.

Guyton, Arthur C., M.D.: *Textbook on Medical Physiology.* W.B. Saunders Company, Philadelphia, 1971. P. 778.

Harvey, A.M., M.D., et al.: *The Principles and Practice of Medicine.* Appleton-Century-Crofts, New York, 1972. Pp. 758, 880.

Innerfield, I., et al., Proc., 123, 871, 1966.

Randolph, T.G.: The Enzymatic, Acid, Hypoxia, Endocrine Concept of Allergic Inflammation. *Clinical Ecology.* Dickey, Lawrence D. (Ed.). Thomas, Springfield, 1976. Pp. 577-596.

Speer, Frederick: *Allergy of the Nervous System.* Thomas, Springfield, 1970.

Weiss, Jules M., and Kaufman, Herbert S.: A Subtle Organic Component in Some Cases of Mental Illness. *Arch Gen. Psy.,* Vol. 25, July, 1971.

Wolf, Max, M.D.: *Enzyme Therapy.* Regent House, Los Angeles, 1972.

RECOMMENDED READING

Clinical Ecology. Lawrence D. Dickey, M.D. Thomas, Springfield, Illinois, 1976.

Allergy and the Cardiovascular System. Sol. D. Klotz, Pp. 184-192.

Cardiac Arrhythmias Due to Foods. Robert W. Boxer, M.D. Pp. 193-200.

The Enzymatic, Acid, Hypoxia, Endocrine Concept of Allergic Inflammation. Theron G. Randolph, M.D. Pp. 577-596.

The Four-Day Rotation of Foods According to Families. William H. Philpott, M.D. Pp. 473-486.

Modern Nutrition In Health and Disease, 5th Edition. Robert S. Goodhart and Maurice E. Shils. Lea and Febiger, Philadelphia, Pennsylvania, 1973.

The Proteins and Amino Acids. Anthony A. Albanese and Louise A. Orto. Pp. 28-88.

Abnormalities in Serum Protein Metabolism and Amino Acid Effects. Marcus A. Rothschild, Murray Oratz, and Sidney S. Schreiber. Pp. 89-98.

Carbohydrates. Rachmiel Levine. Pp. 99-116.

Fats and Other Lipids. Roslyn B. Alfin-Slater and Lilla Aftergood. Pp. 117-141.

Nutrition in Relation to Acquired Immunity. A.E. Axelrod. Pp. 493-505.

Nutrition in Diseases of the Pancreas. Phani Dhar, Norman Zamcheck, and Selwyn A. Broitman. Pp. 819-826.

Allergy and Diet. Vincent J. Fontana and M.B. Strauss. Pp. 924-940.

Textbook of Medical Physiology, Fourth Edition. Arthur C. Guyton, M.D. Saunders, Philadelphia, Pennsylvania, 1971. sylvania, 1971.

Regulation of Acid-Base Balance. Pp. 427-441.

Secretory Functions of the Alimentary Tract. Pp. 753-764.

Digestion and Absorption in the Gastrointestinal Tract. Pp. 765-774.

Protein Metabolism. Pp. 812-820.

Vitamin and Mineral Metabolism. Pp. 852-860.

Enzyme Therapy. Max Wolf, M.D. Regent House, Los Angeles, 1972.

Dohan, F.C., M.D., and Grasberger, J.C.: Relapsed Schizophrenics: Earlier Discharge from the Hospital After Cereal-Free, Milk-Free Diet. *Am. J. Psychiatry,* 130:6. June, 1973. Pp. 685-688.

Dohan, F.C., M.D.: Schizophrenia: Possible Relationship to Cereal Grains and Celiac Disease. In *Schizophrenia — Current Concepts and Research.* Edited by Siva Sankar DV. Hicksville, New York, PJD Publications, 1969. Pp. 539-551.